# THE CANCER

# REVOLUTION

## INTEGRATIVE MEDICINE
### THE FUTURE OF CANCER CARE

YOUR GUIDE TO INTEGRATING COMPLEMENTARY AND CONVENTIONAL MEDICINE

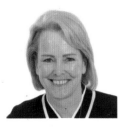

## PATRICIA PEAT
with 37 expert contributors

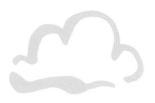

Published by Win-win Health Intelligence Ltd

The Cancer Revolution copyright © Win-win Health Intelligence, 2016

Win-win Health Intelligence
Unit 4, The Energy Centre
Bowling Green Walk
London N1 6AL

All enquiries to: enquiries@win-winhealth.co.uk

Design by Bina Tarulli

Original photographs by Jemma Allett

Printed in China by 1010 Printing with soya-based inks on FSC certified materials

First published 2016. Reprinted with minor amendments 2017

The Cancer Revolution – Integrative Medicine: the future of cancer care. Your guide
to integrating complementary and conventional medicine – Patricia Peat

ISBN 978-1-5262-0032-7

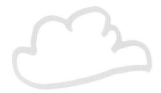

*The Cancer Revolution* is dedicated to the many extraordinary scientists, practitioners and individuals with cancer who have, often at great personal cost, laid down the foundations of Integrative Medicine for cancer.

# CONTRIBUTORS

Principal Author
Patricia Peat

Other Contributors
Lynda Brown

Dr Francisco Contreras

Dorothy Crowther

Jo Daly

Patricia Daly

Dr Rosy Daniel

Lizzy Davis

Dr Gary Deng

Dr Friedrich Douwes

Dr Damien Downing

George Emsden

Dr Chris Etheridge

Jane Fior

Barbara Gallani

Janey Lee Grace

Juliet Hayward

Tom Hoyland

Robert H. Jacobs

Daphne Lambert

Clare McLusky

Dr Henry Mannings

Dr John D. Moran

Dr Maurice Orange

Prof. Jane Plant

David Potterton

Dr Thomas Rau

Jessica Richards

Margella Salmins

Patrizia Sergeant

Shazzie

Prof. Shimon Slavin

Prof. Robert Thomas

Jason Vale

Robert Verkerk

Xandria Williams

Dr Bernard Willis

Dr André Young-Snell

General Editor
Robin Daly

Medical Editor
Patricia Peat

Editorial Consultant
Ruth Thackeray

Editorial Support
Nicki Williams
Kareen Davidoff
Ashley Frayling
Leighanne Manesi
Hilary Martin

Scientific References
Helen Gibson
Arunima Maiti
Xiao Lu

Design
Bina Tarulli

Layout
Bina Tarulli
Geoff Stevens

Photography
Jemma Allett

Proofreading
Ellen Daly
Joanie Speers

Indexing
Jan Ross

# ACKNOWLEDGEMENTS

I owe an enormous debt of gratitude to the many, many people who have contributed to this book. In an extraordinary flood of generosity and intention to help people with cancer, Patricia Peat and thirty-seven specialists have given their contributions completely free of charge, as has our designer Bina Tarulli, our editorial consultant Ruth Thackeray and the many others who have helped bring the project to completion.

By buying this book you will not only be helping yourself or someone close to you, you will also be supporting the work of Yes to Life.

Robin Daly
Chairman and Founder, Yes to Life
yestolife.org.uk

# CONTENTS

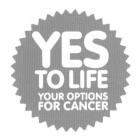

# AND THE CANCER REVOLUTION

## Robin Daly

*The Cancer Revolution* represents the fruition of a long-held dream to pull together the best information on the broadest range of approaches to cancer. We want this book to act as a catalyst for individuals to empower themselves, and to become part of a revolution that promises to change the experience of cancer treatment completely. This revolution, Integrative Medicine, has the power to cut deeply into the devastating survival statistics and the desperately poor quality of life experienced by many following treatment for cancer. Even more importantly, it will help to promote a cultural revolution: the increasingly obvious sources of the ever-rising tide of cancer in the UK point clearly to where the solutions lie.

A sobering statistic:

BY 2020 HALF OF US ARE PREDICTED TO GET CANCER AT SOME POINT IN OUR LIVES [1]

The evidence points to the fact that cancer is largely a lifestyle disease promoted by an 'industrialised' Western style of living: we have become increasingly sedentary; the vast majority of our food is appallingly denatured, adulterated and unsuitable; our environment is dangerously polluted, both at large and in our homes; smoking, stress and alienation can all lead towards cancer; the list goes on.[2] The good news is that, armed with this understanding, we can now choose to avoid many of the factors driving cancer. But in order to do so, we need to know exactly where the threat is coming from. Many of the worst toxins and the most unhealthy choices have been beautifully packaged and fragranced, and seductively advertised to make them as appealing as possible; and we are now relentlessly bombarded with pressure to consume, almost from birth. As predatory market forces get wise to the emerging public awareness of these issues, even complete junk food is starting to be marketed as 'healthy'.

Crucially, taking steps to make choices that are positive and healthy for ourselves simultaneously addresses the root of the problem for all. As more people buy organically produced food, so farming without toxins improves the environment. As sales of junk food decrease, the market is forced to move towards less adulterated products to remain profitable. When we decide to bike to work, we get fitter, while everyone else is exposed to less pollution. This is positive, life-affirming, 'win-win' and just plain good common sense.

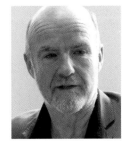

And it is the logic behind a conscious move towards wholesome lifestyle choices that leads naturally to many of the approaches that Integrative Medicine adds to standard treatments, creating a completely novel synthesis of 'what works'. These approaches consist largely of carefully constructed protocols based around targeted and refined lifestyle choices. This book aims to make it clear what those choices are.

Yes to Life was set up in 2004, while my daughter Bryony was in the midst of her third bout of cancer, aged twenty-three. At that time, I was naturally desperate to find anything that had a chance of helping her. My efforts made a few things crystal clear to me:

> There is an enormous amount you can do to help yourself if you have cancer

> Finding out which approaches are genuine, relevant and accessible is a massive and daunting task

> If you do manage to find out, you may discover that they are unaffordable

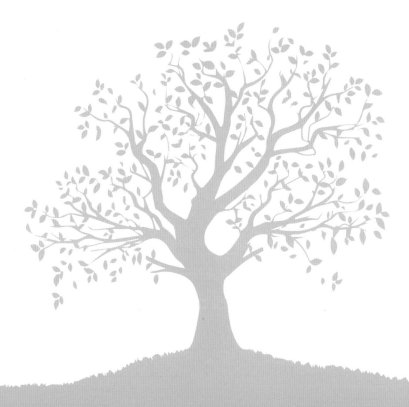

So Yes to Life was conceived as a charity to address this tragic situation. We wanted to create an organisation totally separate from any commercial agendas, focused entirely on helping people with cancer, to give them every chance of surviving and living well.

Now in 2016, I see Britain as poised for a revolution. The evidence base for many approaches that were formerly thought of as 'alternative' or irrelevant is now undeniable. For example, the benefits of an exercise programme to breast-cancer survivors have been shown to be double that of chemotherapy;[3] furthermore it has been shown that something as simple as taking a multivitamin can reduce the likelihood of death for breast-cancer patients by almost one third.[4] These two examples alone are clear indicators of the urgency behind embracing the integrative approach.

Sadly I lost my beautiful daughter, suddenly, before we were really able to begin on the programme we had been devising. We ran out of time. Yes to Life aims to respond quickly with the best information and to do everything possible to ensure no-one ever has to 'go it alone' again.

My hope is that this book will play a significant part in this and in revolutionising cancer care.

YES TO LIFE

YES TO LIFE OFFERS SUPPORT TO PEOPLE WITH CANCER WHO WANT TO TAKE A PROACTIVE ROLE IN THEIR TREATMENT

## Charity Details

Contact Office
0845 257 6950
office@yestolife.org.uk

Helpline
0870 163 2990
helpcentre@yestolife.org.uk

Website
yestolife.org.uk

Charity No
1112812

Yes to Life Radio Show
ukhealthradio.com

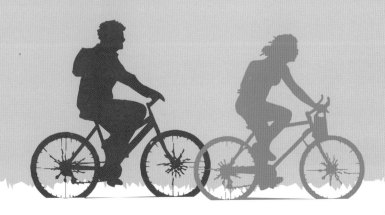

# ABOUT THE AUTHOR:
## PATRICIA PEAT

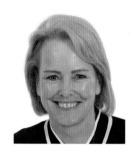

Robin Daly

Patricia Peat spent many years as a nurse working in
NHS oncology wards, supporting people through standard
treatments – surgery, chemotherapy and radiotherapy.
She always set great store by the 'therapeutic relationship'
between patient and caregiver, but, in common with other
staff, had little interest in Complementary and Alternative
Medicine (CAM). That was until she began to notice that
many of those integrating a range of other therapies into their
regime were actually managing rather better than expected.
She simultaneously became aware of their intense frustration
at finding their doctors not only unable and unwilling to
engage in constructive dialogue about their options, but
unsupportive of their choices.

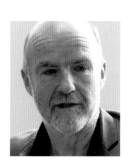

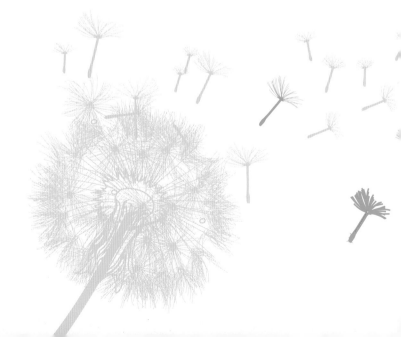

Inspired by these pioneering endeavours, Patricia set up Cancer Options in 1998 to support people with cancer in taking charge of their situation, in exploring the widest possible range of treatment options and in building their own integrative treatment programme based around their personal choices. Passionate about encouraging the safe integration of complementary therapies with standard treatments, she has developed Cancer Options into a unique service at the forefront of integrative cancer care in the UK.

Patricia has added – and continues to add – to her experience and knowledge of standard cancer treatments through her extensive research into the evidence base for all CAM approaches in use, both in the UK and abroad. She has developed a deep understanding of the methods of many of the top integrative practitioners and clinics in the world. Additionally, she has made it her business to be right up to the minute with new techniques being pioneered within the NHS and other health services abroad.

Fifteen years of close work with all types of cancer have provided her with an unparallelled overview of what is helpful at each stage of each cancer. She still finds that the UK is lagging far behind some other countries in acceptance of integrative methods, but hopes that this book will play a part in moving things forward.

Patricia is a medical adviser to Yes to Life and the Integrated Healthcare Trust, also a patron of the charity CANCERactive. She is a respected public speaker and writer on the subject of Integrative Medicine and empowering people to make their own health decisions.

CANCER
OPTIONS

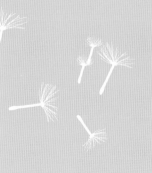

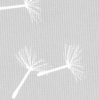

# INTRODUCING OUR CONTRIBUTORS

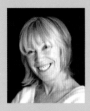

### Lynda Brown, BA (Hons)

An award-winning food and cookery writer, Lynda has a lifelong interest in nutrition, organic food and farming as well as kitchen gardening. She is the author of eight major books, including *The Cook's Garden* and the landmark *Shopper's Guide to Organic Food and Farming,* and *Organic Living.* Lynda has been actively Involved with the organic movement since the mid-1990s; she writes regularly for the Soil Association, contributes the 'Food in Depth' column to *Living Earth*, and is currently working on her next book.

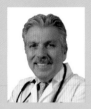

### Francisco Contreras, MD

Dr Contreras is Director, President and Chairman of the Oasis of Hope Hospital, Playas de Tijuana, Mexico. A distinguished oncologist and surgeon, he is renowned for integrating conventional and alternative cancer treatments with emotional healing and spiritual care to provide patients with outcomes superior to those of conventional methods alone.

After graduating from medical school at the Autonomous University of Mexico, Dr Contreras specialised in surgical oncology at the University of Vienna in Austria, where he graduated with honours. He is the author or co-author of more than fifteen books concerning integrative therapy including *50 Critical Cancer Answers*, *Beating Cancer, Hope, Medicine & Healing*, and *The Hope of Living Cancer Free.*

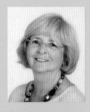

### Dorothy Crowther, BSc (Hons), RGN, RCNT, RNT, FRCN

Dorothy Crowther is Chief Executive of Wirral Holistic Care Services, which she founded in 1988 and has been the driving force behind that organisation's many developments and achievements ever since. Her degree in science and qualifications in nursing have led her to work in the field of therapeutic cancer care for most of her professional life. While studying in the USA, she also trained in Gerson Therapy at the Gerson Institute in San Diego, California.

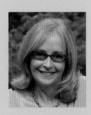

### Jo Daly, CCH

Jo Daly has been practising as a homeopath since the 1980s. Having lived, trained and worked in the UK, in 1989 she moved to the USA. She has been a founder and developer of two schools of homeopathy, first in California and later in New York as Dean of Education at the School of Homeopathy. Besides teaching elsewhere in the USA, UK and Japan, she also writes, supervises students, runs on-going study groups and is currently on the faculty at the Berkeley Institute of Homeopathy. Jo is a member of WISH (the World Institute for Sensation Homeopathy), which integrates practices based on those of Dr Rajan Sankaran.

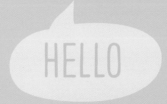

HELLO

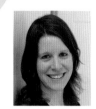

### Patricia Daly, Dip NT, BA (Hons), ITEC, MBANT, MNTOI

Patricia Daly is a fully qualified nutritional therapist based in Dublin, Ireland. Following her cancer diagnosis, she started studying nutrition and specialising in the area of integrative cancer care. She has taken a particular interest in the ketogenic diet and has written two books on this subject. As a native Swiss, she regularly attends training courses in Switzerland and Germany, for instance at the renowned Tumour Biology Centre in Freiburg. She is also a member of the British Society for Integrative Oncology. While her clinic is based in Dublin, she does phone/Skype consultations for clients who live elsewhere.

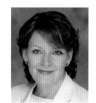

### Dr Rosy Daniel, BSc, MBBCh

Dr Daniel is Founder and Medical Director of Health Creation, and she also works as an Integrative Medicine Consultant at the Apthorp Centre in Bath. She provides consultations for those with cancer who are seeking advice on how to integrate alternative, complementary and self-help approaches to fighting and healing cancer alongside orthodox medical treatment. Having been Medical Director of Bristol Cancer Help Centre (1993-9), she went on to work at the Harley Street Oncology Centre in London (1995-2005). She addresses conferences and seminars nationally and internationally, and is a regular broadcaster. She has written five books, including *The Cancer Directory*, and created the interactive Cancer Lifeline Kit; she also leads the supportive health-coaching programme of Health Creation mentors.

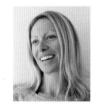

### Lizzy Davis, BSc (Hons) (Cancer Nursing), Cancer Exercise Professional (Level 4), Tripudio Instructor

Lizzy Davis' background is in oncology and palliative care nursing. Her mother's gradual debilitation throughout treatment for lung cancer highlighted the very real and definite need for exercise to be an integral intervention throughout the cancer care pathway. She became an Advanced Personal Trainer and in 2012 successfully completed the first UK REPs (Register of Exercise Professionals) Level 4 accredited course in Cancer Exercise Rehabilitation.

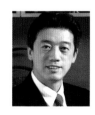

### Dr Gary Deng, MD, PhD

Dr Deng is an Associate Member and Attending Physician at Memorial Sloan-Kettering Cancer Center in New York. His clinical expertise is in cancer supportive care and Integrative Medicine. His clinical practice is one of the few in the USA to be designated a comprehensive cancer centre by the National Cancer Institute (NCI). It focuses on an evidence-based approach to Integrative Medicine and its applications in oncology. Dr Deng has taken a leadership role in this emerging and evolving field. He heads the clinical programmes and the physician education programmes at the Integrative Medicine Service at Sloan-Kettering and in 2011 served as President of the Society for Integrative Oncology. He is a principal investigator of research projects on acupuncture and botanical agents funded by the National Institutes of Health (NIH). Having written review articles, medical textbook chapters and practice guidelines on Integrative Medicine, he is frequently invited to give lectures around the world. He has peer-review responsibilities for professional journals and for NIH grant applications.

Dr Deng received his MD from Beijing Medical University, China, and his PhD in microbiology and from the University of Miami, Florida. He completed his clinical training at the University of Texas Medical School at Houston and research training at the University of Texas M.D. Anderson Cancer Center.

He is a member of the Research Council and the Institutional Review Board at Memorial Sloan-Kettering Cancer Center, and an Executive Board member of the Society for Integrative Oncology. In 2012 Dr Deng was the keynote speaker at the inaugural conference of the British Society for Integrative Oncology (BSIO).

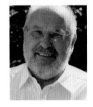

### Dr Friedrich Douwes, MD

Born in Germany, Friedrich Douwes studied at the University of Marburg, receiving his MD in 1962. He then went to the USA and completed an Internship with Philadelphia General Hospital in 1967 and a Fellowship in Haematology and Oncology with Philadelphia's Hahnemann University Hospital in 1970.

Dr Douwes returned to Germany and for almost ten years was on the staff at the University Hospital of Göttingen Medical Department as the Senior Physician in the Oncology Department. He published several articles pertaining to biological and immunological problems of tumours. Not satisfied with the clinical results attained as an orthodox oncologist, he began to integrate alternative methods into his daily work. He founded the first self-help group and the first Psych-Oncological Department in 1980 when he became Medical Director at the Sonnenburg Hospital in Bad Sooden-Allendorf, one of the largest cancer hospitals in Germany.

Between 1981 and 1987 Dr Douwes was involved in developing his integrative cancer concept, a synthesis of conventional and complementary therapies, and in 1991 he started his own cancer hospital, the Klinik St Georg in Bad Aibling, a health resort in Bavaria.

This clinic, with sixteen physicians on its staff, treats around five thousand cancer patients a year. They come from all over the world, and many have had remarkably successful results from the integrative approach to treating all types of cancer, even at an advanced stage.

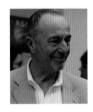

### Dr Damien Downing, MBBS, MSB

Qualifying from Guy's Hospital, London in 1972, Dr Downing has worked in nutritional and environmental medicine since 1980. He is President of the British Society for Ecological Medicine, a founder member of the British Society for Integrative Oncology and was for twenty years the editor of the *Journal of Nutritional and Environmental Medicine*. His book *Daylight Robbery* (1988) was one of the first to highlight the importance of sunlight and vitamin D in healthcare.

Dr Downing practises Ecological Medicine. He explains that this embraces environmental effects on the individual through allergy, toxicology and nutrition, how the biochemical individuality (particularly genomics) of each of us affects our handling of these factors, and how each of us – patient, practitioner and individual – in turn has an impact on and a responsibility for our shared environment.

### George Emsden, ACIB, DipPFS

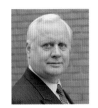

Trained as a banker, George Emsden is Principal at CancerIFA, a London-based financial advisory service to other financial advisers, employee benefit providers and to individuals. In his own words: 'I talk to people about money. After twenty years in financial services, it seems that my real work found me'. His particular expertise comes from having had throat cancer himself in 2007, cured by six weeks of radiotherapy, leaving him with a different outlook on life. He now offers advice to anyone whose life is affected by cancer, whether as patient or as bereaved family member.

### Dr Chris Etheridge, PhD, BSc (Hons) Phyto, BSc (Hons) Chem, MNIMH, MCPP, CChem, MRSC, ARCS, DoIC

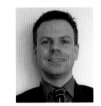

Dr Etheridge trained first at Imperial College, London, and in 1995-9 at the Department of Biochemistry and Molecular Genetics at St Mary's Hospital in Paddington, London. The Department of Chemistry, Imperial College has granted him three patents in Gene Therapy. in 2006 Chris qualified as an accredited Practitioner of Herbal Medicine at the College of Phytotherapy in Epping, Essex.

### Jane Fior, Dip Psych, Dip Couns, MAHPP (Accredited)

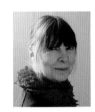

Jane Fior was a founder member of the Cancer Counselling Trust, which has sadly been forced to close due to lack of funds. She remains active as a UKAHPP Accredited Psychotherapeutic Counsellor, UKCP registered with over twenty years' experience in working with cancer issues at all stages of the disease. Based in North London, she has a particular interest in supporting people who choose to supplement their treatment with complementary approaches.

### Barbara Gallani, M Res

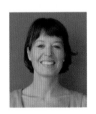

Barbara specialises in yoga for people with physical disabilities and limited mobility and has been working with physiotherapists and carers to provide support to those who are chair-bound or bed-ridden. Barbara began practising yoga in 1995 and obtained a British School of Yoga Diploma in 2005. On attending the Sivananda Yoga Vedanta Dhanwantari Ashram in Kerala, India (2008) she deepened her practice. In 2013 she completed the Yoga for Survivors programme for all types of cancer and all phases of survivorship. Barbara teaches at the London-based Life Centre, which has branches in Islington and Notting Hill, and also runs private and group yoga classes.

### Janey Lee Grace

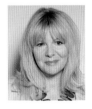

Renowned as an expert on natural health and wellbeing, Janey Lee Grace has written five best selling books on holistic living. She trained as a vocalist and appears regularly as a popular presenter on BBC Radio 2. In 2005 she founded *Imperfectlynatural.com*, a consumer website with a thriving forum.

### Juliet Hayward, BA (Hons), MA, DNN

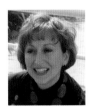

Juliet Hayward originally worked as a nutritionist at the Nutri Centre in London, where she set up a helpline. She now works in private practice, supporting cancer patients and people suffering from other challenging illnesses. Since 2010 she has been involved in consultancy work and lecturing for the Really Healthy Company and is now also part of the Academy of Nutritional Medicine in London.

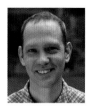

### Tom Hoyland

Tom qualified as a reflexologist in 1999 and set up his private practice in a North London clinic, where he offers reflexology, holistic massage, Thai massage and Reiki. Alongside this he has also run monthly clinics in companies, including Selfridge & Co and Reader's Digest magazine. From 2007 until 2013 he worked at University College Hospital within the Complementary Therapy Team, on the cancer wards for adults, teenagers and young children. Tom is a member of the Federation of Holistic Therapists and also a full member of the Association of Reflexologists.

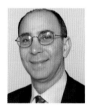

### Robert H. Jacobs, NMD, PhD, HMD, D Hom (Med)

Qualified as a naturopath and homeopath, Robert Jacobs now has over thirty years of experience in natural medicine. He is the driving force behind the Health Natural Ltd clinic in London and the Society for Human Development in Los Angeles. A member of the General Council and Register of Naturopaths and the Homeopathic Medical Association in the UK, he is also a member of the American Naturopathic Medical Association. He specialises in Functional and Nutritional Medicine, promoting optimum function in the cells and systems of the body. These range from immune, digestive, detoxification, energy creation and hormone-balance systems to those involving brain, cardiovascular and anti-ageing functions. He works from the principle that imbalances in the body's functional systems create symptoms and illness.

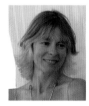

### Daphne Lambert, Dip NT

As a chef, nutritionist and writer, with her company Greencuisine Ltd, formed in 1995, Daphne has developed a series of nutrition-based programmes and retreats. She also runs a private consultancy practice to cater for individuals and organisations. In 2010 she founded Greencuisine Trust, an educational charity focused on 're-thinking' food. Daphne has journeyed with those who have decided to follow the Gerson Therapy, assisting them in the preparation of food. She has also spent time at the Hippocrates Institute in Florida studying nutritional ways of healing. The author of two books, she provided the column on organic gardening for *Healthy Eating* for three years and regularly contributes to various other magazines. She was a trustee of the Soil Association for ten years.

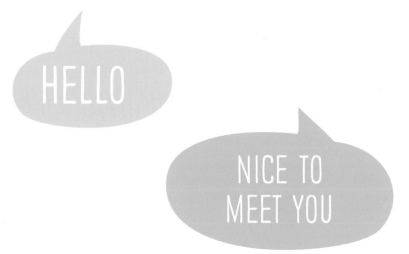

HELLO

NICE TO MEET YOU

**Clare McLusky, BSc (Hons), OT MSc, mindfulness-based cognitive therapy (MBCT)**
A mindfulness teacher based in Oxfordshire, Clare McLusky first started
practising meditation around 2005, following treatment for throat cancer.
Having noticed the profound effect this had on her health and wellbeing,
she was motivated to share this approach with others. In 2012 she graduated
from Oxford University with an MSc in Mindfulness-based Cognitive Therapy.
She is an occupational therapist with extensive experience in mental health
and group work.She began working for Yes to Life as a helpline volunteer
in 2009 and believes wholeheartedly in the philosophy of the charity.

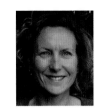

**Dr Henry Mannings, MB, BCh, BAO, MRCP (UK), MSc (Cancer Immunotherapy)**
Dr Mannings qualified at the Queen's University, Belfast, in 1976. He started
his career as a GP. While continuing family practice, part-time, he worked
in hospital medicine as a registrar in general and emergency services. In
1996 he became a specialist doctor in oncology at the Norfolk and Norwich
Hospital but left after a year due to the lack of integrative care and the
ineffectiveness and side effects of many of the chemotherapy regimes.
He returned to part-time family practice and graduated from Nottingham
University with an MSc in Cancer Immunotherapy. He also became an
Honorary Senior Lecturer in Medicine at the University of East Anglia,
tutoring medical students, as well as returning to the James Paget Hospital
in Gorleston to work in oncology.

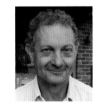

In 2009 Dr Mannings founded the cancer charity Star Throwers in Norfolk,
which offers integrative care as well as immunotherapy and metabolic
therapy. He is aiming to publish scientific studies on cancer-related topics,
including outcomes.

**Dr John D. Moran, RD, MBBS, LDS, RCS, DPsSC, DFFP, MSc, NUTR MED**
Dr Moran is the Medical Director of the privately run Holistic Medical Clinic,
now based in Wimpole Street, London. He qualified in medicine from St
George's Hospital and in dentistry from Guy's Dental Hospital, London. He is
a Diplomate of the faculty of Family Planning and Reproductive Health Care
of the Royal College of Obstetricians an Gynaecologists (RCOG) and holds
post-graduate diplomas in psychosexual counselling, menopause and sexual
dysfunction as well as an MSc in nutritional medicine. Dr Moran has been
extensively trained by Prof. Ben Pfeifer at the Aeskulap Clinic in Switzerland
and is therefore able to treat and advise on prostate and breast cancer
following Pfeifer's protocol.

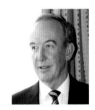

**Dr Maurice Orange, MSc, Clin Oncol**
Dr Orange trained as a GP and in anthroposophic medicine in Holland. He was
Medical Director of Park Attwood Clinic, Worcestershire, a centre for integrative
anthroposophic medical-therapeutic care (now closed), where spiritual,
psychosocial and biological aspects were taken into account in treatment.
Dr Orange's work has focused on integrative cancer care and he lectures and
publishes regularly. His focus of interest and experience include: cancer care;
immunology; mistletoe therapy; whole body hyperthermia; and spirituality in
medical care. He currently holds a senior position in developing Integrative
Oncology at the Ita Wegman Clinic, Arlesheim, Switzerland.

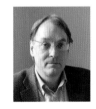

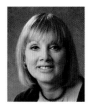

### Prof. Jane Plant CBE, DSc, FREng, FRSM, FRSE, FRSA, FRGS, FIMM, FGS C Eng, C Geol, PhD

One of the world's leading geochemists, Prof. Jane Plant was chief scientist of the British Geological Survey (BGS) from 2000 to 2005, when she became Professor of Geochemistry at Imperial College, London. Having graduated with a Class I Honours degree in geology (special geochemistry) at Liverpool University in 1967, she gained her PhD in geochemistry at Leicester University ten years later. At the BGS she developed the methods for Britain's national geochemical database, with its direct applications in mineral exploration – and most significantly (and at first unexpectedly) in the new field of environmental health: during the 1970s it was her team that helped to identify links between deficiency diseases in livestock and the geochemistry of the land on which they lived. Her personal experiences with breast cancer, and the findings of her research in this field, led her to become an author on the subject. She has published five books on dietary and environmental factors in cancer.

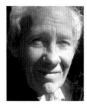

### David Potterton, ND, MRN, MNIMH

David is one of the few practitioners in the UK to be qualified in both naturopathy and herbal medicine. He began his studies in 1969 and in 1975 graduated as a medical herbalist. In 1981 he received a Diploma in Naturopathy from the British College of Naturopathy and Osteopathy, London (later renamed the British College of Osteopathic Medicine).

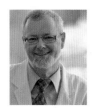

### Dr Thomas Rau, MD

Thomas Rau studied medicine at the University of Berne, the leading medical school in Switzerland, and began his career in rheumatology and internal medicine. In 1981 he became the Medical Director of a rehabilitation clinic in Switzerland, where he treated patients with various degenerative disorders. During that time, Dr Rau first began to notice, as he put it: 'With classical medicine, my patients weren't getting better.' He became interested in alternative therapies, particularly homeopathy and dietary changes, used by those patients whose health was improving. He found his own patients began to show remarkable progress when he treated them more holistically.

Dr Rau became a lifelong student of alternative medical methods, including Chinese and Ayurvedic medicine, as well as of the great holistic practitioners of the Swiss and German traditions. He studied with the leading European practitioners of his age and gradually formed his own method of restoring health to his patients. In doing so he developed theories about detoxification, nutrition, digestion and building up the immune function, resulting in an approach that he calls Biological Medicine.

In 1992 Dr Rau became the Medical Director of the Paracelsus Klinik in Lustmühle. Already recognised as a centre of holistic medicine, Paracelsus has since become one of the premier clinics for Biological Medicine in the world. Dr Rau has continued in his post there, alongside his writing – books, journal articles and conference papers – lectures and teaching.

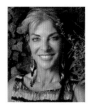

### Jessica Richards, MNCH, Member of the American Council for Hypnotherapist Examiners, Member of the Academy for Chief Executives

Jessica Richards qualified in clinical hypnosis in 1985. As well as training doctors, surgeons, midwives, dentists and anaesthetists for pain control and allied skills, she specialises in personal development and leads Chief Executive workshops and retreats, facilitating rapid change by identifying and resolving self-limiting beliefs, using her highly effective 'Groundhog Day' process (different place, different people but the same situation again). Jessica is a patron of the charity Cancer Active and the author of *The Topic of Cancer*, an inspired and practical guide that will help you take control when faced with cancer. Jessica has recovered from breast cancer through an intensive programme of alternative approaches.

### Margella Salmins, BSc (Hons), TCM, BM (Beijing)

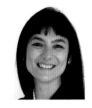

A traditional Chinese Medicine Doctor, Margella Salmins studied at Middlesex University and at Beijing University of Traditional Chinese Medicine. The five-year training included acupuncture, herbal medicine and associated therapies as well as Western medical diagnostic and clinical skills. She also holds certificates in Therapeutic Healing, Advanced Reiki and Macrobiotic Healing.

### Patrizia Sergeant, Journey and Bowen Practitioner, Reiki Healer

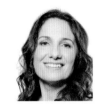

Patrizia's healing work began when she was at a very low point in her life. Financial hardship, a severely prolapsed disc, panic attacks and agrophobia eventually forced her to look deeper into the connection between negative life experiences and emotions that were the underlying causes of these difficulties. Hesitant and resistant at first, she embarked on a journey of self-discovery and healing in an effort to recover her wellbeing. Inspired by the positive results she experienced, she decided to train so that se could offer equally powerful possibilities to others. She aims to support her clients' desire to look deep within to clear old suppressed cell memories, allowing their self-healing potential to be fully activated.

### Shazzie

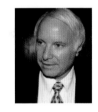

Shazzie has been a vegan since 1986 and a raw foodist since 2000. She is a TV presenter and author of five books. For well over a decade, she has given lectures and workshops around the world at the most prestigious venues, including the Burj Al Arab in Dubai. She is often featured in international media discussing such topics as raw food, superfoods, detox, raw chocolate, breastfeeding and natural parenting.

### Prof. Shimon Slavin, MD

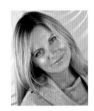

As Medical and Scientific Director of the CTCI, Prof. Shimon Slavin is internationally renowned for his innovative use of cell therapy and immunotherapy in treating cancer and life-threatening non-malignant diseases. Having graduated from the Hadassah Hebrew University School of Medicine in Jerusalem, Israel, Prof. Slavin went on to train in immunology and rheumatology at Stanford University in California and at the Fred Hutchinson Bone Marrow Transplantation Center in Seattle, Washington. His pioneering work in cell therapy of cancer by donor lymphocyte infusions (DLI), post-allogeneic stem-cell transplantation and non-myeloablative stem cell transplantation (NST), or mini-transplant, is now in worldwide use. NST is much safer, less difficult for the patient and more economical than previously developed procedures.

Prof. Slavin has also developed personalised approaches to treat cancer using immunotherapy, mediated by innovative targeted cell therapy and vaccines. He conducts basic clinical research and clinical trials of novel methods to make his patients' immune systems effective in targeting and combating their disease. The world's leading peer-reviewed journals have published over 500 articles of his research. He has written four books on his medical research and innovations.

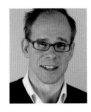

### Prof. Robert Thomas, MRCP (UK), MD, FRCR

A Consultant Oncologist at Bedford and Addenbrooke's Hospitals, Robert Thomas is also a Professor at Cranfield University and clinical teacher at Cambridge University. He treats breast, prostate and bowel cancer with chemotherapy, radiotherapy and brachytherapy as well as biological and supportive therapies; he is also a strong advocate of the role of self-help and lifestyle strategies to improve wellbeing and outcome. His book *Lifestyle and Cancer: The Facts* appeared in 2008 and he is editor of a website about cancer treatment and lifestyle. He has published over 100 scientific papers, including the world's largest prospective trial evaluating lifestyle and prostate-cancer progression. He is chief investigator of the first double-blind randomised controlled trial of a polyphenol supplement (Pomi-T) in men with prostate cancer. Having designed the UK's first level 4 cancer rehabilitation course for exercise professionals, he is also Media Spokesman and Chair of the Macmillan Cancer Support Exercise Advisory Group. In 2001 he was voted 'Doctor of the Year' by *Hospital Doctor Magazine* and in 2007 'Oncologist of the Year' by the British Oncology Association.

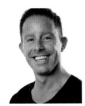

### Jason Vale

Known as the 'Juice Master', Jason Vale has sold over two million books worldwide and is highly regarded as one of the most influential people in the realm of juicing and health. Jason is the author of ten books. Besides appearing in many television and radio shows he has produced DVDs and CDs on juicing, health, fitness and junk-food addiction and is regularly featured in leading magazines.

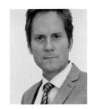

### Robert Verkerk, BSc, MSc, DIC, PhD

Robert is an expert in agricultural, environmental and health sustainability. His MSc and PhD are both from Imperial College, London, awarded before his continuing research for a further seven years at the college's Department of Biology, as a post-doctoral Research Fellow. In 2002 he founded the Alliance for Natural Health International (ANH-Intl), which has become one of the leading non-profit campaign organisations working globally to promote more sustainable healthcare systems through the use of natural and bio-compatible approaches. He is Executive and Scientific Director of the ANH-Intl as well as Co-chair of its Scientific and Medical Collaboration. Around sixty papers by him have been published in scientific journals and conference proceedings, and he contributes regularly to magazines and other popular media. He is also an accomplished and inspirational speaker and communicator on a wide range of issues relating to sustainability.

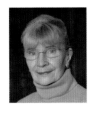

### Xandria Williams, PhD, MSc, DIC, ARCS, MRSC, ND, DBM, MRN

After graduating in chemistry from Imperial College, London, and gaining a further degree from Otago University, New Zealand, Xandria studied naturopathy and botanic medicine in Sydney, Australia. She went on to train in psychotherapy, NLP, EFT and related techniques. She is a member of the Royal Society of Medicine and has worked as a nutritional biochemist and naturopath in private practice for more than thirty years in Australia, the UK and Ireland. She has published more than 400 articles and twenty-one books, has been the head of nutrition departments in several colleges and given many thousands of hours of lectures and seminars in many countries to graduates, post-graduates and general interest groups. During the last ten years or so, she has developed a particular interest in researching cancer as a process, focusing on its early detection and the ways in which nutritional, plant-derived and other natural substances can be used to help restore homoeostasis, cellular chemistry and health. She is a founder member of the British Society for Integrative Oncology.

### Dr Bernard Willis, MBChB, D (Obst), RCOG, MRCGP

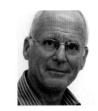

Bernard Willis qualified as MBChB at Leeds University in 1967. After completing his hospital residencies in surgery, general medicine and obstetrics, he left England to work as a private GP in Perth, Western Australia, where he obtained the Diploma in Obstetrics and Gynaecology and Membership of the Royal College of General Practitioners. After three years in Perth he returned to the UK and became a partner in a general practice in Essex. In 1982 he was recruited to become the senior GP at the first private primary care centre in England. In 1991 he and his wife went to Spain, where they spent nineteen years taking care of British and European ex-patriates.

While in Spain Dr Willis became ill with Chronic Fatigue Syndrome (CFS) brought on by a viral infection. This forced him to take time off work, an absence during which he researched and cured himself of the condition through natural lifestyle changes, nutrition, hormones and supplements. This led to the realisation that he could often treat his patients with nutritional therapies, thus avoiding pharmaceutical drugs and their inevitable side effects. He attended many courses on Integrative Medicine and holistic approaches, practising these widely in his clinics in Spain. Subsequently, he ran a busy Integrative Medicine clinic in Auckland, New Zealand for five years and was an active member of the Australasia Integrative Medicine Association (AIMA) and the Australasian College of Nutritional and Environmental Medicine (ACNEM). From early 2016 he will be practising in the UK. His interests currently include nutrition and dietary therapy, herbal treatments, bio-identical HRT and intravenous nutritional therapy for chronic diseases such as CFS, adrenal fatigue, thyroid disorders, male and female menopause and cancer.

### Dr André Young-Snell, MBBS

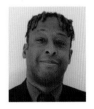

André Young-Snell studied conventional medicine at Guy's Hospital Medical School, London and qualified in 1988. Though specialising in Parkinson's disease, he covered many fields at some of the UK's top hospitals, including Addenbrooke's, Cambridge, Whipps Cross, Barts and Guys, London and Brighton. After much deliberation, in 2002 he decided to set up his own clinic, the Vision of Hope in Brighton, where he could specialise in metabolic protocols. He strongly believes that the patient's mindset is of utmost importance to his or her recovery; he recommends focusing on setting goals, ways of expressing gratitude, making space for relaxation and laughter, all combined with more traditional complementary metabolic protocols.

HELLO

HOPE THE BOOK IS HELPFUL

# HOW TO USE THIS BOOK

The topic of cancer and recovery is huge and can be quite overwhelming. The subject matter of each of the chapters below could easily constitute a book in its own right, so, necessarily, *The Cancer Revolution* is intended to give you a good overview and then to suggest where to look for more information.

Although primarily addressed to someone with cancer, the book is equally intended as a resource for carers, practitioners and anyone interested in living a cancer-free life.

We have designed the book to be easily navigable, and in such a way that, as you learn about yourself and how to build your own programme, you are quickly able to access the information that is relevant and of interest to you.

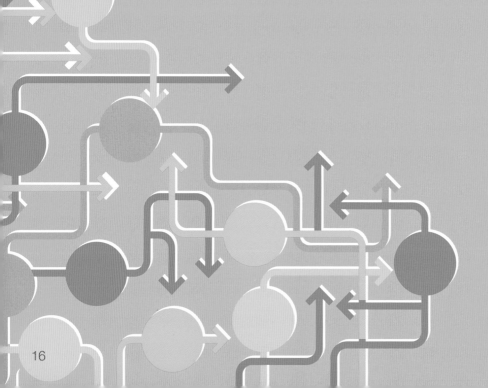

# OVERVIEW

| | | |
|---|---|---|
| **Part One** | is good general reading for everyone, as it lays out the territory, describing and making the case for Integrative Medicine as well as looking at some of the most important resources to help you | 34 to 73 |
| **Part Two** | is devoted to the subject of nutrition, a hugely important element of any integrative programme | 74 to 137 |
| **Part Three** | covers some other equally important aspects of the way we live that will possibly have had a key part in getting you to the point of diagnosis, and that could play an equally important role in restoring your health | 138 to 169 |
| **Part Four** | deals with toxins, an almost unavoidable aspect of modern life, and an important contributing factor to much chronic illness | 170 to 199 |
| **Part Five** | contains useful information about dealing with your medical team and getting the most from testing | 200 to 225 |
| **Part Six** | concludes the main text | 226 to 229 |
| **Part Seven** | consists of four appendices, with information on international clinics, scans, suggestions on how to find appropriate practitioners and how to manage your finances | 230 to 251 |
| **Part Eight** | contains further useful resources | 252 to 293 |

There is no need to read the book from cover to cover. Once you have the **Introduction** and **Part One** under your belt, each chapter stands on its own, and if there is further related information on any given topic elsewhere in the book, it is noted in the text. **Chapter 3, 'Who's who in Integrative Medicine'**, can be used as a reference to give you ideas of practitioners with whom you might want to work on any given issue.

So follow your interests and read the chapters that you feel are the most relevant to you. There is no formula or plan that is ideal for absolutely everyone; furthermore, almost everything varies according to what stage of treatment you are in and what type of cancer you have.

# SUGGESTED READING PLANS

For those who would like some guidance, here are some reading suggestions, dependent on your circumstances. Home in on the topics that are applicable to you.

### Newly diagnosed

If you are newly diagnosed, you are likely to be extremely stressed, as cancer challenges every individual at the deepest level – your very identity is in the balance. You will be dealing with massive uncertainties about your future. A diagnosis of cancer is akin to being dropped on another planet with a strange language, rules that we don't understand, and with absolutely no grasp of how to navigate our way forward. We may go from a sense of ourselves as capable, in control of our lives, directed and responsible, to feeling completely helpless and lost.

All of this is common and to be expected. We are also likely to feel bombarded with more new information than we can possibly cope with, both from a range of experts and from well-meaning family and friends. In these circumstances, you will almost certainly not want to settle down to read *The Cancer Revolution* from cover to cover. What you need is the right kind of support to get you back in the driving-seat with sufficient equilibrium to be able to meet and respond to the choices ahead of you.

In that case, I would recommend that after completing this **Introduction**, you then read:

- **Chapter 9, 'Managing stress'** a chapter that suggests strategies for dealing with the shock, offering a mine of information and intended to inspire you to cope with what is ahead of you

- **Chapter 14, 'Be informed'**, which offers advice on how to work with your doctors: if you are accustomed to being reasonably healthy and therefore unfamiliar with hospitals, specialists and the NHS, this chapter will help you to understand what to expect; furthermore, it will encourage you to prepare yourself and learn how to navigate the system

- **Chapters 6, 7 and 8**, discuss how to support yourself during treatment and explore the ways in which concentrated nutrition and exercise can help you through standard treatments by supporting your immune system, preventing damage or other unwelcome side effects, maintaining your energy levels, and helping you to sustain a positive state of mind through difficulties

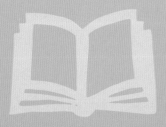

Once you have got a few basics in place and gained some degree of equilibrium, you may then feel ready for:

- Part One, 'Getting to know the territory', a broad look at cancer and the integrative approach, including an overview of the range of practitioners and therapies
- Chapters 4, 'How to buy good food' and 5, 'Diet as the foundation of good health', a careful look at the fuel we give our bodies for survival, which is foundational to any cancer programme; these chapters cover various aspects of food and diet and their relationship to our health and wellbeing

After that, read whatever takes your interest first, as and when you feel it becomes relevant to you. At some point you might find that you want to re-read chapters as your understanding increases, or perhaps you will decide that you are now ready to read the book cover to cover.

**Newly diagnosed**

Summary of recommendation

## Mid-treatment but new to Integrative Medicine

If you are already some way into your treatment, you will probably have found ways to come to terms with the diagnosis, at least to some extent; you might be beginning to become accustomed to living day to day with uncertainty, and you will be somewhat familiar with the 'terrain' of the world of cancer, its language, its range of new and extraordinary experiences.

If you are now feeling the need to look beyond the boundaries of standard treatments to see what else may be available to improve your quality of life and raise your chances of a sustained recovery, then I would suggest reading straight through after completing this **Introduction**:

- **Parts One and Two**: A broad look at cancer, the integrative approach, and the range of practitioners and therapies; the topic of nutrition is a foundational aspect of any integrative programme
- **Parts Three and Four**: There is a lot here and it is probably best to home in initially on aspects that feel important to you and that are most easily addressed in your personal circumstances. Don't try doing everything at once, be kind to yourself – it takes time to make life changes and to form new habits. I strongly suggest that you don't overlook **Chapter 9, 'Managing stress'**, even – or maybe particularly – if you don't think it applies to you
- **Part Five**: By now, perhaps you will feel that you have got the measure of hospital systems and staff, but there might still be a few ideas here that have not occurred to you. As you become more of an expert on your own condition and treatment, **Chapter 15, 'Testing: vital pointers to success'**, could provide you with crucial information that could help validate your choices and progress

**Mid-Treatment new to IM**

Summary of recommendation

8

## Mid-treatment and familiar with basics of Integrative Medicine

If you are already some way along the journey of building and constantly re-evaluating and adjusting your integrative programme, the chances are that you won't need me to tell you what to be interested in! You will probably go straight to the sections that inspired you to start reading this particular book in the first place.

However, as general recommendations, I would say:
• Never forget that an integrative approach is a broad approach – I would never advise putting all your faith in just one of the elements covered in this book. Many people will have personal priorities that they feel are uniquely important to them, but this is not a reason to neglect the others

• Probably the area most often avoided but with a huge amount to offer (particularly to those who seek most to avoid it) is that of our psychological, emotional and/or spiritual wellbeing

• Beware of becoming over-confident in your expertise. Knowledge is a wonderful thing and may even save your life, but it is wise to maintain a healthy respect for the continuing power of cancer to baffle even some of the greatest minds. You can always benefit from the best expert advice

As someone who is already immersed in the world of Integrative Medicine, you will be able to make good use of the Therapeutic Target Icons listed immediately following these suggested reading plans, to locate relevant material.

**Mid-treatment familiar with basics of IM**

Summary of recommendation
Follow your interests

## Facing a recurrence

This is an extremely tough scenario that, tragically, far too many people have to face. You will probably need considerable emotional support and a really good range of options to equip you to move forward with some confidence. *The Cancer Revolution* can help.

If you are new to Integrative Medicine, then – alongside a careful evaluation of any standard treatments that may be offered, based on their predicted outcome and side effects – you have a complete new world of additional resources to explore, both to assist directly with your standard treatments and to work alongside them. After completing the **Introduction**, I would recommend a similar reading plan to those mid-treatment but new to Integrative Medicine, above.

**New to IM**

Summary of recommendation

If you have already been taking an integrative approach, then it is time to take stock of your situation, consider where the gaps might be in your strategy, and also whether it is time to talk to some new practitioners.

As a plan for reading this book, I would recommend that you look through the whole volume with eyes as fresh as you can manage, carefully noting anything that you might not have considered before or that you have perhaps bypassed previously.

As someone who is already immersed in the world of Integrative Medicine, you will be able to make good use of the Therapeutic Target Icons listed immediately following these suggested reading plans, to locate relevant material.

**Familiar with IM**

Summary of recommendation

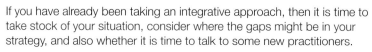

## Given the 'all clear'

If you've bought this book, you probably won't need telling that the very last response to an 'all clear' is complacency. The desire to 'get back to your life' should be an alarm call, as 'your life' was exactly where you got cancer. At this point you have an opportunity to put together a strategy that could well mean taking your life in a completely new direction, or at least replacing many old habitual patterns with new, healthier ones. Once you have had cancer there is never any room for complacency again. Although this may sound like a 'sentence' hanging over you, the good news is that the changes needed are all positive, life-affirming choices.

A certain amount of the book is about working with standard treatments, and that is not relevant to you right now. There is nevertheless a huge raft of useful information on which to build your strategy. At this point I would recommend that you read:

- **Part One**, to gain an appreciation of the territory
- **Part Two**, for a thorough understanding of the essential role of nutrition
- **Part Three**, which contains important information on several other lifestyle factors that are worth examining with a view to making changes
- **Chapter 15**, 'Testing: vital pointers to success', which offers advice on how to evaluate whether your programme is being effective or not; testing can allay some of the worry that is endemic among those who have had cancer

### Given 'all clear'
Summary of recommendation

## At the end of unsuccessful treatment

If you have reached the 'end of the road' in terms of conventional medicine, or if the treatment on offer promises little reward for a great deal of suffering, then Integrative Medicine might still be able to help. If acquiring *The Cancer Revolution* is your first step towards exploring this territory, then I would advise you to read:

- **Chapter 9**, 'Managing stress', for inspiration and, particularly if you are newly re-diagnosed, to help you deal with the shock and stress of your situation. Using this chapter for guidance, find the support you need

- **Parts One, Two, Three and Four,** admittedly most of the book, but there is a need to get an overview of the territory quickly; while there is probably too much information to take in all at once, you will get a broad idea of the types of change you need to make and of the kinds of specialist you could approach; decisive action can have a dramatic effect on a seemingly runaway or hopeless situation

### New to IM
Summary of recommendation

If you have been taking an integrative approach for some time, then I would recommend a reading plan similar to the one outlined in 'Facing a recurrence', on p. 20.

### Familiar with IM
Summary of recommendation

# THERAPEUTIC TARGET ICONS

If you are trying to achieve an objective that has many possible approaches – such as increasing the amount of oxygen in your system – there are icons in the margins of this book that highlight relevant material throughout. A larger icon at the start of a chapter indicates that the entire chapter is relevant. These are briefly described below and also in more detail in **Chapter 1, 'Taking an integrative approach', p. 39.** So a quick flick through the book will lead you straight to relevant information. As a handy reference, there is also a list of the target icons with an index of their locations on the **fold-out back cover flap.**

Here are the icons and a description of the target they each highlight:

 **Detoxification** – changing lifestyle and environment to limit exposure to toxins, and removing toxins from the body, including viruses, bacteria and parasites

 pH **balance** – providing the body with the supportive elements for a slightly alkaline environment within the body, to discourage tumour growth (which favours and promotes an acidic environment)

 **Immune stimulation** – boosting the body's natural defences and assisting them in identifying malignant cells as targets for attack

 **Anti-cancer** – approaches or substances that have clinical evidence of selectively controlling, damaging or weakening cancer cells in some way

 **Oxygenation** – increasing the level of oxygen circulating within the body, or more specifically in tumours, to improve efficacy of treatment

 **Inflammation control** – increasingly, cancer and other chronic diseases are being seen to stem from chronic inflammation; controlling inflammation can determine progress of a cancer

 **Hormone control** – many of the most common cancers in the West are driven by hormones, so survival can depend on the body being able to metabolise them safely

 **Improved absorption** – ensuring that you are absorbing all nutrients and supplements well, and that your gut has recovered from inflammatory effects of drug or radiotherapy treatment

 **Personal resilience** – cancer and cancer treatment are often the biggest challenges that any of us have to face, and they can stretch us to limits physically, emotionally, mentally and spiritually; we need all the help we can get

# ABOUT THE GLOSSARY

Descriptions of cancer and its treatment inevitably contain many unfamiliar words. Getting to understand them is just one small part of the challenge of being dropped on 'planet cancer'. Rather than attempting simply to avoid them, or to explain them repeatedly within the text – an irritation to readers who already understand them – we have provided a Glossary of cancer-specific and other specialised words on the fold-out flap at the back of the book. You can therefore quickly check any terms you need to as you go along. As these words become more familiar to you, I hope that your need to refer to the Glossary will diminish. You will almost certainly reap the benefits of making the effort to learn some of the language of cancer when it comes to talking to and understanding specialists.

Within the Glossary, the primary term is followed by related words in parentheses, in alphabetical order, e.g. alkalise (alkali, alkaline. alkalinity). Words that are included in the Glossary generally appear more than once in the book and are highlighted in blue.

It is worth drawing attention here to a few very common cancer-specific words that have been excluded from the Glossary:

## CAM
the commonly used acronym for Complementary and Alternative Medicine, a broad description for all the approaches to health and wellbeing that fall outside mainstream medicine practised by health service doctors

## Chemotherapy
a standard treatment for cancer, in which toxic substances are administered either intravenously or by mouth, with the aim of damaging cancer cells so that they cannot reproduce and spread

## Oncology, oncologist
the study of cancer and the specialists who work in this field

## Radiotherapy
another standard treatment that relies on high-energy ionising radiation to damage cancer cells so that they die

# BOXED TEXTS

As a way of helping you to home in on the things you are most interested in, several categories of information are set out in 'boxes':

**Self-help boxes** contain instructions for techniques that you can safely try yourself, without needing expert guidance.

**Science boxes** contain fairly technical information that will be of more interest to some readers than others.

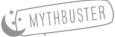

**Mythbuster boxes** highlight common ideas surrounding cancer and Integrative Medicine that have often originated long ago and don't necessarily reflect current research; it is past time to dispel them; all medical approaches are subject to myths and our journey towards understanding often means that early concepts are overturned. If delivered with conviction by a doctor or practitioner, a myth can put you off a strategy that may actually be useful. On top of this, cancer itself has a good few myths built around it that are now seen clearly as untrue; throughout this book, myths relevant to each section are highlighted and 'busted'.

**My story boxes** offer first-hand accounts of those who have experienced situations or techniques outlined in this book.

Other boxes are used occasionally to allow additional material by another contributor to be inserted into a chapter.

# OTHER FEATURES

This book is intended to introduce you to the wider world of Integrative Medicine, and to point you in the direction of the people and places that can help you or someone you are caring for to choose a personalised path to recovering from cancer. We are fortunate that much of this book has been contributed by a formidable range of specialists, both from the UK and from around the world. Sections I have written, or where I have added material to a chapter, are identified by a photo of me.

The thirty-seven further contributors range from media personalities to top scientists. The language used inevitably reflects these different vantage points. In editing the book, we have striven to make every chapter accessible to all readers, while still preserving the 'voice' of each author. Hence, for example, the chapter by Janey Lee Grace, writer and broadcaster on all things non-toxic for your home, is very distinct from that on exercise by Prof. Robert Thomas, a leading UK oncologist. Furthermore, we have left all measurements in the units supplied by each contributor. A conversion table can be found on p. 26.

Occasionally you will come across information from one contributor that does not completely agree with another. In editing the book we were well aware of this – it is simply a reflection of a developing science. There is now a broad consensus about many foundational principles of Integrative Medicine, but as with any new science, there are diverging opinions on some matters. As new research comes in, so people's opinions might change or consolidate according to the latest findings. So, rather than artificially honing the information to conform to a single view, we are occasionally presenting views that differ to enable you to come to your own conclusions.

An important thread that runs through the material is the research that underpins it; the book also includes some relatively undocumented information, for example about therapies and healing techniques that many cancer patients have found helpful and are generally agreed to be unlikely to have any harmful effects.

## Companion website

*The Cancer Revolution* has a companion website (thecancerrevolution.co.uk) that hosts all the scientific references (indicated by superscript numbers in the text), as well as other interesting material related to this book. Many of the contributors were more than generous with their material and it simply wasn't possible to include it all in the finished publication. But you can find it on the website along with other material adding to the background of the authors and the subject matter they present.

## QR codes

Throughout the book there are QR codes (see the example on the right). Provided you have a QR Reader app installed in your smartphone, these will take you directly to a website relevant to the adjacent text. Where there are two or more QR codes on a page, take care to hold your phone close to the page to avoid picking up the wrong code. If you don't have a smartphone, all the website addresses are in **Part Eight**, '**Resources**'.

## Appendices

At the end of this section, I would like to draw attention to the appendices that feature, among other valuable information, descriptions of the approaches taken at a number of the world's leading Integrative Medicine clinics, written by their medical directors or senior physicians. Although they introduce a wealth of new concepts and treatment approaches that you might find a little overwhelming, I hope that the sheer breadth of work being undertaken internationally will start to inspire you to want to 'look outside the box' in relation to your own situation. I also hope that it will provide a desperately needed beacon for our own cancer services, plotting a tried and tested route towards greater success in cancer care.

I hope you find this book a great help and wish you every success.

# UNITS OF MEASUREMENT: CONVERSION TABLE

| | UK (IMPERIAL) | EUROPE | USA |
|---|---|---|---|
| **DISTANCE / LENGTH** | | | |
| 1 mm (millimetre) | 0.039 in | 1 mm | 0.039 in |
| 1 cm (centimetre) | 0.39 in | 1 cm | 0.39 in |
| 1 m (metre) | 39.37 in | 1m | 39.37 in |
| 1 in (inch) | 1 in | 2.54 cm | 1 in |
| 1 yard | 1 yard | 91.44 cm | 1 yard |
| 1 mile | 1 mile | 1.61 km | 1 mile |
| **WEIGHT** | | | |
| 1 mcg (microgram) | 0.000000035 oz | 1 mcg | 0.000000035 oz |
| 1 mg (milligram) | 0.000035 oz | 1 mg | 0.000035 oz |
| 1 g (gram) | 0.035 oz | 1 g | 0.035 oz |
| 1 oz (ounce) | 1 oz | 28.35 g | 1 oz |
| 1 lb (pound) | 1 lb | 0.45 kg | 1 lb |
| **VOLUME** | | | |
| 1l | 1.76 pints | 1 l | 2.11 pints |
| 1 pint | 1 pint | 0.5683 l | 1.20 pints |
| 1 cup | 8 fl oz | 250 ml | 1 cup |
| **TEMPERATURE** | | | |
| ${}^0$C (Celsius, centigrade) see conversion formulae below | ${}^0$F (Fahrenheit) | ${}^0$C | ${}^0$F (Fahrenheit) |
| **AMOUNT** | | | |
| 1 mSv (milliSievert) | 1 mSv | 1 mSv | 100 mrem |
| **CURRENCY** | | | |
| £1 (GB pound sterling)* | £1.00 | EUR1.42 | USD1.50 |
| 1 p (penny, pence)* | 1p | 1c | 2c |

To convert Fahrenheit to Celsius: $x^0 F = 5/9(x - 32)^0 C$
To convert Celsius to Fahrenheit: $y^0 C = (9/5y + 32)^0 F$

*as at Nov 2015

**N.B.:** Many European (metric) units are now in common use in the UK.

# LIST OF ABBREVIATIONS

| | |
|---|---|
| ACE | Academy for Chief Executives |
| ACIB | Associate of the Chartered Institute of Bankers |
| ACNEM | Australasian College of Nutritional and Environmental Medicine, Sandringham, Victoria, Australia |
| ACTM | Association of Chinese Traditional Medicine |
| AFA | aphanizomenon flos-aquae |
| AIDS | acquired immune deficiency syndrome |
| AIMA | Australasian Integrative Medicine Association, Terrigal, New South Wales |
| ALA | alpha lipoic acid |
| AMP-K | adenosine monophosphate-activated protein kinase |
| ANH-Intl | Alliance for Natural Health International |
| AoR | Association of Reflexologists |
| app | application |
| ARCS | Associateship of the Royal College of Science |
| AST | acoustic shockwave therapy |
| ATP | adenosinetriphosphate |
| BA (Hons) | Bachelor of Arts (with Honours) |
| BANT | British Association of Nutritional Therapists |
| BAO | Bachelor of Obstetrics |
| BBC | British Broadcasting Corporation |
| BCh | Baccalaureus Chirurgiae (Bachelor of Surgery) |
| Bcl-2 | B-cell lymphoma 2 |
| BGS | British Geological Survey |
| BM | Bachelor of Medicine |
| BPA | bisphenol A |
| BRCA | breast cancer (used in gene names BRCA1 and BRCA2 that produce tumour suppressor proteins) |
| BSc (Hons) | Bachelor of Science (with Honours) |
| BSIO | British Society for Integrative Oncology |
| C | Celsius (centigrade) |
| CAM | Complementary and Alternative Medicine |
| CBE | Commander of the Order of the British Empire |
| CBT | cognitive behavioural therapy |
| CCH | Certified in Classical Homeopathy |
| CChem | Chartered Chemist |
| CD | compact disc |
| C Dip UTR | Certified Diploma in Understanding Therapeutic Relationships |
| C Eng | Chartered Engineer |
| CFS | chronic fatigue syndrome |
| C Geol | Chartered Geologist |
| CHCHD4 | coiled-coil-helix-coiled-coil-helix domain containing protein 4 |
| Chem BSc | (Hons) Chemistry Bachelor of Science (with Honours) |
| Clin Oncol | clinical oncology |
| cm | centimetre(s) |
| CMIT | Contreras Metabolic IntegrativeTherapy |
| CNHC | Complementary and Natural Healthcare Council |
| CoQ10 | coenzyme Q10 |
| CRF | cancer-related fatigue |
| CT | computerised tomography |
| CTCI | cell therapy and cancer immunotherapy |
| D (Obst) | Diploma of the Royal College of Obstetricians and Gynaecologists |
| DBM | Diploma in Business Management |
| DECT | digital enhanced cordless telecommunications |
| DFFP | Diploma of the Faculty of Family Planning |
| D Hom (Med) | Doctor of Homeopathic Medicine |
| DHT | dihydrotestosterone |
| DIC | Diploma of Imperial College |
| DIM | diindolylmethane |
| Dip Couns | Diploma in Counselling |
| Dip NT | Diploma in Nutritional Therapy |
| Dip Pall | (Postgraduate) Diploma in Palliative Medicine |
| Dip PFS | Diploma in Financial Planning (from the Personal Finance Society) |
| Dip Psych | Diploma in Psychology |
| DLI | donor lymphocyte infusions |
| DNA | deoxyribonucleic acid |
| DNN | Diploma in Nursery Nursing |
| DoIC | Diploma of Imperial College |
| DPsSC | Diploma in Pyschosexual Counselling |
| Dr | Doctor |

| | | | | |
|---|---|---|---|---|
| DSc | Doctor of Science | | HL60 | human promyelocytic leukaemia cells |
| dsp | dessertspoon(s) | | HMD | Doctor of Holistic Medicine |
| DVD | digital versatile disc or digital video disc | | HPV | human papilloma virus |
| € | euro(s) | | HSP70 | 70 kilodalton heat shock proteins |
| ECT | electro cancer therapy | | IARC | International Agency for Research on Cancer, Lyons, France |
| EDTA | ethylenediaminetetraacetic acid | | ICTC | Integrative Cancer Therapy Concept |
| EFT | emotional freedom technique | | IFA | independent financial adviser |
| e.g. | exempli gratia (for example) | | IgE | immunoglobulin E |
| EGCG | epigallocatechin gallate | | IGF | insulin-like growth factor |
| EGF | epidermal growth factor | | IGF-1R | insulin-like growth factor receptor |
| EGFR | epidermal growth factor receptors | | in | inch(es) |
| EINECS | Inventory of Existing Commercial Chemical Substances | | IP-6 | inositol hexaphosphate |
| | | | IPT | insulin potentiation therapy |
| EMF | electromagnetic field | | ITEC | International Therapy Examination Council |
| EMR | electromagnetic radiation | | | |
| EPA | Environmental Protection Agency | | IU | international unit (of mass or volume of various active biological substances) |
| EU | European Union | | | |
| F | Fahrenheit | | | |
| FDG | fluorodeoxyglucose | | kg | kilogram(s) |
| FGS | Fellow of the Geological Society | | km | kilometre(s) |
| FHT | Federation of Holistic Therapists | | £ | pound(s) sterling |
| FIMM | Institute for Molecular Medicine, Finland | | l | litre(s) |
| fl oz | fluid ounce(s) | | lb | pound(s) (weight) |
| FRCN | Fellow of the Royal College of Nursing | | LAPd | lipoic acid palladium complex |
| | | | LDN | low dose naltrexone |
| FRCR | Fellow of the Royal College of Radiologists | | LDS | Licence in Dental Surgery |
| | | | m | metre(s) |
| FREng | Fellow of the Royal Academy of Engineering | | MA | Master of the Arts |
| FRGS | Fellow of the Royal Geographical Society | | MAHPP | Member of the Association of Humanistic Psychology Practitioners |
| FRSA | Fellow of the Royal Society of Arts | | MAR | Member of the Association of Reflexologists |
| FRSE | Fellow of the Royal Society of Edinburgh | | | |
| FRSM | Fellow of the Royal Society of Medicine | | MB | Bachelor of Medicine |
| | | | MBANT | Member of the British Association of Nutritional Therapists |
| g | gram(s) | | MBBCh | Medicinae Baccalaureus, Baccalaureus Chirurgiae (Bachelor of Medicine, Bachelor of Surgery) |
| GcMAF | globulin component macrophage activating factor | | | |
| GCMT | General Council for Massage Therapies | | MBBS | Medicinae Baccalaureus, Baccalaureus Chirurgiae (Bachelor of Medicine, Bachelor of Surgery) |
| GLUT-1 | glucose transporter, type 1 | | | |
| GM | genetically modified | | MBChB | Medicinae Baccalaureus, Baccalaureus Chirurgiae (Bachelor of Medicine, Bachelor of Surgery) |
| GP | general practitioner | | | |
| HBOT | hyperbaric oxygen therapy | | MBCT | mindfulness-based cognitive therapy |
| HerbMed | herbal medicine | | MBSR | mindfulness-based stress reduction |
| HEPA | high-efficiency particulate arrestance | | MCF-7 | Michigan Cancer Foundation-7 (a breast-cancer cell line) |
| HIF | hypoxia inducible factor | | mcg | microgram(s) |
| HIFU | high intensity focused ultrasound | | MCP | modified citrus pectin |

| | | | |
|---|---|---|---|
| MCPP | Member of the College of Practitioners of Phytotherapy | PhD | Doctor of Philosophy |
| MCS | multiple chemical sensitivity | Phyto | phytotherapy |
| MD | Doctor of Medicine | PNI | psychoneuroimmunology |
| mg | milligram(s) | Prof. | Professor |
| MFHT | Member of the Federation of Holistic Therapists | PSA | prostate specific antigen |
| ml | millilitre(s) | PSK | polysaccharide-K |
| mm | millimetre(s) | QoL | quality of life |
| MNCH | maternal newborn and child health | QR | quick response |
| MNIMH | Member of the National Institute of Medical Herbalists | RBAC | rice bran arabinoxylan compound |
| MNTOI | Member of the Nutritional Therapists Organisation of Ireland | RCHM | Register of Chinese Herbal Medicine |
| | | RCNT | Registered Clinical Nurse Teacher |
| MRCGP | Member of the Royal College of General Practitioners | RCOG | Royal College of Obstetricians and Gynaecology, Perth, Western Australia |
| MRCP (UK) | Member of the Royal Colleges of Physicians of the United Kingdom | RCS | Royal College of Surgeons |
| M Res | Master of Research | RD | Registered Dietician |
| MRI | magnetic resonance imaging | REP | Register of Exercise Professionals |
| MRN | Medical Research Network | RF | radio frequency |
| MRSC | Member of the Royal Society of Chemistry | RFA | radio frequency ablation |
| | | RGN | Registered General Nurse |
| MSB | Member of the Society of Biology | RNT | Registered Nurse Teacher |
| MSc | Master of Science | ROS | reactive oxygen species |
| mSv | milliSievert(s) | $ | dollar(s) |
| NCCAM | National Center for Complementary and Alternative Medicine, Bethesda, Maryland, USA | SAD | standard American diet |
| | | SEER | surveillance, epidemiology, and end results |
| NCI | National Cancer Institute (30 divisions in the USA) | St | Saint |
| | | SUKD | standard United Kingdom diet |
| ND | Doctor of Naturopathic Medicine | tbsp | tablespoon(s) |
| NHS | National Health Service | TCM | Traditional Chinese Medicine |
| NIH | National Institutes of Health | TEAM | Traditional East Asian Medicine |
| NK | natural killer | TM2-PK | tumour marker 2 pyruvate kinase |
| NMD | Naturopathic Medical Doctor | tsp | teaspoon(s) |
| nmol/l | nanomoles per litre | TV | television |
| NST | non-myeloablative stem cell transplantation | UCLA | University of California, Los Angeles |
| NTOI | Nutritional Therapists Organisation of Ireland | UK | United Kingdom of Great Britain and Northern Ireland |
| NUTR MED | nutritional medicine | UKAHPP | UK Association for Humanistic Psychology Practitioners |
| ORAC | oxygen radical absorbency capacity | UKCP | UK Council for Psychotherapy |
| OT MSt | Occupational Therapy Masters | UKCTG | UK Clinical Trials Gateway |
| oz | ounce(s) | ULPA | ultra-low penetration air |
| PDT | photodynamic therapy | US | United States (adjective) |
| p | penny, pence | USA | United States of America |
| P53 | tumour protein/antigen 53 | UV | ultraviolet |
| PEG | polyethylene glycol | VEGF | vascular endothelial growth factor |
| PET | positron emission tomography | VOCs | volatile organic compounds |
| PFOA | perfluorooctanoic acid | WISH | World Institute for Sensation Homeopathy |

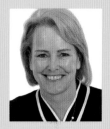

# INTRODUCTION
## INTEGRATIVE MEDICINE:
## A REVOLUTION IN CANCER CARE

Patricia Peat

There is a revolution taking place in the way we think about cancer, how we treat cancer and how we recover from it. This book is intended to give you the information and tools you need to become a part of this revolution and to give yourself the best possible opportunity to prevent and treat cancer, and to recover in a way that is not achievable with standard orthodox approaches alone.

Integrative Medicine is the name of this revolution, integrating the best that medical science has to offer with a comprehensive, holistic approach that supports your body through whatever treatment you choose. You then emerge with a fully functioning immune system, ready to move on to your recovery plan, aimed at detoxifying the effects of treatment, supplying the body with the nutrients which enable DNA repair, and changing the lifestyle and environment that allowed the cancer to take hold in the first place.

Integrative Medicine, or more specifically Integrative Oncology, is the title for an approach to cancer care that encompasses the widest spectrum of methods. It includes all the elements of standard care along with a vast range of therapies that, as a group, have been termed Complementary and Alternative Medicine, or CAM.

As the different sections of this book reveal, there is much more to developing and recovering from cancer than just passive 'treatment'. Integrative therapy is 'holistic', a word that is now bandied about a great deal. But what does it mean for someone who has developed cancer? In my work it is about making the body whole again, right down to the cellular level. It is about far more than just treatment, supplements, diet and exercise. It is about *you*, the whole you, the real you, in relation to your life, your environment, your stresses – what depletes you, what nourishes you, what makes you fearful, what makes you joyful.

INTEGRATIVE MEDICINE IS ABOUT POSITIVE, HEALTHY CHOICES IN DEALING WITH CANCER. IT IS ABOUT YOU DISCOVERING WHAT MADE YOU ILL AND WHAT MAKES YOU WELL AGAIN. IT IS YOUR JOURNEY TOWARDS BECOMING YOUR OWN HEALER.

This book offers you the tools to embark on your journey of discovery towards renewed long-term health. The word 'tools' used here covers a multitude of approaches: chemotherapy is a tool; nutrition is a tool; fresh air and exercise are also tools. These are all important, and should all be considered as valid methods for improving your health.

Probably the most important thing, however, is to bring together the practical and physical approaches with the psychological, spiritual and healing elements that are common to us all and that we need to embrace in order to thrive. These elements are the ones that often become neglected in our frantic and stressful lives; we not only lose touch with them but with the skills needed to use them. This book aims to show you how important it is for you to re-embrace all these elements.

Remember – it is all important!

One-dimensional approaches and magic bullets that take cancer away simply do not exist. Many factors come together to cause cancer, and many elements have to come together in order for anyone to regain full health – which is entirely possible. In my experience I have been lucky and privileged to have been drawn to an integrative approach to dealing with cancer; time and time again, I have worked with people who have far outlived any expectations of their medical team, some ridding themselves of cancer altogether.

The common traits of people who successfully embrace an integrative approach are that they believe in themselves and in their right to make their own decisions, to do things their way. The most important person when it comes to cancer is *you*; the person who should be in charge is *you*; the person who needs to become the expert on you and your survival is *you*.

If you have experienced sitting in a busy oncology unit waiting-room, waiting for your next round of chemotherapy or appointment to see your oncologist, the thought of being an expert in charge of what is happening to you might seem a distant dream, or even a little nonsensical. But that is exactly what people who embark on their own integrative plan achieve. They become:

- knowledgeable
- empowered
- in touch with themselves physically, psychologically and spiritually

Everyone develops a personal plan and lifestyle that encompasses all the elements required for them as an individual to enable recovery to take place – never mind what anybody else has done. All the strands of these programmes harmonise and reinforce the body, so that the resulting whole becomes greater than the sum of its parts. By taking this comprehensive approach, you maximise your potential for healing.

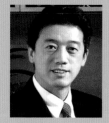

# THE FUTURE OF CANCER CARE

## Dr Gary Deng

For more than a decade, Integrative Oncology has been gaining momentum in the USA. Increased awareness of patients' needs, and the recognition of corresponding room for improvement in current cancer care, have contributed to this movement. Clinical and research resources are now more readily available to study whether and how certain modalities may be suitable components of Integrative Oncology.

Most major US academic medical centres now have an Integrative Medicine programme to provide clinical services, conduct research and to educate healthcare professionals and the public. The NIH allotted close to $110 million in 2011 each to the National Center for Complementary and Alternative Medicine (NCCAM) and the NCI for research in this area. The number of nonprofit organisations that focus on research and education in this field is also growing.

Patients have a desire to participate in the success of their own treatment programmes, and physicians are more receptive to the possibility that this engagement can reduce adverse symptoms and increase the ability to adhere to treatment regimens. More rigorous research will generate the data necessary to guide the practice of Integrative Oncology so that patients can receive the most benefit in the most effective, efficient and economic way.

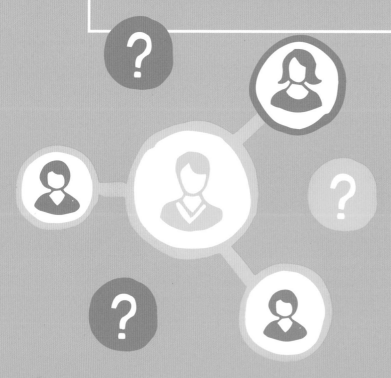

# INTEGRATIVE CANCER CARE IN THE UNITED KINGDOM

Traditionally the UK has had a less comfortable relationship with CAM therapies than is the case in Europe and elsewhere in the world. Have you ever been on holiday and noticed the quantity of herbs and homeopathy available? Their use as a tangible and supportive element is well accepted. In England, however, the medical profession has been more resistant to integrative approaches.

Why is that? In many instances it is because medical professionals do not want people to be exposed to poor practice, charlatans and bad research – and quite right too! The development of the internet has brought us easy access to vast quantities of information, including increased knowledge about cancer. But it has also exposed us to people making outrageous claims about the efficacy of their products – as if a single magical elixir could instantly turn cancer around.

There is also evidence that some CAM therapies will interfere with treatment, which is undesirable to say the least. There are four main points I have found in my conversations with doctors and nurses about CAM:

- They want to make sure that their patients are safe and not subject to poor advice
- They are keen to know ways in which they can increase the support they offer
- They are largely uninformed about how things have developed in Integrative Medicine
- They are not aware of where to go for good information and whom they can trust

Combine these with the business and the stress of running busy oncology clinics and hospitals, and it is not surprising that we have reached an impasse when it comes to safe integration. Lack of funding and the evolving nature of how we learn about cancer are also partly responsible. It is one of the aims of this book to make some progress towards changing that. It is intended both to offer common sense and to stand up to scientific scrutiny. Although not everything about becoming well can be measured scientifically, there are many people who have the knowledge and skills to help you on your way.

In developing Integrative Medicine in the UK, we are fortunate to be able to follow the model of some excellent and well-established integrative clinics in Germany, Israel, Mexico, the USA and elsewhere (see **Appendix 1, 'Integrative clinics around the world'**). The Society for Integrative Oncology has been pushing forward the agenda for integration in the USA since 2003 and has now inspired the founding of the British Society for Integrative Oncology. The BSIO is quickly establishing itself as the primary professional reference point for the best information and practices in Integrative Oncology.

SIO

BSIO

# PART ONE

## GETTING TO KNOW THE
# TERRITORY

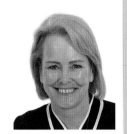

# INTRODUCTION TO PART ONE

Patricia Peat

This introductory part of our main text begins to explore the integrative model of cancer care, along with some of the practicalities of setting out on this path. We cover the current understanding of what cancer is, and how and why we get it. We look at the way that it develops and then at the many pathways through which Integrative Medicine can influence this. Taking an integrative approach in the UK has its own special challenges, so we go into these as well as some sound strategies for finding our way through. Hormones are being implicated in an increasing number of cancers, so we focus on understanding their key role. Importantly, we look at the underpinnings of Integrative Medicine, the evidence for its safety and effectiveness.

Part One ends with a round-up of many of the types of specialist you are likely to encounter in the field of Integrative Medicine, what they do, and how their expertise might help you.

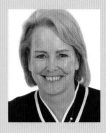

# CHAPTER 1

# TAKING AN INTEGRATIVE APPROACH

## Patricia Peat

### What is cancer?

Cancer is a process whereby normal body cells begin to transform and mutate from a controlled regular state into an irregular one. This is not an unusual occurrence in the body, as millions of body cells are produced every day. We have a highly developed immune system designed to identify the rogue cells, and then to either repair the DNA deficiency or perform what is known as apoptosis. This way the cells are not allowed to mature and mutate further.

If for some reason this process fails, cells are allowed to multiply unchecked and begin to develop the potential to form a tumour, and in the fullness of time to metastasise. This is a fairly long process in most cases. Early on, cancer cells are a bit like children, full of potential, but not mature enough to know how to survive in the wider world. As time goes on, if left unchecked, they develop the following signature qualities of malignant cells:

- They manage to avoid detection by the immune system
- Their physical appearance starts to change (called dysplasia)
- They lose the 'stickiness' which causes normal cells to stick together
- They stop communicating with the other cells around them. Normally cells preserve their uniformity by making sure they are in the right place at the right time, and that they die when they are supposed to. Much communication takes place among cells to keep the body in order (there is communication between normal cells trying to influence cancer cells as well, an area attracting the interest of cancer research)
- The altered cell and its dependants divide more often than they should
- They don't recognise their boundaries and start to infiltrate other cells
- Over time, or if the mutation of cells is taking place very quickly, the cells develop the means to travel into the lymphatics and blood system to develop a metastatic tumour elsewhere

This involves a multi-complex cascade of chemical switches and growth factors in the body beyond the scope of this book. Interfering with those growth signals is the focus of much of orthodox medicine's current research.

## Why do we get cancer?

It is thought that in many cases the onset of cancer is 'a perfect storm' of multiple factors coming together, allowing cellular aberration to take place. The elements we may contribute to the storm ourselves are:

- poor nutrition, particularly dairy and sugar-based foods
- obesity
- alcohol
- stress
- lack of exercise

These can affect the body's normal methods of dealing with cells that have damaged DNA.

Proving that something causes cancer directly is difficult, so most of the elements that have been identified are described as 'causal links'. Smoking, for example, has been accepted as a causal link, beyond doubt. Among the many other things with varying amounts of evidence for having causal links are:

- viruses
- trauma
- food additives
- asbestos
- chronic inflammation
- environmental hormones
- stress
- genetics
- radiation
- bacterial infections
- obesity
- industrial toxins

## METASTATIC SPREAD

*SCIENCE*

### Patricia Peat

This occurs at what is known as the extracellular capsule. Cancer cells will try to invade normal cells by excreting matrix metalloproteinases that are capable of degrading all kinds of extracellular matrix protein. Research beginning in the 1980s has shown that, rather than a purely aggressive occupation of the normal cells, a lot of communication backwards and forwards between the cells takes place. There is potential for normal cells to prevent the infiltration by the cancer cells and to hold them in check, something that obviously happens when someone is in remission after all chemotherapy has left the body. It is also possible for the normal cells to influence genetic upgrade in the cancer cells, i.e. to induce them to revert to normal cells – if they are in a healthy enough position to do so.[1]

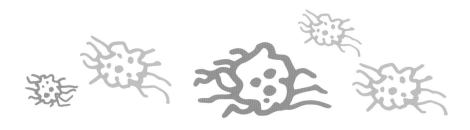

## Integrative Medicine: the best of both worlds

Approaches to treating cancer have, until recently, developed along two parallel paths, based on two different views of cancer. Orthodox medicine has focused on the destruction of tumours and cancer cells and in this has had some extraordinary successes, as can be seen clearly in a few specific cancers which have become largely curable, in the field of acute medicine with complex life-saving surgical techniques, and in survival, with some of the newer targeted drugs. Furthermore, recent developments hold the promise of non-toxic alternatives to chemotherapy and radiotherapy for some patients (see **'Frontier NHS treatments'**, **p. 208**, in **Chapter 14, 'Be informed'**). But at this point, NHS doctors give little attention to overall physical and psychological condition and to the factors that could have led to an immune system becoming sufficiently depleted to allow cancer to develop. This deficiency is usually compounded through standard treatments, leaving people at the end of treatment with a severely damaged immune system, armed only with the hope that they will not relapse.

Meanwhile, Complementary and Alternative Medicine (CAM) has given most of its attention to strengthening what is the most sophisticated known defence against cancer – our own immune system. CAM views cancer as a disease of the whole body that needs addressing in a holistic manner if a lasting cure is to be established. What has been realised is that the same factors that are needed to sustain a healthy life are even more necessary for people whose defences are so weakened that they have succumbed to cancer. Hence many CAM treatments are based on concentrated nutrition and healthy lifestyle choices, in combination with specific strategies to avoid and remove toxins. The vast majority of CAM methods are 100 per cent non-toxic.

Both these approaches have their place and their strengths. The good news is that the impossible 'either/or' choice between the two is now being supplanted by a scientific synthesis of both, under the banner of Integrative Medicine or, more specifically to cancer, Integrative Oncology. This new discipline is growing apace in some parts of the world, and adds the following possibilities over and above standard treatment:

- significant reduction in damage and side effects from standard treatments
- improved action of standard treatments
- improved tolerance of, and recovery from standard treatments
- decreased relapse rates after treatment
- increased life expectancy
- improved quality of life at every stage

It is clear that many people are benefiting enormously from this synthesis, and there are great strengths in a combined protocol.[2] For example, some of the best integrative clinics regularly combine low, and therefore far less toxic, doses of regular chemotherapy with hyperthermia, a heat technique that increases the effect of the chemotherapy, together with intravenous vitamins and minerals to sustain the body's defences. This method can achieve the same level of tumour shrinkage as regular chemotherapy alone, but with minimal toxicity and side effects.

# THERAPEUTIC TARGETS

The Therapeutic Target Icons that appear throughout this book are intended to highlight specific aims that could form the basis of an overall approach. One of the great strengths of an integrative programme, and the aspect that makes it revolutionary, is its ability to work simultaneously with several or all of these targets, and to thereby maximise the total anti-cancer effect. This is in contrast to standard treatment methods, which generally target just one or a very few of the mechanisms of cancer spread. Here I want to spend a little time explaining each target individually, so that you can understand its importance in relation to you and to building your own programme.

## Detoxification

One of the 'side effects' of modern lifestyles is that we are bombarded with toxins which our bodies have to deal with continually. As Robert Verkerk shows in **Chapter 11**, the cumulative effect leaves us vulnerable to cellular change which can lead to cancer development. Research is showing us, for example, that underlying HPV virus not only influences the transition of cells to malignancy, but it can also influence the potential for cancer recurrence following successful treatment.

Detoxification to reduce the burden can be undertaken in different ways and to different extents, depending on your circumstances and preferences. Juicing for example is an excellent form of detoxification; oxygen therapy is another. Liver flushes and coffee enemas can also form part of a home programme.

Integrative practitioners can help with testing (see **Chapter 15, 'Testing: vital pointers to success'**), to establish if there are any underlying imbalances or toxins in your body and can devise a suitable programme to address these. Where appropriate, you could attend a clinic that specialises in intravenous support and more intensive detoxification. The ultimate detoxification approach is provided at some European clinics, where people spend several weeks undergoing intensive therapy; this of course comes with a substantial price tag.

## pH Balance

Every part of the human body is, at any time, weighted towards one side or the other of the acid /alkali balance. The level of alkalinity or acidity is expressed as the pH. Alkaline solutions (pH over 7.0) tend to absorb oxygen, while acids (pH below 7.0) tend to expel oxygen. For example, a mild alkali can absorb over 100 times as much oxygen as a mild acid. Therefore, when the body becomes acidic (below pH 7.0), oxygen is driven out. As discussed below (under **Oxygenation**; see also **'The dangers of glucose', pp.85-6**, and **'The** ketogenic **diet', pp. 90-93** in **Chapter 5, 'Diet as the foundation of good health'**), cancer cells obtain their energy from glucose (sugar), unlike normal cells which depend on oxygen for energy. It follows that allowing the body to become acidic and low in oxygen creates the perfect environment for cancer to thrive.

All body fluids, except for stomach and urine, are supposed to be mildly alkaline (pH 7.4). Stomach fluids must remain acidic to digest food, as must urine to remove wastes from the body. Blood, however, must always remain alkaline (pH 7.4) so that it can retain oxygen. With adequate minerals from diet, the blood is supplied with the crucial elements required to maintain this alkaline state.

It is desirable to keep your body as alkaline as possible through your programme. Oxygen therapies can help with this, as can excercise and taking sodium bicarbonate. Maintaining a high proportion of vegetables in the diet will also help you achieve it. There are supplements available which alkalise the body, although some of these should be viewed with a healthy degree of scepticism – always check with your practitioner.

## Immune stimulation

Stimulating the immune system is vitally important, particularly when undergoing chemotherapy or radiotherapy, both of which deplete it. Ultimately, long-term survival after cancer depends upon the body controlling the situation itself, as people cannot survive being given chemotherapy interminably. Many natural compounds have immune stimulating properties which will prevent excessive damage during treatment, promote repair afterwards, and destroy cancer cells. Most good natural foods contain many of these compounds and they are also available in supplement form. Japanese mushrooms and rice bran are two immune stimulants with much clinical research behind them.[3]

## Anti-cancer

Research is identifying an increasing number of natural compounds that have direct anti-cancer effects on cells. Many are derived from food, but in order to reach the therapeutic level (the concentration at which they have their desired effect) need to be taken in more concentrated form, as supplements. As with detoxification, more intense regimes are available in clinics in the UK and abroad. The huge range of possible choices, supported by an increasing evidence base, now means that an effective programme can be devised even on a low budget.

## Oxygenation

Cancer cells have a complicated relationship with oxygen, a fact that was not fully appreciated until recently. Blood vessels that deliver oxygen to rapidly expanding tumours struggle to keep up with demand, resulting in oxygen starvation of the cancer cells. This would spell death to normal cells, but cancer cells have a protein called HIF which they 'switch on' in response to this, which turns on other cell molecules. The 'HIF response', as this is called, promotes the formation of new blood vessels from the surroundings into the tumour, and helps the tumour to adapt to the lack of oxygen by using another method of energy production.

A normal cell relies on the mitochondria to generate energy, using oxygen as the fuel for chemical reactions. A protein called CHCHD4 checks that oxygen levels are adequate and activates the HIF response if levels drop too far. Laboratory studies have shown that blocking CHCHD4 stops the HIF response and prevents cancer cells from growing and from developing blood vessels.[4] Conversely, the HIF response was promoted by increasing CHCHD4 in cells in a low-oxygen (hypoxic) environment, creating the conditions necessary for the cells to be able to survive.

A lot of work is currently being done to develop drugs to interfere with this signalling sequence and thereby to prevent cancer cells utilising hypoxia in this fashion. Scientists are increasingly ascribing current levels of treatment failure and recurrence to this survival mechanism, as it has been found that cells in hypoxic regions of tumours are resistant to standard chemotherapy treatments. Hypoxia also destabilises genes and promotes mutations. This can lead to drug resistance.

The effects of low oxygen in the body include:

- treatment-related fatigue
- build-up of toxins
- poor transport of nutrients to cells

Benefits of high oxygen levels in the body include:

- reduced radiation damage from radiotherapy
- increased speed of healing following treatment

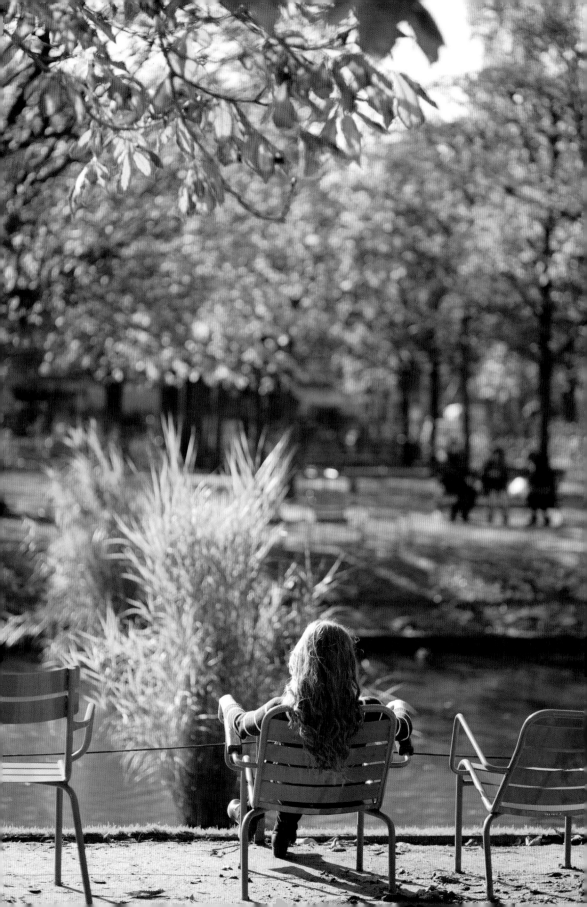

- reduced lymphoedema
- reduced resistance to chemotherapy and radiotherapy
- an alkalysing effect on the tissues

## Inflammation control

Inflammation is often a precursor to the onset of cancer. For example, in a condition known as Barrett's oesophagus, gastric acid splashes back into the oesophagus wall, which is not designed to withstand it. It becomes inflamed, and over time the constant assault on the cells causes DNA damage and they become malignant.

This is an area in which cancer has a lot in common with many other chronic diseases such as arthritis. Inflammation causes changes to the cellular environment, and when this becomes inflamed, several further problems may result. A key message underlying every page of this book is:

> IF YOU CAN PREVENT INFLAMMATION OCCURRING IN YOUR BODY YOU MAY WELL AVOID THE FIRST STEP ON THE ROAD TO CANCER.

Chemotherapy and radiotherapy both cause a tremendous amount of inflammation. Body cells can become chronically inflamed, a state in which they actually perpetuate the level of inflammation. I don't find it unusual to be approached by someone months after chemotherapy still suffering from chronic diarrhoea because the bowel wall has become chronically inflamed.

Good diet prevents inflammation, as do exercise and increased oxygen levels. Some of the most powerful natural anti-cancer compounds such as turmeric and boswellia have strong anti-inflammatory elements. Interestingly, some pharmaceutical anti-inflammatories are also linked with treating cancer, although they unfortunately often have detrimental effects on the liver. When devising a programme, anti-inflammatories should play a large part.

## Hormone control

We are now beginning to realise the very significant role that hormones can play in cancer (see **Chapter 2, 'The crucial role of hormones'**). We have found that they can be part of the driving force of many cancers, not only breast and prostate. How well our bodies metabolise the toxic hormones that we are exposed to in the environment, and stop them contributing to the development of cancer cells, can be of great importance.

The toxic exposure that our bodies struggle to cope with comes mainly from dairy foods, tap water and plastics. The safe metabolisation of these depends on the functioning of the gut and the liver, as well as good nutrition – particularly cruciferous vegetables – regular exercise and reduction of stress. Our endocrine system is finely balanced: if one of its elements is knocked out (as can happen to the adrenals, for example, as a result of prolonged stress) this can lead to a failure to methylate hormones down the correct metabolic pathways.

## Improved absorption

Most holistic practitioners will tell you that the gut is where everything starts. It is our first line of defence against every toxin that may be detrimental to our health. Our gut flora is a fine balance of microbes, and indeed includes a tumour suppressor, discovered in 2013, doubtless the first of many to be found. When I first started researching CAM, I was introduced to the concept of leaky gut: under assault, the gut wall becomes increasingly permeable, which allows toxins to enter the blood stream. It also causes the intestinal lining to become inflamed, and the microvilli (the hair-like membranes that line the gut and absorb nutrients) become damaged or altered. The damaged microvilli cannot then produce the necessary enzymes and secretions that are essential for healthy digestion and for the absorption of nutrients, the very building blocks for healthy DNA. The balance of bacteria is key to a healthy gut, as is lack of inflammation to a vital healthy balance.

Antibiotics and chemotherapy destroy bacteria. Replacement of good bacteria is therefore essential to restore healthy gut function as quickly as possible. When I first came across leaky gut, it was an alien concept in the general understanding of factors that contribute to health. It is interesting to note the increasing number of television and online advertisements for probiotic foods and drinks, showing how an underlying truth has gradually found its way into the mainstream to become an established fact.

## Personal resilience

Resilience is the ability to adapt well in the face of adversity. It is something you need to develop to carry you through to surviving cancer. It involves behaviours, thoughts and actions that anyone can learn and develop. You need it in bucketfuls to cope with the shock of diagnosis, the emotional turmoil of the journey and to confront crucial decisions.

There is a physical side to resilience too. Cancer, and particularly the standard treatments for cancer, take an enormous toll on the body, so it is vital to do all you can to improve your body's ability to tolerate these challenges and to bounce back. There are many strategies, both nutritional and physical, for achieving this.

Following an integrative path requires even greater resilience: the people I meet constantly use the words 'confusing' and isolating' to describe their experience of cancer. 'Resilient' is probably not how you were feeling when you had the rug pulled from under your feet by diagnosis, but it's something you should work towards developing. Being resilient does not mean that you don't experience difficulty or distress, but that you adapt to it and take what you have learned with you.

It may be that 'defiance' is a good word too! You could just meekly accept the cancer world as it stands, with its single strategy of killing cancer cells and the associated poor prospects of survival; you could just deem that to be your fate. Alternatively, you could choose to learn how to walk your own path, supported by your family, friends and/or carers, all those who provide you with the emotional and physical tools to become your own healer.

To do this:

- Accept that change is necessary
- Find strategies to deal with the fear; don't let it paralyse you or you will not grow
- Learn that there are no experts on your cancer; become your own expert on yourself
- Listen to the people who support and nurture your road to health; ignore others who would dissuade you or are negative about what you want

Be prepared for a bumpy road. You need resilience to cope with the occasional knock-back; people rarely recover their health without a few stumbles along the way. It's like playing chess, you keep strategies in mind if things need to be altered, and you must be versatile.

Above all believe in yourself. We all have the ability within us to cope, to adapt, to heal – these capacities are what define us as humans.

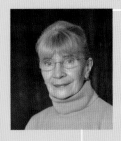

# THE SCIENCE BEHIND INTEGRATIVE MEDICINE

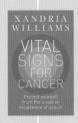

XANDRIA
WILLIAMS

## Xandria Williams

It is often said of unconventional, alternative or complementary medicine that it is unproven, that it is based on hearsay or anecdotal results and that there is little or no evidence of any benefits. From this it is then concluded or assumed that by using Complementary and Alternative Medicine (CAM) methods you could be wasting your money or changing your lifestyle unnecessarily. Further, it is assumed that if this in any way lessens your use of conventional medicine you are putting yourself at risk. My aim here is to show that there is an immense body of evidence for the benefits that can be obtained from adding some CAM methods to whatever other treatments you choose; you could even use them instead of certain medical approaches.

Two things have to be considered in the adoption of any CAM approach: safety and efficacy. The assessment of both of these should be based on sound evidence. As a measure of evidence I have chosen to focus on research papers and studies published in peer-reviewed medical and scientific journals.

### The two approaches to healthcare

An orthodox medical system, built largely around drugs, is intended to treat symptoms and aims either to eradicate or at least manage them, thus restoring some level of wellbeing. The second approach is based on using substances that are common to the body; it aims to make good deficiencies, to support the body's own healing mechanisms and to correct metabolic faults. This is variously known as alternative or complementary medicine and also as naturopathy.

Orthodox medicine has developed excellent solutions to many acute conditions, but it is often poor at resolving or even managing chronic disease. CAM, on the other hand, has resolutions or improvements on offer for many chronic conditions; unfortunately, however, it is seldom equipped to meet an emergency.

### Safety/toxicity

It is now important to discuss the place for 'double blind placebo controlled trials', often referred to as the 'gold standard' for medical trials. In the testing of pharmaceutical drugs, for example, which always have side effects and often involve considerable risks to health, a rigorous testing system is entirely appropriate. Almost no medical drug is found naturally within the body. All medical drugs have at least some adverse toxic effects, many have more serious and often as yet unknown dangers, both on their own and in combinations. It should not be assumed, however, that any procedures or treatments recommended by your doctor have undergone this testing process. In most cases they have not, and in many where they have, it is unfortunately becoming apparent that pharmaceutical company fraud has been involved in the results. If there are serious risks involved in a suggested treatment, it is worth asking questions before you begin. When making important treatment decisions it is well worth talking to an Integrative Medicine practitioner to ask for advice on a balanced approach to your particular situation. Once you understand the types of supportive programme that may alleviate some of the side effects, you will be in a position to make a more informed choice.

Because almost all the substances used in CAM are non-toxic and can be utilised, metabolised, broken down and eventually eliminated in or by the body, there is little danger in using them. There are very few evidenced reports of harm with them compared with those produced when medical drugs are used. In fact, compared with nutritional supplements, an individual is about 900 times more likely to die from food poisoning and nearly 300,000 times more likely to die from a preventable medical injury during a hospital stay in the UK (these figures are on a par with the individual risk of dying that active military personnel face in Iraq or Afghanistan). Adverse reactions to pharmaceutical drugs are 62,000 times more likely to kill you than food supplements and 7750 times more likely to kill you than herbal remedies.[5]

From these data, collected from official sources in the UK and EU, it is clear that CAM remedies, food supplements, nutrients, plant remedies and phytonutrients can be regarded as essentially safe. The risk of death from their consumption is less than one in ten million. To put this in perspective, the risk of being struck by lightning or drowning in your bath is far greater than that.

The latest figures in the USA show similar levels of safety. There was not a single death from vitamin supplements in 2010.[6] Given that Americans consume more than sixty billion doses of nutritional supplements every year, the fact of not even one death is a powerful indication of the lack of toxicity in such supplements.

While there are many arguments supporting the unsuitability of standard medical trials to CAM, the single factor of relative safety is in itself sufficient to justify a simpler, cheaper and more relevant way of testing CAM approaches.

## Efficacy

Many of the suggestions for CAM that are made to people with concerns about cancer are relatively inexpensive, especially when compared with the cost of medical treatments; these are generally easy to fit into individual lifestyles yet they can make a huge difference to the effectiveness of whatever other therapies are chosen.

It is important to look at the evidence for efficacy. In stark contrast to the picture often portrayed of CAM, there has been a considerable amount of research, within peer-reviewed, medical and scientific papers, for the benefit of diet-based and other phytonutrient approaches to cancer. A good resource for evidence is GreenMedInfo's website. This website references research-based material and studies that have been published in public domain Medline, a biomedical and health database consisting of over twenty million records from approximately five thousand selected peer-reviewed publications. This means that these are not anecdotal studies, or indications passed from one person to the next, possibly altering in the process. They have passed technical scrutiny prior to publication.

GREENMED

MEDLINE

## Summary

There is clearly a substantial evidence base from which to build an integrative programme with a degree of confidence. This is currently given little credence by the medical authorities in the UK, but change is clearly on the horizon. The evidence continues to build, as forward-looking programmes for chronic disease, known as 'lifestyle interventions' are being developed; health insurance companies in the USA are finding these to be both effective and economic.

### How best to manage communications

Until the level of integration in the UK matches that being enjoyed elsewhere, communication between practitioners is likely to remain difficult to manage. There are two polarised viewpoints on how to deal with cancer. Many doctors do not appreciate the benefits of looking closely at individual cases and of exploring a wide range of strategies. Nor do they have a unified opinion on the subject. So the level of co-operation, understanding and communication you get on any issue will vary largely, depending on your doctor's views. This can be stressful if you have a doctor who is either very opposed to your using anything that he or she has not prescribed, insisting that you will be just wasting your money; another type of doctor makes definitive statements designed to put you off what you are doing, passing his or her views off as an 'expert opinion' when the doctor in fact has little or no knowledge of it.

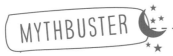

MYTHBUSTER

## "THERE'S NOTHING YOU CAN DO ABOUT YOUR GENES. FOR BETTER OR WORSE, THEY'RE FIXED FOR LIFE"

Genes respond to the emotional and physical environment in which they exist, which is of course constantly changing. Our understanding of genes and our influence upon them is still in its infancy. This is the new science of epigenetics. Some genes we know are highly likely to lead to the development of cancer, for example BRCA1 and 2, which signal susceptibility to breast or other cancers. If genes are deprived of the basic building blocks of DNA through poor nutrition for example, or subject to stress, then they are more likely to become faulty, which can lead to malignancy.

Some natural compounds such as turmeric have been shown to affect the genetic upgrade of cancer cells directly and thus to maintain the health of non-cancerous cells.

In these circumstances it may be challenging and hard work, but here are some suggested ways to organise your team so that communication is as good as it can be:

- Ask your oncologist (or relevant secretary) for copies of all scan results, biopsies, blood results and letters; although some doctors may consider this unusual, you have a right to access this information; the request should therefore not present a problem

HEALTH RECORDS

- If you wish to ask your oncologist's opinion on a treatment option that he or she may not be aware of, send some information about it, along with your questions, before the consultation; in a busy clinic, no-one likes being given a wad of papers and asked to come up with an answer on the spot

- Ask your integrative practitioner to write to your oncologist outlining the aims and methods of the approach that are being followed, thus opening up communication channels; it appears unprofessional if this is not done, and even if the communications are ignored, it is on record that your doctors have been informed

- Assign a friend or relative as collator of information and research; you will easily be overwhelmed by the sheer quantity of information there is to wade through, and that can be exhausting and off-putting

- Try to be analytical if possible; write down each of the elements you want in your programme, which strategy is going to achieve it and how that will be evaluated

- Make sure that all the people involved in your health-care, your team, know that you are in charge, and that nobody has the monopoly on your treatment; each person has a contribution, but no-one should be trying to influence you too much or to be evangelical about particular beliefs in what various treatments can achieve

Keeping the overview on what you are learning about yourself, what influences your body, and how much of each element you need at any one time, is only achievable by you.

Become the expert on yourself!

N.B. For more on how to work with your medical team, see **Chapter 14, 'Be informed'**.

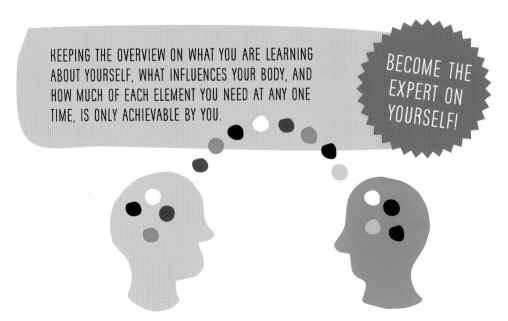

KEEPING THE OVERVIEW ON WHAT YOU ARE LEARNING ABOUT YOURSELF, WHAT INFLUENCES YOUR BODY, AND HOW MUCH OF EACH ELEMENT YOU NEED AT ANY ONE TIME, IS ONLY ACHIEVABLE BY YOU.

BECOME THE EXPERT ON YOURSELF!

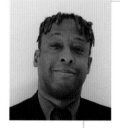

# INTEGRATION IN PRACTICE IN THE UK

## Dr André Young-Snell

**VISION OF HOPE**

At the Vision of Hope Clinic in Brighton, we feel it is essential that people facing a challenging medical condition are empowered. For this they need to feel that their physical, psychological and spiritual needs are being met. Increasing numbers of patients are being drawn towards taking a broad, integrative approach to dealing with their new situation, an approach that inherently respects individual choice and that supports empowerment.

This is not yet considered a standard approach in the UK as it is increasingly elsewhere. In Germany or Mexico for example, and in forward-looking clinics in the USA, patients can have chemotherapy and radiotherapy alongside complementary treatments such as hyperthermia, intravenous vitamin C and ozone therapies. Clearly, in such clinics, patients who favour complementary approaches are fully empowered.

Since there is no option in the UK to have a complete integrative programme of treatment at one clinic, it is ideal if you can find an open-minded, forward-thinking oncologist who is willing to work with you and with your personal choices. That person becomes a key member of your 'core team' of experts and you will need him or her to support the various strands of your programme.

Treatment programmes can be broken down into three broad groups:

- psychological, including mental and emotional
- nutritional i.e. dietary
- oral supplements and external treatments

For a good outcome it is absolutely vital that the patient tackles the first group. This can be achieved by the patient on his or her own in several ways: set yourself powerful goals; be assertive and learn to say 'No'; stand by what you truly believe in; make time to have fun, to laugh and to love. Some of you will appreciate the support of a life coach (see **'The mentor/life coach'**, p. 68 in **Chapter 3, 'Who's who in Integrative Medicine'**, p. 68, and **Chapter 9, 'Managing stress'**) in making changes of this type. All patients who have had successful outcomes in my clinic have taken this essential first step seriously.

As emphasised in **Part Two** of this book, nutrition is very important. It has been established that certain acidic foods can encourage ill-health, whereas an alkaline body supports the healing process.[7] Organic green vegetable juices and plenty of water (preferably reverse osmosis filtered) I think are essential. Nutrition for cancer is now becoming such a sophisticated discipline that a nutritionist is a key member of your team. While there are many good books on the subject of nutrition, most attempts at 'DIY' fall far short of what is possible under expert supervision. Although nutrition is an essential strand of any integrative programme, it is important that your chosen regime will not cause undue stress and that you will not beat yourself up if you have the occasional treat.

Exercise is also vital. If possible, at least four times a week patients should be doing half an hour of aerobic exercise that gets you out of breath and needing a shower afterwards. Exercise does many positive things: it pumps lymph and thus moves toxins to organs for elimination; it increases oxygen intake, stimulates toxin removal via the lungs on expiration and releases 'feel good' endorphins, thus also promoting relaxation, releasing anger, frustration and other pent-up negative emotions. If taken outside, it is an opportunity to connect with nature. Again, some of you will find it easy to build your own programme, while others will benefit enormously from a specialist coach (see 'The physical trainer', p. 61, in Chapter 3, 'Who's who in Integrative Medicine', and Chapter 8, 'The benefits of physical activity after diagnosis').

Expert help is a requirement for the third group. Although it can prove a steep learning curve, and will involve you in doing some research of your own, having a fair idea of what elements you want in your treatment programme before approaching a clinic or practitioner is a tremendous advantage; this will put you firmly in control and significantly increase your confidence. Organisations such as Cancer Options and Yes to Life can help with this challenging process (see Part Eight, 'Resources').

In my experience, oral vitamin C, with or without intravenous vitamin C, is a very important treatment for many cancer patients. Ozone and hyperthermia, both of which can be carried out at home if desired, are also key treatments. Ozone is a powerful oxidising agent and can be introduced into the body through the skin, vaginally, rectally and even via the ears for the head and neck area. My treatment programmes also include immune-boosting agents such as RBAC, cordyceps or cat's claw along with antioxidants such as salvestrols and glutathione. These should all be taken under expert supervision.

MYTHBUSTER

# "CAM DOESN'T REALLY WORK – IT CAN'T KILL CANCER CELLS"

This is a complete misunderstanding. CAM is not trying to replicate the cancer-killing techniques of chemotherapy. It takes the fundamentally different approach of changing the body's environment and getting your immune and other systems working optimally.

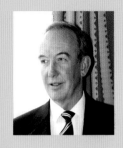

# CHAPTER 2

# THE CRUCIAL ROLE OF HORMONES

Dr John D. Moran

HOLISTIC
MEDICAL

There has been an exponential increase in breast and prostate cancers in industrialised nations over the past fifty years. Arguably the prime causes for this are the toxins outlined in Part Four, 'Avoiding or reducing toxins'. Some of these hormone disruptors are now commonly found in the food chain (fish and animal products) and others in household dust and public water supplies.

The world has developed an environment that exposes us to toxic levels of hormones every day. It is becoming clear that some people are better able to survive this toxic assault than others, and for those of us whose bodies struggle to metabolise and excrete the toxins, the risks of developing cancer are higher. For those who don't, the effect on the cells of the body is to create the potential for genetic change; over time may this enable a cancer whose growth is influenced by toxins in the environment.

While breast, prostate, testicular, ovarian and endometrial (uterine) cancers are the most likely to be driven by hormones, some forms of lung, colon and brain cancer may also be hormone dependent. Indeed the list of cancers in which hormones are implicated is growing steadily as our understanding increases.

The ability of the liver to detoxify oestrogens is relevant to the cause and prevention of breast and prostate cancer.[1] A twenty-four hour urine test measuring the metabolites of oestrogens and the ultimate excretion in the urine via methylation (i.e. measuring the by-products of oestrogen that the liver has failed to detoxify) can identify a possible cause, and may help in prevention and treatment of breast and prostate cancer. Nutritional products are now able to treat and regulate some of the metabolic pathways that are not functioning.

Genetic testing to assess the risks of developing cancer is available. Medication, change of diet and nutritional supplementation can all contribute to changing gene expression, as can reduced exposure to environmental pollutants.[2] This is Integrative Medicine at its best, offering the latest treatments and investigations that are least harmful, often combining orthodox and complementary treatment. Identifying the breast-cancer genome and targeting treatment on an individual basis have become the principal aims in some centres.

Low vitamin D3 levels are relevant to the risk of many cancers, including prostate and breast, and vitamin D is able to alter gene expression. Therefore levels of vitamin D need to be above 80-100 nmol/l to decrease the risk, and much higher levels are required to treat cancer.[3] (For further information on the vital role of vitamin D in cancer, see **Chapter 10, 'Sunshine and vitamin D'**).

Most studies on breast cancer have not addressed the possibility that exposure to phyto-oestrogens early in life, or over several decades of life, may confer protective changes. The weight of evidence in humans supports a protective role for soya – which contains high levels – in breast-cancer risk.[4] A low-fat/high-fibre diet, combined with a phyto-oestrogen diet from birth, results in a lower incidence of breast cancer.[5]

**Ways to reduce your risk from hormones include:**

- reducing toxic exposure
- reducing dietary intake of saturated fats
- filtering your water supply (with a reverse osmosis filter; see **'The importance of water', pp. 94-5**, in **Chapter 5, 'Diet as the foundation of good health'**)

- exercising
- maintaining or achieving an optimal weight
- optimising gut and liver function
- supplementing with vitamin D3

Other integrative strategies for correcting hormone imbalance include a non-dairy diet (see **'The problem with dairy', p. 99**, in **Chapter 5, 'Diet as the foundation of good health'**), stress reduction, infrared sauna use (see **'Detoxing at home', p. 197**, in **Chapter 13, 'Detoxifying your body'**), pomegranate, red cherry, Pfeifer Protocol (protocols formulated by Prof. Ben Pfeifer for prostate and breast cancer, containing a wide variety of phytochemicals, phytonutrients and immune stimulants). These approaches can be used as complementary treatments alongside existing orthodox medicine, or instead of 'active surveillance', an increasingly common approach to non-aggressive prostate cancer.

PFEIFER

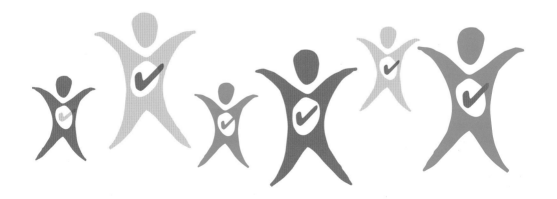

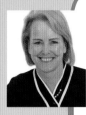

# HORMONE-RELATED CANCERS AND ORTHODOX HORMONE TREATMENTS

There is an epidemic of hormone-related cancers in Britain, and indeed across the developed world, and we are finding that more cancers than we previously thought can be encouraged by hormones. How the body metabolises hormones into non-harmful substances is very individual – unfortunately orthodox treatment is not.

The problems with orthodox hormone therapy in a holistic sense are:

- It does not address the treatment side effects, which many people find extremely debilitating
- If it isn't working properly, doctors have no way of analysing this
- It does nothing to address the underlying issues. Once treatment stops, or cancer evolves to the point where it is ineffective, the original problem re-emerges unchanged

Integrative Medicine has strategies. We talk a lot about identifying contributory factors. Developing a hormone-related cancer gives you the opportunity and motivation to fundamentally reassess your lifestyle choices. This will enhance your potential for positively influencing the outcome. I hope that you will go on to be among those who become healthier as an outcome of diagnosis. Diet, liver function, endocrine function, gut symbiosis and stress are the main causes of poor hormone methylation and all are well within your influence. Don't miss the opportunity.

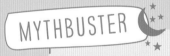

MYTHBUSTER

# "WE DON'T KNOW WHAT CAUSES CANCER"

We certainly don't know all the triggers, and it will be many years before we do. But we do know a great many of the factors that can come together to create the 'perfect storm' for an individual, and that by identifying and rectifying them we can contribute to recovery.[5]

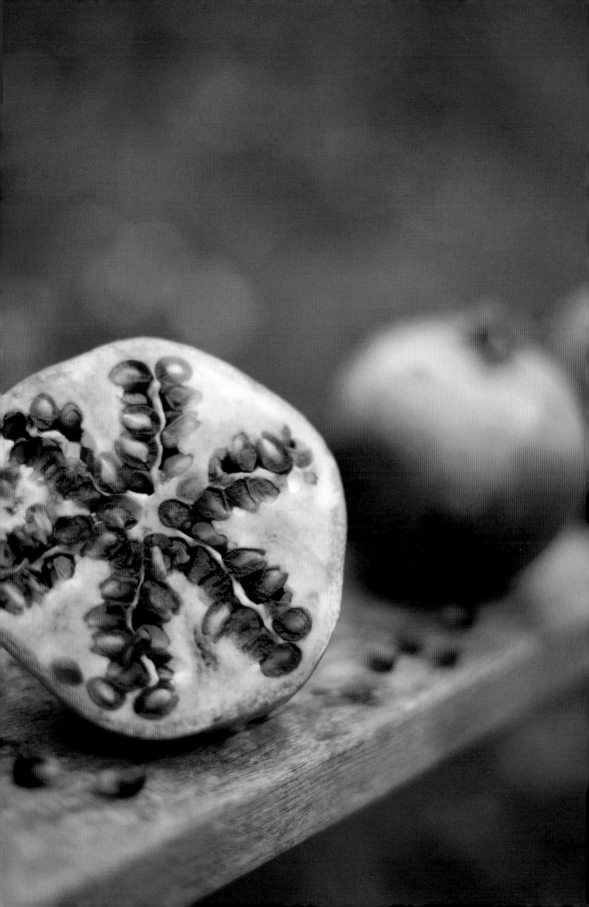

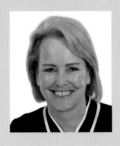

# CHAPTER 3

# WHO'S WHO IN INTEGRATIVE MEDICINE

Patricia Peat

An enormous range of treatment options is now available from around the globe, some recently developed, others from traditional approaches thousands of years in the making. In time, you will find those that are key to your recovery, including particular practitioners who will come to form an essential part of your 'team'. I suggest you start by using your intuition to home in on what interests you most. This chapter aims to give a broad idea of who is offering what in Integrative Medicine.

One of the main points we hope to bring out in this book is the importance of taking a multi-faceted approach to recovery, one that draws on approaches detailed in all the chapters below. For this, you will need to build yourself a personal 'team' that reflects an equally broad range of expertise.

It is worth noting that many of the mind/body approaches are non-invasive and therefore unlikely to be risky; this means that you can afford to be fairly 'experimental' in this sphere. A low level of evidence is not necessarily a reason not to try a supportive therapy, if you think it could help. However I do always advise finding a practitioner with at least a couple of years' experience of working with cancer, due to the complexities of cancer and cancer treatments.

Whether or not you decide to work with an integrative doctor will depend on where on the spectrum of Integrative Medicine you choose to centre your personalised strategy. For example, if you have decided to centre your care around standard treatments, but are looking for some supportive therapies to help you cope with the resulting stresses, then you probably won't need an integrative doctor. As you move along the spectrum towards equal reliance on standard treatments and integrative approaches, it becomes increasingly important that you establish a good working relationship with an integrative doctor. Clearly, if you are depending more, or even entirely, on non-standard approaches, then an integrative doctor is essential.

There is pretty much always a strong case for getting the support of a nutritionist (or other practitioner with nutritional expertise) who is experienced in working with cancer patients, to help you. However, which other types of practitioner become part of your team will be completely dependent on your choices, your intuition and the particulars of your situation.

Communication between members of your team can be vital at times to ensure the best results, although this is not always possible. It is desirable to have at the least one person, other than you, who is keeping an eye on how you are progressing with your programme. You will certainly get to know your medical team at the hospital (who are covered in more detail in **Chapter 14, 'Be informed'**) and your GP. This chapter offers an outline of some of the integrative practitioners most commonly consulted by people with cancer. They have been grouped into types of therapy to help you find what you are looking for quickly. Some of the material has been contributed by specialist practitioners.

## The integrative doctor

This professional title is applied to a medically trained specialist who promotes the use of natural compounds and herbal and homeopathic preparations in preference to, but not excluding pharmaceutical compounds. Such doctors aim to establish underlying factors which may have contributed to a state of ill-health. They can offer a wide range of approaches to help the body to return to a state of balance. The basic approach is holistic, embracing physical, psychological and spiritual elements of medicine to empower you in your own healing journey. With your oncologist, they can form a powerful collaborative part of your team.

YES TO LIFE

Approaches used include:

- intravenous replacement of vitamins and minerals
- high-dose intravenous vitamin C
- hyperthermia

CANCER OPTIONS

- ozone therapy – introducing additional oxygen into the body
- thermography – non-invasive complementary scanning
- nutritional therapy

- detoxification
- chelation – removal of toxic heavy metals from the body

For help with finding a suitable doctor, contact Yes to Life or Cancer Options; you could also consult LIFE>, the Yes to Life searchable web directory.

LIFE>

## The nutritionist

### Juiet Hayward
Nutritional therapy is a good adjunct to the mainstream approach to cancer, as it focuses on the terrain in which the tumour grew in the first place, while the oncologist works on the tumour itself, endeavouring to shrink and destroy it. Used together, the two approaches can complement one another.

Nutrition can bolster immunity, improving the body's ability to form a co-ordinated immune defence against cancer and helping the immune cells to communicate with each other. Glyconutrients, RBAC and vitamin D3 all help to improve this dialogue between the cells, thus reducing tolerance towards cancer cells (see **Chapter 7, 'Supplements and natural compounds'**).

This approach can help to address nutritional deficiencies that may originally have had a role in cancer development. For example, those with cervical cancer commonly suffer from low folic acid and beta-carotene. Nutritional therapy can ameliorate some of the side effects of chemotherapy, including mouth ulcers, vomiting, diarrhoea, constipation, nerve tingling, a low white blood-cell count and lack of energy.

Good nutrition can help balance blood sugar levels, thereby helping to prevent sugar excess from fuelling cancer growth (see 'The dangers of glucose', p. 85, in Chapter 5, 'Diet as the foundation of good health'). It can improve hormonal balance, helping women with oestrogen positive breast cancer to metabolise oestrogen in a much safer form. Supplements such as coenzyme Q10 and liquid oxygen can oxygenate the body, creating a hostile environment for cancer cells. And don't forget that when the orthodox treatment is over, nutrition can help with repair.

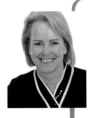

## FINDING A NUTRITIONIST

When choosing a nutritionist, it is essential to find one who has long experience in supporting people with cancer. It is an extremely specialised field and requires an expert to advise on how to help the body control cancer, to assist with symptoms and to deal with the side effects of treatment.

Good places to start when looking for a suitable practitioner are Yes to Life (and LIFE>, the Yes to Life searchable web directory), Cancer Options or your integrative doctor; see also Part Eight, 'Resources'.

YES TO LIFE

# ALTERNATIVE MEDICAL SYSTEMS

This section examines traditional or other medical systems based on a particular view of the human body.

LIFE>

### The naturopath

David Potterton

Naturopaths are alternative medicine practitioners who use a combination of natural methods to help people regain their health. They have been doing this for well over a century. So successful are their methods that in the USA and Canada, naturopaths are licensed as Naturopathic Doctors and often work alongside medical teams within the established state health systems.

The National Occupational Standards defines naturopathy as a philosophy and holistic healthcare system that recognises the healing power of nature present in all living things. That authoritative source states: 'As a healing system it aims to promote and restore health by employing various natural treatment approaches that may include: naturopathic nutrition, lifestyle advice, detoxification techniques, hydrotherapy, physical therapy, naturopathic psychosocial support and other appropriate techniques.'

CANCER
OPTIONS

Most naturopaths in the UK have further professional qualifications in addition to the core naturopathic training, such as homeopathy, herbal medicine, osteopathy or wholefood nutrition. They treat the patient rather than the disease, recognising that optimum health is the achievement of emotional, nutritional and musculo-skeletal wellbeing.

For patients with a current or past cancer, a gentle, multi-modality naturopathic approach can complement conventional cancer treatment. Naturopaths aim to enhance the body's healing power and immune system in order to reduce side effects of orthodox medical treatment and to prevent recurrence. By using modalities in combination, such as organically produced wholefoods, herbal and homeopathic medicines as well as therapeutic exercise, naturopaths believe that a healing synergy is created to help optimise the body's defence and immune systems. They encourage their patients to follow an all-round health regeneration regime and to use non-invasive, non-drug modalities, many of which are supported by clinical evidence, to improve the body's own innate healing abilities. They frequently work as part of a team in alternative and complementary medicine clinics as well as in private practice. They may also be found as part of the team at cancer help centres.

## The homeopath

### Jo Daly

For well over two centuries homeopathy has been used as a popular means of treating the symptoms of disease naturally, effectively and without unpleasant side effects. It is based on the principle that 'like cures like'; a principle that modern medicine also employs in some cases. For example Digitalis, made from the foxglove plant that, if ingested, can have a toxic effect on the heart, is used as a drug to treat heart disease and also in homeopathy as a remedy. A significant difference is that homeopathic doses are as small as possible, nevertheless producing a deep healing action.

JO DALY

Homeopathy is a holistic form of treatment in that it takes into account symptoms of both mind and body, no matter what your diagnosis. Homeopaths can treat a wide range of ailments; even in cancer, relief can be obtained by homeopathic treatments such as those that combat the side effects of conventional ones. During a consultation, a homeopath will listen carefully to your personal description of symptoms and history, aiming to provide a course of treatment that is matched to your individual needs.

Your homeopath may have a background in conventional medicine or have been trained specifically at one of the homeopathic colleges and accredited by the Society of Homeopaths. Either way it is recommended that you seek a referral. Remedies can be obtained from homeopathic pharmacies and can sometimes be obtained on prescription.

SOH

Look for a homeopath on the Society of Homeopaths website or, if you are looking for a medical homeopath, consult the British Homeopathic Association.

BHA

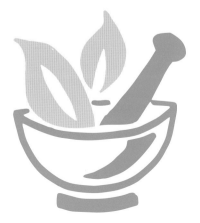

# SELF-HELP HOMEOPATHY

Jo Daly

Homeopathic remedies have a great deal to offer during the treatment of cancerous tumours and also in mitigating the side effects of conventional drug treatments. It is advisable to consult a trained homeopath for in-depth care. However, there are a number of over-the-counter homeopathic remedies that can be used at home for alleviating pain and assisting the healing process:

- *Aconite*; for sudden fevers with chills; also useful in calming fears
- *Arnica montana*; invaluable after all types of surgery or invasive procedures to assist recovery
- *Arsenicum album*; for weakness and relief of pain especially when there is great restlessness of mind and body accompanied by chilliness; also useful in nausea from chemotherapy
- *Hecla lava*; when there are metastases in the bones and after bone-marrow transplants
- *Hydrastis*; for pain and weakness in those with stomach, intestine and pancreatic cancers
- *Mercurius solubilis*; for ulceration, mouth ulcers
- *Nux vomica*; for nausea, vomiting and constipation
- *Radium bromatum*; for side effects of radiation, especially burning pains
- *Thuja*; for bladder and prostate support
- *Bellis perennis*; for healing after mastectomy operations
- *Staphysagria*; after abdominal surgery

All of these remedies should be used in a 30C potency and repeated up to three times a day.

## The Traditional Chinese Medicine doctor

Margella Salmins

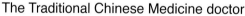

MARGELLA
SALMINS

Chinese Herbal Medicine, one of the oldest and most widely practised medical traditions in the world, focuses not on cure but on the relative balance of yin and yang, in other words, maintenance of cellular homeostasis. It treats the root cause of the problem not just the resulting disease. It is often used in combination with acupuncture. Its use of polypharmacy (the administration of combination of herbs to address several issues) is central to its success in helping with the multi-faceted disease process of malignancy.

### The aims when creating a herbal formula for an individual are to:

- strengthen immunity and optimise the body's own mechanisms, in order to resist invasion and resolve the disease
- nourish and strengthen the blood and promote good blood circulation
- eliminate inflammation by removing the source

- soften and dissolve hard masses
- use cytotoxic herbs targeted at particular cancers

Modern Chinese medicine, TEAM or TCM, is essentially an amalgamation of Chinese classical medicine and modern biomedicine. The pharmacological understanding of herbs allows for a fully integrative approach with conventional therapy and a number of possible points of intervention for its use:

- post-diagnosis, before treatment
- supportive treatment related to chemotherapy, radiotherapy or surgery
- on-going health promotion treatment following conventional intervention
- supportive treatment for people living with cancer
- palliative care

RCHM

A list of fully qualified registered and insured UK practitioners may be obtained from both the Register of Chinese Herbal Medicine (RCHM) and the Association of Traditional Chinese Medicine (ATCM).

ATCM

## The acupuncturist

Acupuncture is a Chinese approach to healing, in use for thousands of years, and one of the mainstays of Traditional Chinese Medicine. TCM views the body as containing a network of meridians or pathways through which the body's energy, qi (pronounced 'chi'), flows. These energy flows can be accessed through over 350 specific acupuncture points. Good health is seen in terms of balance between the interdependent opposing forces of yin (e.g. passive) and yang (e.g. active). It can be promoted through the use of fine needles inserted into acupuncture points to remove blockages in the energy flow, which can result from a wide range of physical and mental stresses or traumas.

Western science uses neuroscience to explain acupuncture's mechanism of action, and it has been the subject of a considerable amount of research. This has established it as a useful way of tackling nausea or neuropathy from chemotherapy, dry mouth or hot flushes; it can also help to reduce pain and anxiety, as well as contribute to improved sleep and general wellbeing.

You can find a practitioner through one of the associations listed in **Part Eight, 'Resources'**. Acupuncturists are also often available at specialist complementary cancer care centres. This can be a good option as the practitioners there will be particularly experienced at working with the issues faced by people with cancer and will also have an excellent understanding of the situations in which acupuncture can be unsuitable (see LIFE>, the Yes to Life searchable web directory, for a full listing of UK centres).

LIFE>

## The Ayurvedic practitioner

Ayurvedic medicine is one of the longest surviving medical systems. It originated in India, purportedly at least five thousand years ago, as an entirely undocumented oral tradition. This practice views us as consisting of three doshas (life forces). The balance and interdependence of these, along with our connection to the cosmos, directly affects our health, and the practitioner will work to restore and establish this balance. Ayurveda is an all-encompassing or holistic view of health, concerned primarily with disease prevention and the promotion of wellbeing. Patients are expected to be active participants in this, and are often asked to make changes to their diet and lifestyle.

Ayurveda employs a range of techniques and substances to cleanse the system of toxins or other sources of disease. There is a heavy reliance on herbs, plants, oils and spices, and there are hundreds of established formulae in use. It can be combined with massage, meditation, yoga and other practices as part of a patient's programme.

Many people find the Ayurvedic approach helpful and supportive in meeting the physical, emotional and mental challenges that cancer can present. However it is important that any use of herbs is carefully assessed by an expert for possible negative interaction with standard treatments.

## The herbalist

### Dr Chris Etheridge

DR CHRIS
ETHERIDGE

I see herbal medicine (phytotherapy) as an essential part of any integrated cancer regime. It is particularly useful for supporting the body before, during and after aggressive conventional treatments such as surgery, chemotherapy and radiotherapy. Herbal medicine is safe to use, as long as it has been prescribed by a fully qualified medical herbalist. Despite the concerns raised by some medical doctors, herbal medicine will not interfere with conventional treatments if it is used according to a trained herbalist's instructions.

As part of a cancer support regime, herbal medicine is particularly useful to:

- decrease inflammation levels in the body (cancer is now recognised to be an inflammatory disease)
- increase the strength of the immune system to fight cancer, particularly after chemotherapy and radiotherapy
- increase circulation in the body to ensure that cancer-fighting immune cells, oxygen and nutrients can get to the cancer, and waste products are quickly eliminated
- increase detoxification (to remove toxins from the body)
- increase the body's vitality and resistance to disease by promoting balanced health in the body
- decrease stress levels and increase coping mechanisms in the body, so that it can deal efficiently with the effects of physical and psychological stress

For example, the herb Siberian ginseng (*Eleutherococcus senticosus*) is an adaptogen, a herb that helps the body resist the effects of stress. It also has a balancing action that helps to maintain a healthy, efficient immune system. When given to cancer patients, it has been shown to minimise the side effects of chemotherapy, radiotherapy and surgery, improving recovery times, immune-system function and general quality of life.[1]

A significant amount of research has shown how effective herbs can be. As additional high-quality research is published, I am confident that more conventional doctors will realise that herbal medicine can make an invaluable contribution to any integrated cancer regime.

# PHYSICAL ACTIVITY

This section explores active forms of physical intervention (see **Chapter 8, 'The benefits of physical activity after diagnosis',** for more on exercise and cancer).

## The physical trainer

### Lizzy Davis

I believe that physical activity is the 'hidden wonder-drug'. I developed the organisation CanExercise to bring this knowledge direct to those living with cancer. Evidence is now growing to support the role of physical activity, both during and after cancer treatment. Through keeping active you can preserve or improve physical function and psychological wellbeing.[2] It has also been proven that exercise can help to reduce the negative impact of some treatment-related side effects. Compelling research data also suggest that regular physical activity can potentially reduce the risk of cancer recurrence, increasing longevity.[3]

CAN
EXERCISE

In fact, regular exercise can help with everything you feel and do. It can make you feel stronger or more flexible, relieve tension, help you sleep better and help you to maintain an ideal body weight and composition. The focus is to live well and keep moving, and more importantly to find an activity that you enjoy.

It's your body and your health that you are fighting for, so make exercise part of your recovery. Working with cancer survivors at all stages of their diagnosis, we celebrate the fact that we 'can exercise' to be active against cancer.

## Yoga

### Barbara Gallani

There is a growing body of evidence showing that yoga, as a complementary therapy to conventional treatments, can help those affected by cancer. It can reduce anxiety and improve the quality of life of cancer patients, cancer survivors and their carers.[4] Yoga classes can be specifically tailored to support those affected by cancer. Specialist classes for cancer survivors include plenty of gentle stretches, breathing exercises and restorative poses, as well as sequences developed to improve lymphatic flow. The range of movement can strengthen the body and mobilise the joints without depleting energy reserves or causing exhaustion.

BARBARA
GALLANI

Every type of patient can benefit from specialist yoga classes for cancer survivors. Yoga classes are suitable at any phase of treatment and can help alleviate treatment-related symptoms such as post-surgical pain, a limited mobility range, as well as fatigue, sleep and digestive problems. Because of a strong focus on body awareness, mindfulness, relaxation and meditation, yoga can greatly assist people feeling isolated and emotionally affected by their cancer diagnosis or in search of a new balance.

Group sessions are indicated for people who are reasonably mobile and can move independently, after all surgical incisions have healed. Private sessions are suited to bed-bound patients or people gradually building up the confidence to include exercise and physical activity as part of their healing process.

Here are two examples of what cancer patients say about yoga:

- I'm doing yoga to maintain physical fitness and emotional equilibrium. The most significant thing I get from yoga is maintaining a positive relationship with my body; regular yoga is also helping me to deal with anxiety - *Kate*

- Yoga has been a weekly anchor to help negotiate the cancer journey - *Jessica*

Specialist teacher-training courses equip experienced yoga teachers with the knowledge and skills required to develop classes that are not just safe but also beneficial for different types of cancer and different stages of survivorship.

# YOGA BODY SCAN

Barbara Gallani

Practising the exercise below can help you feel connected with all parts of your body.

It is the middle of the day. Things have been quite hectic since the morning. You have attended a hospital appointment, queued in the rain outside the GP clinic for a prescription, and received one call after another from friends and family checking how everything is going… It is time to close the door, switch off the phone and find a quiet corner where you can safely let go of all tension and anxiety and connect with your body in the present moment.

To prepare yourself:
- Lie comfortably on your back
- Wear warm clothes and socks and cover yourself with a blanket (unless the room is comfortably warm)
- You can have a folded blanket under your head and shoulders and a cushion under your knees to help release any tension

THE CANCER
REVOLUTION

This is a body scan that you can do on your own, reading the whole piece and then mentally going through it with your eyes closed; or guided by a friend, who can read this out for you, slowly and softly. It is also on thecancerrevolution.co.uk.
- Become aware of your body and start relaxing your muscles, melting into the floor and becoming completely still
- Close your eyes
- Detach the tongue from the roof of the mouth
- Breathe slowly and naturally

You are now going to bring your awareness to different parts of your body, without the need to move any of them. We are going to start from the feet and work our way up:
- Bring your awareness to the feet, ankles, lower legs, knees, thighs, hips, buttocks
- Then gradually focus on the pelvis, lower belly, lower back, waist, thorax, chest, middle of the back, upper back, shoulderblades, shoulders, upper arms, elbows, forearms, hands
- Still working upwards, now focus on the neck, throat, face, forehead, back of the head, top of the head
- The whole body is still, heavy and relaxed

What do you notice most about your body today?:
- Are your feet warm or cold?      • Are your hands relaxed or tense?
- Are both shoulderblades pressing equally against the floor or is one heavier than the other?

How does your body feel as a whole?:
- Do you feel heavy or light?      • Do you feel comfortable or tight?
- Is there a part of the body that feels particularly comfortable or uncomfortable?

Remember that there is no right or wrong. There is just your ability to find stillness, to observe your body and to connect with it deeply:
- Slowly deepen your breath      • Bring some movement into your fingers and toes
- Stretch your arms above your head      • Turpn onto one side and open your eyes

Welcome back. *Namaste*\*

See also 'Yoga exercises for you to try', p. 148, in Chapter 8, 'The benefits of physical activity after diagnosis'.

\* This ancient Sanskrit greeting remains in common use in India and Nepal. Rough translations include 'From my heart to yours' or 'The spirit within me salutes the spirit in you'.

## Qigong

Pronounced 'chi gong', Qigong is an ancient Chinese practice involving movement, breathing and meditation. TCM (see **p. 58-59** above) views the body as a network of meridians or channels through which our life force or qi (pronounced 'chi') flows. Free flow of qi leads to a healthy balance of the opposing interdependent forces of yin and yang (e.g. positive/negative, active/passive).

Qigong can play an important role in regulating respiration and in increasing oxygen levels in the body. It is also useful as a means of creating and maintaining mental and emotional stability, a key to implementing any integrative programme. This can be further enhanced by practising Qigong as part of a group. Many people are inspired by the example of others, particularly their successes.

### Qigong can:[5]

- have a direct effect on the immune system
- lower stress and calm the nervous system
- lower blood pressure

- improve energy
- improve digestion
- improve blood circulation

# BODYWORK

This section focuses on passive physical interventions.

## The Massage Therapist

### Tom Hoyland

There are many types of massage, some of which are covered below. In most techniques the therapists will use their hands to work the soft tissue of the body; however other techniques use certain tools, for example hot stones. In Shiatsu and Thai massage thumb and finger pressure is used to work into specific points on the body. All therapists will use varying degrees of pressure, depending on the client's needs. In most cases a light pressure is chosen for patients diagnosed with cancer.

TOM
HOYLAND

Massage can help to ease muscular tension, thus promoting relaxation. It also helps to increase delivery of blood and oxygen to the treated areas. A treatment can involve the whole body or work on specific areas. Most treatments are given with the patient on a massage couch, though sessions are also given with the patient on a futon mattress. Oils are sometimes used directly on the skin to help with different techniques. Massage is used for a variety of reasons but is primarily seen as a way to reduce stress and anxiety, to relax and to reduce pain.[6]

People with cancer may have specific reasons to be cautious in relation to massage. For example, areas that have been treated recently with radiotherapy should be avoided altogether, or if lymph nodes have been removed, resulting in a buildup of fluid (lymphoedema), this requires a specialised massage technique called lymphatic drainage.[7] As with all complementary therapies, it is always best to find a practitioner who has at least a couple of years' experience working with cancer, as they will know exactly what to look out for.

GCMT

A good place to find a massage therapist with the right experience is at one of the many specialist CAM centres for people with cancer. LIFE>, the Yes to Life searchable web directory, has a full listing of UK centres. The GCMT, CNHC and FHT websites are also good places to look.

CNHC

FHT

### The reflexologist

Tom Hoyland

This form of healing is thought to have been practised since ancient times in Egypt, China and elsewhere.

CNHC

Modern reflexology is based on the work of Dr William Fitzgerald, who was doing research on something he called zone analgesia in the early 1900s. Dr Fitzgerald's theories were picked up by a physical therapist, Eunice D. Ingham, who in the 1930s worked extensively with her patients mapping out the reflex points of the feet. Using this map, reflexologists apply gentle pressure to the reflex points of the feet to help bring about balance in the systems and organs of the body. Pressure can also be applied to the hands if the feet cannot be worked.

AOR

Most people find that a session of reflexology is deeply relaxing. It is one of the most frequently requested therapies on offer at CAM cancer centres in the UK and is valued for its ability to relax and calm the body and mind, to help with pain relief and induce feelings of wellbeing.[8]

Reflexologists can be found through the Complementary and Natural Healthcare Council (CNHC). Other good resources are the Association of Reflexologists (AoR), and the Federation of Holistic Therapists (FHT).

FHT

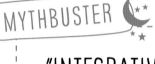

# MYTHBUSTER

## "INTEGRATIVE MEDICINE IS ONLY FOR THE WELL OFF"

Looking outside the NHS can certainly be expensive. But there is a great deal that you can do to help yourself without breaking the bank. Apart from looking at the many low-cost options discussed throughout this book, you could contact Yes to Life or Cancer Options, both of which offer help in developing a low-budget programme.

YES TO LIFE

CANCER OPTIONS

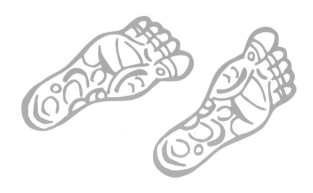

# PROGRESSIVE MUSCULAR RELAXATION

Tom Hoyland

All self-help advice given, including that below, should be done within your own limits and practised in a safe and secure way. Do not over-exert yourself. If you feel that the advice is not working for you or if it makes you feel uncomfortable, stop.

### Progressive muscular relaxation (PMR)

This is a useful exercise to help you reduce muscular tension and to cope with stress.

Find somewhere quiet to lie down and practise PMR at least once a day so that you can begin to recognise and then let go of tension in your body. For each of the muscle groups, tense your muscles for 5 seconds and the release/relax for 10 seconds. Repeat once.

Muscle groups and how to tense them:

- feet: pull toes apart
- calves: point toes towards head.
- thighs: point toes away from head
- buttocks: clench
- abdomen: pull in towards back
- back: arch
- shoulders: shrug upwards towards ears
- arms and hands: stretch wide apart
- face: shut eyes and clench jaw
- whole body: tense all muscle groups together

Before getting up at the end, give yourself a few moments to reflect on how your body feels.

### Controlled breathing

Controlled breathing is a useful way of helping to restore the balance of oxygen (that we breathe in) and carbon dioxide (that we breathe out).

Controlled breathing should be done through the nose and with appropriate movement of the abdomen.

Practise this for 2 minutes at a time at least three times a day:

Place one hand on your abdomen and the other on your chest. Make sure that your abdomen does most of the movement while breathing. It should move out when you breathe in and move in when breathing out.

- empty your lungs by breathing out fully
- breathe in fully and slowly for 3 seconds; do not hold your breath
- breathe out slowly and fully for 5 seconds

N.B.: If you are experiencing any breathing difficulties, consult your primary healthcare professional before trying this technique.

### The Shiatsu practitioner

CNHC

SHIATSU
SOCIETY

Shiatsu is derived from traditional Japanese massage, and its name means 'finger pressure'. It is another form of treatment, like acupuncture, that is based on the principle of a network of energy meridians that conduct our life energy, or qi, around the body. Blockages in the flow of qi are thought to lead to imbalance and disease. These can be removed by application of pressure to selected points along the meridians.

Shiatsu has been shown to be helpful in dealing with pain, nausea, poor sleep and low energy – often one of the worst side effects experienced during standard treatments. The anti-nausea wristbands commonly sold for travel sickness make use of a pressure point in the wrist.[9]

Shiatsu practitioners can be found through the Complementary and Natural Healthcare Council or the Shiatsu Society website.

### The aromatherapist

In aromatherapy essential oils are combined with massage. There are around 400 essential oils that are used, although with cancer, in practice, a limited range is used, for example lemon, peppermint, jasmine, geranium, marjoram, rosemary, lavender, ylang ylang, eucalyptus and chamomile.

IFPA

CNHC

There are two different suggestions about how aromatherapy achieves its effects. First, that it is by direct absorption through the skin; second, that it is via our sense of smell. Both may be true, but it seems that the resulting effects are on the brain, in particular the hypothalamus that controls hormones. In theory at least, this could be how some of the reported improvements to anxiety and stress levels are achieved. Other reported benefits include improved wellbeing, and the reduction of nausea and depression.

Aromatherapy is much in demand by people with cancer, but although it may seem a fairly innocuous therapy, it is a mistake to attempt a DIY approach without some professional guidance.

Professional aromatherapists can be found at the International Federation of Professional Aromatherapists or the Complementary and Natural Healthcare Council.

# MIND AND SPIRIT THERAPIES

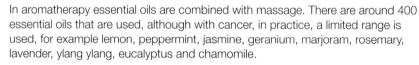

MINDFUL
CHOICE

The approaches discussed in this section can have a huge effect in countering stress and the mental and emotional challenges of cancer and cancer treatment.

For more on stress and cancer, see also Chapter 9, 'Managing stress', p. 152.

### The mindfulness meditation teacher

#### Clare McLusky

It is inspiring to realise that the way we approach illness may affect not just our happiness, but also our body's innate capacity to heal. Mindfulness training enables us to change our relationship to our thoughts, feelings and sensations. By learning to pay attention with kindness and curiosity to whatever is present, we begin to see the connection between the different elements of experience. This allows us to break old habits such as avoidance, negative rumination or catastrophic thinking. As we learn to pay attention in this way and to settle in with our minds, we are able to live more fully in the moment, rather than filling our minds with thoughts about the past or the future. Mindfulness is intentional and helps us create the space to choose consciously how we respond to the stresses and challenges of life. This re-empowerment is particularly welcome on receiving a diagnosis of cancer, a vulnerable time in our lives when we may feel things have slipped completely beyond our control.

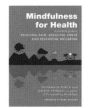

OMC

The proven benefits of mindfulness-based cognitive therapy (MBCT) and mindfulness-based stress reduction (MBSR) courses on cancer treatment are substantial:[10]

- reduced stress symptoms
- improved sleep quality
- enhanced quality of life
- increased immune function
- changes in cancer-related cytokine production

But it goes beyond that: practising mindfulness usually makes personal growth and spiritual healing possible; you will learn to get below the surface of fear, anxiety and depression, and to alleviate the difficulties of living with a chronic illness like cancer, dealing with loss and one's own mortality.

For further reading recommendations, visit the Oxford Mindfulness Centre website; see also the book by Vidyamala Burch and Danny Penman, *Mindfulness for Health*.

# TRY MINDFULNESS

### Clare McLusky

While mindfulness may be notoriously difficult to describe in words, it is nevertheless a simple skill that anybody can learn, often with profound effects. If you would like to try it now:

Notice how your body feels, sitting here. Notice the weight of your body sitting on the chair, the sensations of your feet on the floor, feelings of warmth or cold. Notice whether you are holding any tension in the body, maybe in the shoulders, the face. When you are ready, bring your awareness to your thoughts, noting whether they are calm or racy and where they might be focused (worrying, planning). Then notice how you are feeling right now (peaceful, anxious, joyful, sad). Now become aware of your breathing. How does your breath feel in the body? Resist the urge to change or control your breath, allow the body to breathe itself, simply noticing any sensations as the breath moves in and out of the body. Allow yourself a few moments to sit in stillness, being with the sensations of the breath in the body. Always remember, as Jon Kabat-Zinn says, 'if you are breathing, there is more right with you than wrong with you'*.

* Jon Kabat-Zimm developed mindfulness-based stress reduction (MBSR) in the 1970s.

BE
MINDFUL

LIFE>

To find a class, visit the Be Mindful website. Mindfulness-based approaches are beginning to be offered within hospital settings and at cancer resource centres (see LIFE>, the Yes to Life searchable web directory).

## The mentor/life coach

### Jessica Richards

Having lived with a cancer diagnosis for over six years, I know first hand that managing cancer is a full-time job. Anyone who has been through cancer knows that it is a long-term project and one never really feels as if it is 'all over and done with'. Whatever pathway of care one chooses, a plan and a mentor can go a long way to assist in recovery or prevention.

In my experience, the most common personality characteristic shared by cancer patients is one of selflessness: always putting the needs of others first; always being last in line and taking care of others' needs and feelings at the expense of our own. Addressing this aspect of one's life is vital for prevention as well as recovery. Being selfish is the greatest gift we can give ourselves and others. No-one really wants our help at the expense of our own wellbeing.

JESSICA
RICHARDS

Having a mentor can help one to remain focused during the long years of treatment and recovery; it can provide inspiration to keep going when we've had enough. Or when we're having a 'bad day', it can help change our life-negating mental and emotional habits. A mentor can help with developing a plan. A plan enables us to remain present and therefore to imagine and work towards the desired outcome. In this context, imagination is more important than knowledge. A plan will keep us going even if we run out of reasons. A plan is empowering and keeps hope alive. With a plan we 'get busy living' and each day we awaken knowing exactly what we're doing and why we're doing it, which in turn enables us to focus on the present and remain present.

A coach or mentor who helps you develop, maintain and carry out your plan is truly life-enhancing, not only during your recovery, but as a means of enabling you to remain well over the long term, perhaps even to prevent cancer in the first place. Whatever your situation, a plan means there's always hope, so 'start the revolution from your bed' if you have to.

CNHC

## The healer/Reiki therapist

### Tom Hoyland

Healing comes in many forms. Reiki and therapeutic touch are two that are in common use in specialist CAM centres for cancer around the UK and that have proved popular with patients. Healing is an 'energy therapy' that is generally described as a conscious channeling of universal energy by the practitioner to the person they are supporting. Reported benefits include peace of mind, reduced stress, pain relief, lowered anxiety and blood pressure, and improved sleep. It can help people cope better with the rigours of standard treatment.

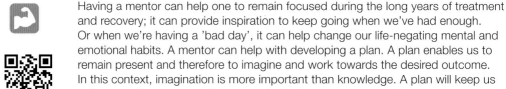

REIKI
COUNCIL

A study in 2012 explored how healing techniques can help women who have been undergoing long-term hormone therapy. The side effects of the latter are often challenging enough to prompt women to stop treatment. The results were impressive: reduced side effects; improved energy levels, wellbeing, and emotional relaxation.[11]

HEALING
TRUST

Healers can be found through the Complementary and Natural Healthcare Council (CNHC), the Reiki Council and the Healing Trust.

## The aromatherapist

Aromatherapy is a specific form of massage often used to combat psychological difficulties; see **p. 65** above.

## The hypnotherapist

There are several ways in which hypnotherapy, the use of hypnotism with a therapeutic goal, can help people with cancer. The side-effects of standard cancer treatments are many and often severe, and hypnotherapy has been shown to help with several of them, including nausea after chemotherapy and hot flushes. It can also assist with managing the side effects of the disease, such as pain, insomnia and fatigue.

An important area in which hypnotherapy can make a difference is the way in which it deals with the life-size existential issues. Confronting death has become inseparable from the topic of cancer. A hypnotherapist can also help you to face major adjustments to your self-image, whether caused by the debilitating effects of the disease or the treatment. Interestingly, hypnotherapy was found to have a significant effect on the way a group of women coped with and recovered from surgery.[12]

During hypnotherapy, although you are in a trance state induced by one of several methods, you are in control at all times. Ultimately you are the one who chooses whether or not to implement the positive suggestions made by your therapist.

You can find a professional hypnotherapist through the Complementary and Natural Healthcare Council (CNHC) and through several other websites. See **Part Eight, 'Resources'**.

CNHC

## Guided imagery/the visualisation therapist

### Patrizia Sergeant

Visualisation shares some common ground with hypnosis, but does not involve a trance state. The therapist provides support in guiding you to visualise positive scenarios and outcomes. First the aim of the session is established. It may range from changing an undesirable feeling, such as terror, to imagining chemotherapy having a devastating effect on a tumour. The therapist leads the client step by step to the imagined goal. This approach has been shown to help with anticipatory nausea (experienced by some people at the thought of having chemotherapy), mood improvement, reduced anxiety (e.g. regarding new experiences such as radiotherapy) and hot flushes. It can also lower pulse, blood pressure and breathing rate.[13]

PATRIZIA
SERGEANT

Visualisation is used extensively in a method known as The Journey, which was developed by Brandon Bays when she had cancer; it is now used worldwide to help people with cancer. Experiencing and learning the tools of a Journey Process can help us regain abilities we all possess but, through a life time of conditioning, have forgotten how to use. It is the teaching of re-connecting the mind, body and spirit, so that they can work together, keeping all three in perfect balance and health. One of the foundations of a state of good health is the maintenance of our connection to the light that is in every single cell of our bodies. Scientists believe that the light (or biophoton) -emission level is directly related to the health of the cells.[14] In areas of the body where there is disease, this light has faded from the cells, enabling unhealthy cell growth to take place. A Journey Therapist sees the absence of this light as usually the result of a negative experience or trauma, when emotions were suppressed. This could have been for a variety of reasons. We are all able to restore this light to our cells by releasing our unhealthy experiences, enabling transformation to take place.

JOURNEY

# A VISUALISATION EXERCISE

Patrizia Sergeant

Here is an exercise you could do by yourself or with a person you trust: settle yourself comfortably, either sitting or lying, somewhere that is quiet and where you will not be disturbed. Close your eyes and spend a few moments relaxing, consciously letting go of tension and busy thoughts.

Place your hand on the unhealthy area of your body. Ask yourself the question: 'What has created this absence of light in my cells?' Allow any memory or negative emotion to come up. Be patient with yourself while learning how to communicate with your body. Usually the emotions that have been stored inside the cells are feelings like pain, anger, fear or resentment.

Now allow your cells to feel those emotions by sitting in them, consciously. If you have a partner working with you, he or she can ask you what emotion it is. Name it, feel it, then let it wash over you. If another negative emotion comes up, feel that too. All your companion has to do is to ask what emotion is here now. Keep doing this until you start feeling lighter.

While this is taking place, a memory usually appears of people who have hurt you in the past. Now visualise a strong white light going through your hand into that area of your body. As you do so, see everybody, including yourself and your cells, bathed in that light. Speak the words: 'I forgive you from the bottom of my heart', visualising dark memory connections being cut to set everybody free. Know that by holding onto anger, we accumulate toxins, which take the light from our cells, making them unhealthy. By forgiving others, we set ourselves free, back into a healthy state of mind. We might not approve of the initial hurt, but we can turn it into a positive experience by learning from it. It is our choice whether to allow past experiences to hurt us for ever, or to let go of them so that we can be free again.

## The emotional freedom technique (EFT) practitioner

EFT is a widely used self-help technique that is easy to learn and can be used any time to help with difficult emotional circumstances or emotional blocks. It can help you to deal with your response to pain as well as negative emotions. EFT uses the energy meridians that form the basis of much Traditional Chinese Medicine (see **pp. 58-9** above). Rather than inserting needles or applying pressure to points on the meridians, EFT consists of tapping the points with the tips of the fingers, while simultaneously focusing on the problem and voicing positive affirmations.

ACEP

Many people have succeeded in learning the technique from reading or from internet videos, but you can also get help from a trained professional (see ACEP website). Users report a high degree of success with this strikingly simple therapy. As a self-help technique, EFT is a valuable tool that you can use anytime, anywhere, to meet some of the many challenges you may find yourself facing.

# EFT SELF-HELP EXERCISE

Perhaps you are worried about an imminent consultation with your oncologist. This might be having a detrimental effect on your sleep and general wellbeing.

Remove your watch and glasses (if you usually wear them), and, using two or three fingertips, tap firmly but not hard with both hands around five to seven times on each of the spots indicated below, or for about the time it takes for one full breath in and out. Don't tap with both hands simultaneously; keep them slightly out of synch.

While tapping, say (preferably out loud): 'Even though I am very worried, I deeply and completely accept myself.' This can be modified as appropriate, e.g. 'Even though I am very depressed...'. It doesn't matter if you believe what you are saying or not, but it can help to say it with as much conviction as possible.

**01  Top of the head (TH)**
With fingers back-to-back down the centre of the skull

**02  Eyebrow (EB)**
Just above and to one side of the nose, at the beginning of the eyebrow

**03  Side of the eye (SE)**
On the bone bordering the outside corner of the eyelid

**04  Under the eye (UE)**
On the bone under an eye about an inch below your pupil

**05  Under the nose (UN)**
On the small area between the bottom of your nose and the top of your upper lip

**06  Chin (Ch)**
Midway between the point of your chin and the bottom of your lower lip (even though it is not directly on the point of the chin, we call it the chin point because that is descriptive enough for people to understand easily)

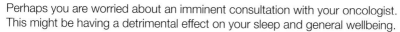

**Collarbone (CB)  07**
The junction where the breastbone (sternum), collarbone (clavicle) and the first rib meet

This is a very important point and in acupuncture is referred to as K (kidney) 27. To locate it, first place your forefinger on the U-shaped notch at the top of the breastbone (about where a man would knot his tie). From the bottom of the U, move your forefinger down toward the navel an inch and then go to the left (or right) an inch. This point is referred to as CB even though it is not in fact on the collarbone

**Under the arm (UA)  08**
On the side of the body, at a point even with the nipple (for men) or in the middle of the bra strap (for women); about 4 inches below the armpit

**Wrists (WR)  09**
The inside of both wrists

N.B.: We are indebted to Dr Joseph Mercola for some of the information above which is from his 'Basic Steps to Your Emotional Freedom', available (with further details) on the Mercola website (see **Part Eight, Resources**).

### The counsellor

CCL

#### Jane Fior

Seeing a trained counsellor or psychotherapist, one who has experience of working with cancer patients, can help you and others close to you to deal with the emotional impact of a cancer diagnosis. Most of you will benefit from professional support if you are struggling to make sense of your feelings.

Talking to a trained counsellor who is not personally involved has helped many people to gain fresh insights and has been an important first step in regaining control of their lives. They often discover a new strength and previously unrecognised inner resources, which has helped them to make choices about treatment decisions and the appropriate way forward.

After receiving a diagnosis of cancer, people can understandably feel out of control and anxious. Even those surrounded by loving and supportive family and friends often feel isolated and can find relief in speaking to someone about their true feelings in a confidential and non-judgemental environment. Being able to express painful or angry feelings, without fear of being judged or upsetting those close to you, can bring a great sense of relief; it can also help to alleviate many distressing symptoms such as depression, sleep disturbances and anxiety. This in turn can reduce tension and stress and help you to regain a sense of control as well as to reduce feelings of loneliness and isolation.

LIFE>

You can see a counsellor at any stage; at diagnosis, during treatment or when treatment has finished. You may sometimes be offered counselling support as part of your medical care. However, if this is not available, you can self-refer. Check that your therapist is experienced working within cancer issues. Some clinics and individual practitioners offer telephone consultations and home visits, so do check this when you first contact them.

A full listing of qualified UK practitioners and organisations, experienced in working with cancer, is available within LIFE>, the Yes to Life searchable web directory.

### Support groups

Joining a support or self-help group can be an important step for many people following a cancer diagnosis. Apart from providing a safe place in which to share the many and varied difficulties that cancer presents, both as an illness and in its treatment, it can also be a forum in which to receive and share useful information, hope and inspiration.

MACMILLAN

Talking to others who are further down the road and who have found ways to adjust to the new realities of their lives can give enormous reassurance. The insights gained over time can be very hard to come by early on in the journey. A diagnosis of cancer is akin to being dropped on another planet, so great are its effects on people, and so much is unfamiliar and stressful. Sharing the simple practicalities involved in dealing with everyday difficulties such as hair loss, mouth ulcers, or even how to manage friends and relatives, can be hugely rewarding, and can combat the feelings of isolation that almost everyone reports.

CANCER
ACTIVE

Possibly the most significant aspect of group work is its capacity to inspire. Survival and the workings of the immune system are directly linked to our will to live and our hopes for the future. Simply working with others facing the same challenge has been proven to increase survival.[15] Some groups are led by a trained facilitator. It is important to find a group that reflects your needs – this could be based on cancer type, particular challenges and interests. Crucially, your group must be uplifting and inspirational to you. Word of mouth can be a great way to find something suitable; you can also explore the Macmillan and CANCERactive websites.

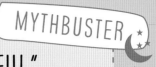

# "CAM IS COMPLETELY NON-HARMFUL"

While this is largely true, there are potential dangers in any approach, and cancer is an extremely complex condition. Make sure you have a reputable practitioner and don't rely on what you read on the internet.

## Supportive complementary therapies: an overview

### Dorothy Crowther

Integrating medicine with complementary therapies gives patients the support to take back control in their lives. Using therapies such as acupuncture, reflexology and aromatherapy not only helps the patients with their fears and anxieties, but also assists in alleviating some distressing symptoms.

WIRRAL
HOLISTIC

Acupuncture, for example, is beneficial for frozen shoulder, which can occur after breast surgery. The patient often has a problem coming to terms with not only the cancer diagnosis, but another health issue that needs addressing, such as painful joints due to arthritis.

Unfortunately patients do have side effects due to their medical treatments: chemotherapy, for example, often results in nausea, hot flushes and sleeping problems. This is where complementary therapies will help greatly. Acupuncture and reflexology can reduce and alleviate nausea and hot flushes. Aromatherapy is extremely good for relaxation, which in turn will help the patient to have a better night's rest. Aromatherapy is ideally used after the person has completed a full treatment course of chemotherapy.

Although I have mentioned aromatherapy, reflexology and acupuncture, there are other commonly used complementary therapies: these include Indian head massage, Reiki and hypnotherapy, all of which are equally beneficial.

LIFE>

A full listing of the UK centres specialising in CAM therapies to support people with cancer can be found in LIFE>, the Yes to Life searchable web directory.

## Summary

This is by no means an exhaustive list of possible therapies to consider as part of an integrative treatment programme. A few others that you may want to consider are art therapy, music therapy, journal writing, relaxation and deep breathing, biofeedback and T'ai Chi (see **Part Eight**, 'Resources').

You may need to try a few different approaches to any given need before settling on the one that works for you. Use this chapter together with **Parts Two**, **Three** and **Four** of this book to build a team around you that gives you the confidence to know that you are doing everything you can to achieve the best possible outcome.

# PART TWO

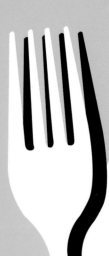

# NUTRITION

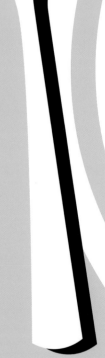

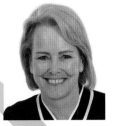

# INTRODUCTION TO PART TWO

Patricia Peat

In this part of *The Cancer Revolution* we go on to look at one area of life that anyone who wants to avoid cancer, who wants to control cancer or who seeks to avoid a recurrence simply cannot afford to ignore. The topic of nutrition is so vital that it merits the whole of Part Two to itself.

It is a central issue, and it promotes passionately polarised points of view that are fed to the public every day, which, in turn, can lead to stress and confusion. The good news is that, although there are certainly still wildly divergent views on many aspects of diet within Integrative Medicine, a growing ground of agreement is developing on which to build.

Apart from looking at basics such as buying and preparing good food, Part Two investigates specific areas such as sugar, dairy products and specialist diets, including juicing and superfoods; weight loss due to cancer and supplementation and its role in cancer are also discussed in detail.

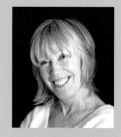

# CHAPTER 4
# HOW TO BUY GOOD FOOD

Lynda Brown

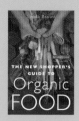

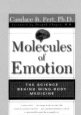

Taking care of our daily diet – what foods we choose to buy, cook and eat – is fundamental to saying 'Yes to Life'. For good food nourishes body, mind and soul on many levels, and brings that all-important healing joy and pleasure into our lives at every meal. Only good food provides the vital nourishment that our bodies need. Nor is there a better way to show ourselves that we love ourselves: as Candace B. Pert illustrated in her groundbreaking book *Molecules of Emotion*, this has immediate positive effects for our immune systems.

Feeding ourselves well empowers us in many other ways, increasing self-respect and confidence, reconnecting us with nature and the seasons, and opening up a whole new world of positive benefits. For example, buying food in supermarkets is fundamentally an alienating and negative experience, which, ultimately, is a drain on the immune system. When we change to buying food from farmers' markets, food shopping immediately becomes a positive, empowering and happy experience. Similarly, cooking or sharing a simple home-made meal rather than reheating a ready-made one has the same beneficial effects; both boost rather than drain our immune systems; both stimulate 'feel good' not 'feel bad' feelings. Simplifying our shopping, buying and cooking habits can have profound positive effects on our lives. Such goals are easy to achieve.

## What are 'good' and 'bad' foods?

As far as everyday eating goes, there are two main types of food:
'Good' foods are those that nature provides. They can be eaten raw or cooked. 'Natural' or 'real' foods include meat, fish, dairy, eggs, fruit, vegetables, nuts and seeds, grains, pulses, sea vegetables and so on. Traditional artisan and fermented foods such as natural leaven breads, sauerkraut, yoghurt and kefir, also fall into this category.

'Bad' foods are devitalised, processed foods, of which 'junk' foods – those laden with additives, salt, sugar, processed carbohydrates and hydrogenated fats – are the worst.

The first step, then, is to remove processed foods from our diets (as a rough guide, if you don't recognise anything on the label as food, don't buy it). General health improves immediately because our systems no longer have to 'fight' foods made from ingredients which are detrimental to health, or in the case of artificial additives, are 'foreign' to our immune systems.

The second step is to learn a little more about how food is produced, for the quality of the food we eat will only be as good as the care that has been taken in its production. With this in mind, the books and websites listed in **Part Eight, 'Resources'**, have been chosen specifically to help you understand, source and buy better food.

The single most important factor in a good diet is to avoid industrialised food. Apart from the negative effects it has on the environment and wildlife, intensive farming methods for both crops and animals require heavy use of pesticides. Artificial fertilisers are required for crops; and extreme stocking densities for animals, which in turn require constant use of routine medication and antibiotics. This results in pesticide residues, depleted vitamin and mineral content in food crops, and poor-quality meat.

High-quality food, by contrast, is produced using traditional extensive (as opposed to intensive) or organic farming methods that work with nature, avoid pesticides and artificial fertilisers, and practise high animal welfare standards – for example, low stocking densities where animals are raised primarily outdoors and given diets based on natural foodstuffs instead of concentrates. Food produced by artisans can also be of high quality. Good food will always have provenance and integrity.

## Cheap versus expensive food

Inevitably, the cheaper the food, the less one will want to know about how that food has been produced, and the less true nutrition it will contain. High-quality food not only tastes good but also turns out to be relatively cheap at the price, in terms of its beneficial effects on the environment and on us. Unfortunately, for many cost can be a key determining factor in food choices, especially if illness has led to loss of employment. In these circumstances, the best choice may not always be possible. But this chapter aims to clarify that some choices are better than others. Simply aim to make the best choices you can. As a rule it is better to eat less and to eat really well than to have plenty of poor-quality, toxin-laden food.

## Fake high-quality food

Expensively packaged food, novelty breads, fashion fads, up-market ready meals and expensive low-fat substitutes are not high-quality foods but merely added value foods. They represent poor value for money, which would be better spent on genuine food where the cost reflects its production, not its packaging.

## Labels: organic, biodynamic, free range, artisan

All these have come to denote quality foods, and it's useful to know the difference between them.

### Organic

Organic farming principles are founded on the belief that a healthy soil begets healthy plants, in turn begetting healthy animals, and healthy people. Care of the soil, animal welfare and human health is thus paramount. This is why organic farming systems build natural fertility, forbid nitrogen fertilisers and all but a tiny handful of approved pesticides; they also ban the use of genetically modified crops and ingredients, and reject intensive farming methods. Organic processing standards forbid the use of hydrogenated fats and almost all food additives. To qualify as organic food, foods must be certified as complying with their standards set by an approved body such as the Soil Association.

SOIL
ASSOC

### Biodynamic

This is a highly specialised system of self-sufficient organic farming, which employs herbal preparations and operates in parallel with the lunar calendar. It consistently produces the most health-full food, with maximum vitality and harmony.

BIO-
DYNAMIC

### Free range

A term used mainly for pigs and poultry (table birds) – hence also eggs. Truly free-range animals are intended to have unlimited access to outside and to fresh grass; in reality this is rare, and the concept of free range is usually a compromise between the number of animals on a given piece of land and access to limited space permitted under law. Soil Association standards stipulate lower stocking densities and more outside space than other free-range standards.

### Artisan

Genuine artisanal foods are foods produced on a small scale, using traditional time-honoured methods of production. As with organic and biodynamic foods, provenance and integrity are their hallmarks. Classic examples are artisan cheese, breads, olive oil and olives, smoked and salted foods, and charcuterie; in terms of flavour and authenticity, they can be very fine. However, rather like 'free range', or 'local', not all foods labeled artisan are worthy of the description, and need to be chosen with care. Those on a tight budget will often find that the premium price tag commonly attached to artisan foods puts them out of reach. Given that many of these items could reasonably be categorised as 'nice to have', or even as luxuries, this is not a great concern.

### Natural fats versus processed fats

This is another important issue that impacts directly on food quality for dairy products and meat. There is a considerable body of evidence emerging that natural animal fats and cholesterol do not cause heart disease and are not harmful but vital for good health (they play a critical role in many functions);[1] it now seems that the real culprits are hydrogenated fats and refined vegetable oils. Healthy nutritious natural fats are animal fats, butter, cream and unrefined cold-pressed oils as well as coconut butter (both butter and virgin coconut cream consist largely of short-chain saturated fatty acids, which our bodies need and do not readily store as body fat). Avoid margarines and low-fat butter substitutes at all cost: both are highly processed fats made from cheap highly refined ingredients.

### Fresh produce

Wherever possible, buy and eat home-grown seasonal crops that exude freshness and vitality, produced using non-intensive growing methods, be that local, organic or biodynamic. A box scheme (see **'Where to buy good food', p. 82** below) is a good option; supermarkets can be useful for organic fair-trade bananas, organic mushrooms, citrus fruit and staple vegetables such as organic carrots.

### Red meat (beef and lamb)

As with all free-range products, the key to quality is that the animal has been grass- or pasture-fed, preferably from slow-growing traditional breeds, allowed to grow to full maturity (twelve to thirty months for beef; six months or more for lamb). New research also shows that levels of CLA (conjugated linoleic acid, a valuable omega-6 fat) are significantly higher in grass-fed animals. The same applies to milk (which is why organic milk is acknowledged to be more nutritious). If you eat red meat, therefore, choose organic, or meat sourced from traditionally reared grass-fed herds from farmers' markets or high quality butchers. Lamb generally is less

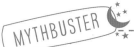

MYTHBUSTER

# "SUGAR DOESN'T PROMOTE CANCER"

Many oncologists in the UK are still stoically maintaining this view, while simultaneously relying on cancer's appetite for glucose as the mechanism for one of their primary diagnostic tools - the PET scan (see Appendix 2, 'Understanding scans').

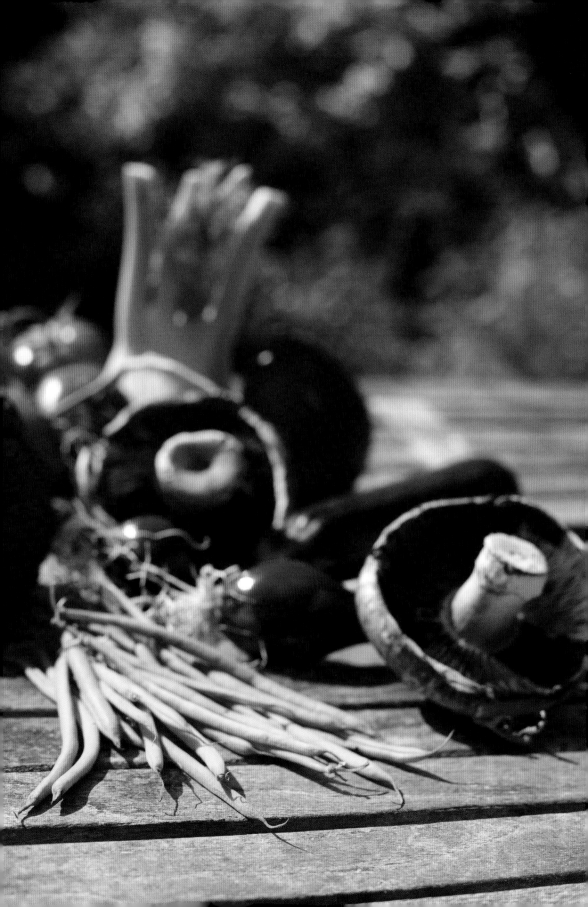

intensively reared; hill, Manx and salt-marsh lamb are examples of traditionally produced, high-quality meat, all well known for their superb flavour.

Once slaughtered, both need to be aged properly (dry aged is best): beef for two to three weeks or more, lamb for seven to ten days.

## Poultry and pork

With these meats especially, you get what you pay for. Choose free range as a baseline level, and organic where possible. Look for traditional slow-growing breeds, (chickens of eight to twelve months; pigs of six to eight months) that have been raised in small numbers. Both chicken and pork should have proper covering of fat and firm flesh; avoid flabby, pale, insipid or watery looking meat; both also benefit from proper ageing.

## Breads

For bread to be digestible, it needs to be allowed to ferment and prove slowly. This rules out the majority of breads, including bake-off breads, which are all produced using modern quick methods, aided by an array of chemical dough improvers and other additives.

Choose breads made with organic flour as a minimum standard (pesticide residues in wheat regularly exceed legal limits). Wherever possible, buy artisan breads made from natural leavens or minimum yeast, using traditional slow-rise methods. Organic pumpernickel-type breads using whole fermented grains, such as Biona, are also excellent. If budgetary restrictions are a bar to buying the best, you may want to consider buying good ingredients and baking your own, which is not as daunting as many believe.

## Dairy

The quality of dairy products depends on the scale of manufacture (small versus factory-produced). This involves not only the question of freshness, but how much processing milk has undergone, whether the product is made from a general milk pool or a single farm. In the case of cheese, quality depends on whether it has been aged or 'affined' correctly. Milk from herds raised on grass is healthier (see '**Red meat**', above, **p. 78**).

### Milk

Clean raw (green top) milk from pasture-fed cows is generally acknowledged by nutritionists to be a far superior product to pasteurised milk; it contains an array of beneficial bacteria, anti-microbial agents, enzymes and other micro-nutrients which make it easy to digest and which strengthen the system. Pasteurisation kills most of these and also reduces milk's intrinsic nutritional value. Homogenisation is another technical process that subjects milk to further heat treatment and unnaturally forces the fat cells to be distributed throughout the drink. This is why unpasteurised dairy products – milk, cream, butter and cheese – are worth seeking out, and can contribute positively to health. Wherever possible therefore, choose organic, non-homogenised full cream milk (this is not fattening!); Guernsey and Jersey milk are good choices; raw/unpasteurised/green top milk is best. Avoid skimmed milk, which is an impoverished product.

### Cheese, cream and butter

Again, where possible, choose unpasteurised artisan farm-made cheeses, cream and butter. Avoid processed cheeses, cheap commercial cheeses, cream or butter, ready-grated cheeses, and made-up cheeses with added flavourings.

### Yoghurt

Natural yoghurt, i.e. milk fermented by lactic bacteria, is one of nature's simplest health foods. Most yoghurt on sale is not true yoghurt but effectively processed yoghurt-like gloop, made with skimmed milk, added milk proteins, stabilisers, preservatives, added sweetened fruit and more. These are not healthy products. Choose organic natural yoghurt made from full cream milk. Probiotic yoghurts are expensive but to be valued. Home-made kefir qualifies as a natural super probiotic and superfood, and largely makes itself (see **Part Eight, 'Resources'**).

## Eggs

Eggs are a wonderful food: they are highly nutritious, easy to cook and digest, but sadly much debased. The difference between a first-class egg, which will have a deliciously rich yolk and creamy clean-tasting white, and a cheap one is a revelation. The colour of the yolk is no indication of quality – the egg producer can choose from a range of preferences. It is determined by the feed. The colour of good free range-eggs will vary throughout the year, depending on the quality of the grass to which the hens have been exposed: by early summer the eggshells will be deep orange, in winter much paler. Eggs keep very well: they can last for two or three weeks; longer for first-class eggs. Choose organic or true free-range eggs from small flocks. Backyard eggs produced from hens that lay naturally (i.e. given no unnatural daylight) are generally superb.

## Grains

Choose organic for preference, and biodynamic where possible. This is to avoid commonly detected contamination of non-organic grains with pre- and post-harvest pesticide residues.

## Nuts

The fresher the nuts you buy, the better; choose unshelled nuts when in season and shelled whole nuts rather than pieces, which are more easily subject to oxidation. Avoid stale-looking cheap nuts, which often have a slightly tell-tale rancid/oxidised flavour, and check the sell-by date. Organic nuts, especially almonds, tend to have a deeper, richer flavour than non-organic ones.

## Oils

Most oils are highly processed and refined, including olive oil. Cold-pressed oils are usually best: choose extra virgin olive oil; cold-pressed 'virgin' coconut butter (this has a high smoking point, making it an excellent cooking fat as well as an extremely healthy one); cold-pressed nut oils are excellent in salads.

## Grow your own

To make your own salads from vegetables and fruit that you have grown yourself- even in a taster patch – is perhaps one of the most health- and life-enhancing things to do. It provides a benchmark of truly good food, radiating a vitality that you can see and taste. The rewards, satisfaction and pleasure it brings are beyond measure. This is clearly a great option if you are on a tight budget but have some space for growing.

You do not need a large – or even a small – garden, nor do you need to be self-sufficient: a few pots, a window sill, or a small purpose-built box filled with compost will provide fresh herbs, salad ingredients, sugar-snap peas, French beans and strawberries. Orchard fruits grafted onto dwarf rooting stocks grow well in large pots, too. The golden rule is to grow what you like and what you find easy. Buy young plantlets and dot them around the garden or grow in pots.

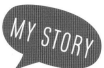

### Melissa Sharp
36 at diagnosis, triple-negative breast-cancer survivor

*It's astonishing how few people have any idea of the life-changing benefits of a healthy diet, and not just for those who are unwell. But that was me too, until I decided to combat my cancer and the toxic side effects of my treatment with a super healthy diet that has since become the best hobby I've ever had. And now I even work in nutrition!*

Here are some ideas of what to grow and where:

### Beetroot
Superfood and the easiest root to grow, this vegetable takes up little space.

### Climbing French beans and runner beans
These are unbeatable value. They can be trained on a trellis or made into a wigwam of canes around a large pot to provide a climbing structure. Water every day in summer. Keep picking; feed with an organic liquid feed, and the beans will crop well into autumn.

### Cut and come again seed mixtures
Sow and cut these instant salads as seedlings of three to four weeks (when their vitality and vitamin content is at their highest). Then leave to re-grow and cut again.

### French beans
These delicious and prolific greens crop well into autumn. Dot among flowers or grow in pots.

### Garlic
Related to the onion, garlic is the easiest superfood to grow: pop cloves into a pot and use the shoots; or plant them in the ground in autumn and harvest the bulbs in early summer.

### Herbs
Rosemary, sage, thyme, bay leaves, parsley, basil, dill, chervil, sorrel and chives are all beneficial to your health; they also enhance your cooking and the life of bees. Some herbs, including lemon balm can be infused in boiling water and enjoyed as a tea (tisanes or herbal infusions).

### Lettuce
This basic salad ingredient is perfect for growing in a small garden: Little Gem is the best all-rounder.

### Tomatoes
Choose cherry varieties (sweetest and highest in vitamin C) and give them the sunniest and most sheltered spot you can find.

### Sugar snap peas
This variety of pea is sweet and crunchy, high in vitamin C and grows prolifically. For an instant superfood, pick the shoots when 5-7.5 cm / 2-3" high (an ordinary packet of marrowfat peas is perfect for these).

### Swiss chard
This dark green vegetable crops over several months and is always delicious. It requires no preparation and cooks in two to three minutes.

## Where to buy good food

The best places to buy good food are farmers' markets and farm shops, where you can buy direct from the producer, together with independent shops who have the know-how and can help you choose: traditional butchers, artisan cheesemongers, fishmongers, greengrocers, specialist delis, artisan breadmakers, health- and whole-food shops and so on.

For organic food, there are plenty of options, including specialist organic outlets, farm shops, supermarkets and online. Joining a local organic box scheme is one of the best and cheapest way of buying organic vegetables; if that's not possible, there are excellent online box schemes that can also provide organic meat, dairy, groceries and more (see **Part Eight, 'Resources'**).

Buying locally produced food has many advantages: it involves fewer food miles, fresher food, and you can get to know the producer and how they produce their food. A local food tag on its own, however, is no guarantee of quality, especially if it has been intensively grown. So always check that the food meets the quality criteria.

# CHAPTER 5

## DIET AS THE FOUNDATION OF GOOD HEALTH

### Daphne Lambert

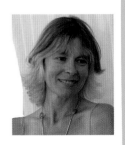

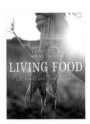

There is little dispute that nutritional measures strengthen cells and help prevent cancers from forming. Opinions differ considerably, however, around the role that nutrition plays in enabling the body to reject established cancers. Furthermore, even among those who know that nutritional therapy can be effective in eliminating cancer from the body, there is a wide variance in what is considered the 'right' diet.

GREEN-CUISINE

Many different diets are available for those with cancer. Some have clinical trials behind them, like the treatment protocols of Dr Nicholas Gonzalez, while others do not. All of them demonstrate, in one way or another, that the food you choose to eat can help you reclaim a healthy body.

Here are three brief outlines of well-known cancer diets:

- Dr Nicholas Gonzalez, who practised in New York, evolved his diet treatment from the extensive studies and work of Dr William Kelley, who determined healing diets based on the function of the autonomic nervous system. He named this method metabolic typing. The prescribed diets are quite variable, and can range from nearly vegetarian to diets requiring red meat two or three times a day. Each patient receives individualised dietary recommendations.

- The Budwig Diet uses cottage cheese and flaxseed with a minimally processed vegetarian diet. Dr Johanna Budwig (1908 -2003) was a pharmacologist, chemist, physicist and a leading authority on fats and oils. Qualified in Germany, she made in-depth studies on the effect of hydrogenated and other denatured fats upon human health, finding this to be disastrous. She discovered the truly healing effect of essential fatty acids on all manner of degenerative diseases, including cancer.

- Gerson Therapy is a dietary therapy that aims to provide optimum nutrition in the form of an abundance of minerals, enzymes and vitamins. Only organic fruit and vegetables are used; some of the vegetables may be cooked very slowly with a minimum of liquid, stewed fruit, potatoes and oatmeal. The diet centres on freshly made juices of vegetables, fruits and leaves, consumed within twenty minutes of preparation to avoid losses in enzyme effectiveness. By combining hypernutrition and concurrent detoxification it aims to rebuild the immune system, thereby enabling it to tackle the malignancy.

Further reading on specialised diets is listed in **Part Eight, 'Resources'**.

Along with many others, these demonstrate that different diets work for different people. Every individual is different, so we all respond differently to the foods we eat. To find an eating plan that works for you, seek advice and coaching from a qualified nutritionist.

While there are many conflicting ideas, cancer-healing diets do have some common ground. Sourcing food from a system that maximises nutrition and minimises toxins, eliminating processed foods and eating a wide range of leaves, vegetables and fruits – a colourful rainbow diet – are basic guidelines.

## Food from a natural farming system

For foods to be healthy and naturally vibrant, the way nature intended, we need to look at their source. The food we eat is a product of the soil. Healthy, life-giving food needs a vibrant soil ecology, teeming with microbial life. Organisms that underpin the fertility of the soil are the foundation of human health. Through over-farming, soil gradually loses its mineral content. As many of the minerals that pass from plant to our bodies are not needed to make the plant grow and appear healthy, there is not always an incentive for growers to add these minerals back. On the whole, industrial farming concentrates on adding nitrogen, phosphate and potassium to the soil; although this encourages growth, it leaves the plants deficient in many important and essential minerals as well as other nutrients vital to human health.

Sustainable farming maintains humus and soil fertility, maximises the nutritional value of food and minimises toxins. For a healing diet, it is fundamental to source food that is grown naturally, food that comes from a growing system such as biodynamic or organic.

## Processed foods

WESTON
PRICE

If we eat food that has been split apart and refined, the concomitant lack of wholeness diminishes both the quantity and quality of nutrients, making them less likely to nourish us. Nutritional researchers such as Dr Weston A. Price and Dr McCarrison studied the diets of indigenous cultures and found that when their diets were comprised of natural, unprocessed, locally grown foods, the people had no tooth decay or signs of degenerative disease. When the same cultures began to use denatured, processed foods such as white flour and sugar, canned foods and insufficient amounts of fresh, raw foods, they found that the people began to suffer from dental decay and degenerative diseases. Regardless of the composition of the diet, whether it was exclusively vegetarian, lacto-vegetarian, predominantly meat or largely dairy based, if the foods were natural and unprocessed, with a good proportion eaten raw, the people maintained good health.

Raw whole milk, whole wheat grain, grilled fish and nuts in their shells are examples of whole foods. By contrast, pasteurised skimmed milk, white flour, fish fingers and ground nuts have all been 'altered'. The more you eat food that has been altered as little as possible, the more healing your diet will be, thus helping to return you to and maintain vital, energised health.

Two processed foods that wreak havoc in the body are refined sugar and altered fats.

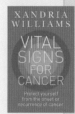

# THE DANGERS OF GLUCOSE

## Xandria Williams

A patient recently said to me: 'I have been told to give up all sugar and all grains, but surely that is ridiculous. I've looked into it, and the case for sugar is not proven, and surely wholemeal bread and brown rice can't be bad?' The truth is that they are dangerous foods for you if you have cancer, and there is a clear biochemical and physiological foundation for these statements.

XANDRIA
WILLIAMS

The reasons why follow:

Just as the human body contains organs, each with their specific function, so the cell contains much smaller, individual, organelles with their own specific function. The organelle that is of interest here is the mitochondrion. Each of your cells has thousands of these mitochondria, and they are unique, within your cell, in that they contain oxygen, whereas the rest of your cell and all the other organelles are anaerobic, or oxygen-free.

It is the mitochondria that contain the necessary materials and the mechanisms for releasing the energy that is locked up in the food that you eat. It is in the mitochondria that you 'burn up' the fats, proteins and most of the carbohydrates that you eat, releasing the energy that they contain. This energy is then available for the cell to use. Effectively all of the energy that you obtain from proteins and fats is released here, and arguably around 90 to 95 per cent of the energy from carbohydrates.

IN 1924 THE EMINENT PHYSIOLOGIST OTTO WARBURG DEMONSTRATED THAT THE CAUSE OF CANCER WAS A LACK OF OXYGEN AND FAILURE OF MITOCHONDRIAL FUNCTION;[1] HE EVENTUALLY WON A NOBEL PRIZE FOR THIS WORK IN 1931.

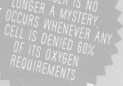
...THE CAUSE OF CANCER IS NO LONGER A MYSTERY, IT OCCURS WHENEVER ANY CELL IS DENIED 60% OF ITS OXYGEN REQUIREMENTS

He stated that: 'The cause of cancer is no longer a mystery, we know it occurs whenever any cell is denied 60% of its oxygen requirements'; also that 'Cancer, above all other diseases, has countless secondary causes. But, even for cancer, there is only one prime cause. [...] the prime cause of cancer is the replacement of the respiration of oxygen in normal body cells by a fermentation of sugar.'[2]

$O_2$

If cancer cells do not have mitochondrial function, it follows that they cannot obtain energy from fats or proteins and so become desperate for carbohydrate in the form of glucose as an energy source. Glucose feeds cancer. Keep that firmly in mind as you choose your foods.

So let's find out where glucose comes from in the diet. Sugar is made up of glucose and fructose joined together to form a dimer or double molecule. In your body this fructose is changed to glucose, so, essentially, when you eat sugar you are adding to the glucose level of your blood and providing fuel for any cancer cells that may be present.

Starches are large complex molecules made up of thousands of glucose molecules joined together. The arrangement of these glucose chains varies within individual foods. This glucose composition is true of the starches in all grains and similar starchy foods, for example potatoes, starchy root vegetables and bananas (which also contain sucrose). It is also true of the starch in above-ground vegetables, but these contain much less starch than root vegetables, much more fibre and a large number in substantial amounts of many vital nutrients. Most fruits contain fructose which is, again, converted to glucose. Berries, however, are relatively low in starch, low in sugars and very rich in beneficial nutrients and are therefore highly recommended.

What about physiological proof of this? Cancer cells have been shown to have a three to five fold increase in glucose uptake compared with healthy cells.[3] In fact, so desperate are cancer cells for glucose that they have many more receptor sites (entry portals) for glucose than do normal healthy cells. There are various estimates as to the number, ranging upwards from six times as many.[4, 5]

Insulin is needed to increase cellular uptake of glucose, so it is not surprising to find that cancer cells have many more receptor sites for insulin, compared with healthy cells.[6] Furthermore, cancer cells have devised another clever tool to take in glucose and feed their insatiable appetite for it. They have developed special channels called epidermal growth factor receptors (EGFR) which stabilise a protein that channels a constant supply of glucose into the cancer cells.[7] To improve their chances of getting the lion's share of the glucose in your bloodstream, cancer cells actually make their own insulin, the hormone that is essential for, and encourages, cellular uptake of glucose. Not only does glucose feed cancer, but it has been argued that most cancer cells would die if starved of glucose.

So how can you plan your diet? First, as my patient discovered and I endorsed for her, give up all sugars, grains, beans and other high-starch foods. Beans are good sources of protein, it is true, but there are other ways of fulfilling your protein needs. If you still want to eat legumes, then sprout them. This will turn the starch into cellulose and other non-digestible carbohydrates that support the growing plant structure but do not break down within your digestive tract; your uptake of glucose is therefore not increased. Sugars come in many different guises, such as dextrose, malto-dextrin, agave, corn syrup and so on, so become sugar-wise and learn to read labels. If this is too much for you, first give up all sugars, then give up refined grains, then all grains.

Of course you cannot go on a totally glucose-free diet, but by focusing on above-ground vegetables, good-quality protein, nuts and berries, you can avoid the floods of glucose that would result from eating sugars (of all sorts), grains and other starchy foods.

## Altered fats

Altered fats are especially detrimental to health and healing. Cooked oil is a major cause of free radical damage in the body. Free radicals are oxygen molecules that have lost an electron, becoming unstable and reactive. These radical oxygen molecules steal electrons from healthy molecules, thus causing damage and creating more free radicals in the process. Light, air and heat turn polyunsaturated fats (corn, safflower, sunflower, walnut, flax and hemp) into trans-fatty acids and free radicals which are linked to cancer. Keep polyunsaturated fats in small dark bottles in the fridge, do not cook with them, but use as salad dressings or add a spoonful to a smoothie.

## Meat, fish, eggs and milk

If you decide to include meat and fish in your diet, there are two key considerations – the quality and the quantity. Meat quality is dependent on the life the animal led before it was killed. There is a vast difference between eating the meat of a wild deer and eating the flesh of a non-organic chicken reared in a 'broiler' system. While we might not have the option to eat animals caught in the wild, we can and must avoid non-organic flesh for a healing diet. Chickens, for example, reared in an intensive farming system, are bred to develop quickly, reaching slaughter weight in just forty-two days. They spend their entire life indoors, are routinely fed antibiotics and other anti-microbials. In addition to the medications condensed in their flesh will be pesticides, herbicides and other toxic substances used in raising their feed crops. If the addition of a little meat in your diet makes you feel better, to limit toxins, choose organic and eat small portions.

The most nutritious fish are wild-caught, small oily fish like sardines and herrings. Wild Alaskan salmon is another possibility. Farmed salmon, due to overcrowding and diet, have weakened immune systems and are prone to parasites, bacteria and viruses. Organic farmed salmon is slightly better, although all farmed fish have more saturated fat than wild fish, due to their largely stationary existence.

Organic eggs contain high-quality proteins, fats, vitamins, minerals and antioxidants. Exceptionally easy to digest, they provide a wonderful boost to the immune system. Raw eggs are nutritionally superior to cooked ones. If you find the texture a problem, it is easy to pop them into a smoothie.

Modern ways of producing milk – pasteurised, semi-skimmed and homogenised – have negative effects on our health. In general, I recommend that dairy products are avoided. However, from time to time there can be benefit for some people in small amounts of organic, raw, unpasteurised kefir and curd cheese (see 'The problem with dairy', on p. 99).

The most important foods to include in any cancer diet are plants, and if you choose a colourful rainbow of vegetables and fruits, you will optimise your ability to overcome cancer with a wide range of anticancer nutrients and phytonutrients. Phytonutrients are plant chemicals which have been produced by plants as part of their means of survival. The constant biological challenge of being exposed to direct sunlight and ultraviolet rays all day forced plants to form powerful free radical scavenging antioxidant polyphenols in order to protect themselves. When we eat a diet rich in fruits and vegetables, we harness the powers of these phytonutrients into our diet. The level of phytonutrients within any plant varies depending on the species of plant, soil conditions and many other environmental factors. Research shows that organic plants have more phytonutrients than non-organic ones. Phytonutrients are powerful protectors and fighters against cancer. They contain antioxidants to quench free radicals, anti-proliferative nutrients to slow tumour growth and foods that stimulate the immune system.

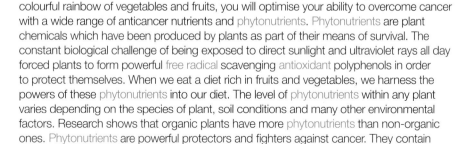

## Pros and cons of a vegetarian/vegan diet

In his practice Dr Nicholas Gonzalez found that some patients have a metabolism that functions most efficiently with the specific combination of nutrients that are found in fruits, vegetables, nuts, whole grains and seeds, and with minimal or no animal protein. Other patients, however, do extremely well with a diet based on animal products and fewer plant-based foods. There may be an argument in some cases to include a little naturally reared animal protein. As a general rule, both vegetarian and vegan diets have been shown to lower blood cholesterol levels and decrease the risk of various disorders such as high blood pressure, stroke, heart disease, diabetes, rheumatoid arthritis, osteoporosis, kidney diseases, gallstones and cancer.

If you choose to follow a vegetarian diet consisting of vegetables, nuts, cereals, seeds, beans, grains, eggs, dairy and fruit, it will be rich in fibre; it will also include an array of vitamins and minerals that are essential for a healthy body. Beans, yoghurt, eggs and seeds are all good sources of protein. Vegetables contain phytonutrients which support our immune systems and green leafy vegetables are a rich source of healing chlorophyll and antioxidants. A vegan diet not only omits meat and fish, but dairy and eggs as well. In planning a vegan diet, take care to ensure that all the essential nutrients are included.

Although vegetarian and vegan diets can provide all that is necessary, there are certain nutrients that are higher and more bio-available in meat or fish. Nutrients of special consideration in a vegan/vegetarian diet are iron, zinc and vitamin B12. Plant sources contain a significant amount of iron, but in non-heme form. Heme iron is primarily found in red meats and is more readily absorbed. The iron found in plants is difficult to absorb but cooking tends to increase iron availability. Some iron-rich foods have other compounds that render the iron less absorbable. However, a diet rich in a variety of vegetables providing vitamin C will neutralise the effect of these compounds.

Whereas non-vegetarian diets seem to enhance the absorption of zinc, vegetarian and vegan diets do the exact opposite – they inhibit it. Generally this is due to high phytate levels, but you can reduce phytates by sprouting some of the seeds that contain high amounts of zinc like mung beans and sunflower seeds, thus making zinc more available.

Many vegetarians lack vitamin B12 simply because it is not thought to exist naturally in any non-animal forms. There is some suggestion that you can obtain B12 from chlorella, but this is not a reliable source. It is possible that organisms in the small intestine may synthesise vitamin B12, which does seem likely in a healthy person. Several foods are fortified with a synthetic form of the vitamin, including most yeast extracts. Probably the best way for vegans to ensure that they maintain adequate levels of the vitamin is to take a food-state vitamin B complex or vitamin B12 supplement.

## Raw versus cooked foods

Eating a diet of natural foods is relatively simple, but there is the more complex question: should we eat them raw or cooked? Views on this can be pretty polarised. But it is not as black and white as a cooked-food diet versus a raw-food diet; not all cooked food is detrimental to health and not all people are able to digest a raw diet. While the vibrancy and aliveness of raw food has huge benefits, there is understanding in the ancient tradition of Ayurveda which acknowledges that some people have compromised digestive systems, making it difficult for them to 'burn' their food. This process can be aided by cooking the food. (For more on raw foods, see 'What is a raw-food diet', pp.112-16, in Chapter 6, 'Concentrated nutrition: juicing, raw and superfoods').

Technically, cooking is the heating of foods to a high temperature, originally by exposure to fire. The heat accomplishes several things. When plant foods are cooked, the heat causes the starch inside the cell to swell. This ruptures the tough cellulose wall of the plant cell that locks in the nutrients, thereby liberating the cell's contents to become accessible to the digestive process. In the case of meats, the heat converts the connective tissue.

Inevitably, with all these methods, some nutrients will be destroyed. This includes the B vitamins, especially thiamine, folic acid and biotin. Vitamin C losses through cooking are up to 80 per cent. Cooking does not destroy minerals, but they will leach into liquid, so always use the cooking liquid. Cooking does, however, disrupt mineral absorption, due to coagulating bioactive mineral and protein complexes.

Even if you decide to eat more cooked food than raw, anyone looking at a healing cancer diet should include at least one green juice and smoothie every day. Packed full of goodness, fresh green juices are quick, easy and satisfying, and an incredibly dense source of important nutrients, which are easy to absorb and do not tax impaired body systems (see '**Juicing for cancer**', pp. 102-8, and '**Smoothies and blenders**', pp 110-11, in **Chapter 6, 'Concentrated nutrition: juicing, raw and superfoods**').

In addition, fresh, raw plant foods, and especially green leaves, are vibrant with high electron energy which provides oxygen to our cells. For discussion of the crucial role of oxygen generally, and specifically in cancer, see '**Oxygenation**', pp. 40-41, in **Chapter 1, 'Taking an integrative approach'**.

## Good foods to fight cancer
The cancer diet needs to include a variety of foods to tackle the whole cancer process, from delivering a full spectrum of minerals and vitamins and boosting the immune system, to oxygenating cancer cells, attacking cancer cells and reducing inflammation.

### All dark green leaves, wild and cultivated
Two of the best are kale and nettles. Kale has the highest levels of 'good-for-you' nutrients among green leafy vegetables, per calorie of energy. In addition to the wide array of vitamins and minerals, researchers have found forty-five antioxidant, anti-inflammatory and anti-cancer nutrients in kale.[27] Nettles are highly alkalising and rich in minerals; they are useful to help purify the blood. In addition to being a potent antioxidant, nettles have immune-boosting, anti-inflammatory and anti-fungal properties.

Other important greens include watercress, parsley, dandelion, barley and wheatgrass, spinach, rocket, Chinese leaves and chard.

### Vegetables
Plan to have as many varieties, according to season, in store as possible. Choose from asparagus, celery, Brussels sprouts, cauliflower, cucumber, fennel, green and red cabbage, peppers – red, green, yellow and hot – courgettes, tomatoes, parsley, kohlrabi, lettuce, leeks, turnips, avocado (actually a fruit!), carrots and beetroot.

### Sea vegetables
All sea vegetables are a good source of minerals and vitamins. Brown seaweed has anti-oestrogenic effects, and may help to stop the growth of breast cancer.[28] Fucoidan, found in kombu and wakame seaweed, helps to promote cancer-cell death and also to stimulate the immune system.[29] Alginate, found in sea vegetables, is a natural absorbent of radioactive elements, heavy metals and free radicals. Edible sea vegetables include nori, kombu, wakame, arame and dulse.They can be used in soups or salads.

### Garlic
Garlic promotes circulation and the growth of healthy intestinal flora; it also eliminates unfavourable bacteria and yeasts as well as toxins from the body. Use garlic daily. Add to juices, soups and salad dressings. Try slow roasting the whole bulb; squeeze out the sweet garlic and toss with steamed vegetables.

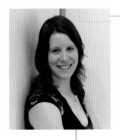

Patricia Daly

PATRICIA
DALY

# THE KETOGENIC DIET

## Patricia Daly

Ketogenic diets have been effective for seizure control in epileptic children for almost a century and since the 1960s they have been widely recognised as one of the most common methods for treatment of obesity-related disorders.[8, 9] Researchers are investigating the ketogenic diet as a cancer therapy mainly because cancer cells rely on glucose to fuel their metabolism.[10] This characteristic is the basis for tumour-imaging using labeled glucose analogues (FDG-PET scans) and has become an important diagnostic tool for cancer detection and management [11] (see Appendix 2, 'Understanding scans', p.244).

The cornerstone of a ketogenic diet for cancer patients involves severe restriction of carbohydrates (3-4 per cent of total calorie intake) to minimise the effect on blood glucose. Carbohydrates are replaced with high amounts of fat (75-85 per cent of total calorie intake) in the form of coconut oils, avocados and oily fish, for example, and adequate intake of vegetable and animal protein (12-20 per cent of total calorie intake).[12] Excessive protein consumption can also result in elevated blood glucose levels through a process called gluconeogenesis.[13] A ketogenic diet causes the body to enter a state of ketosis, in which ketone bodies are produced by the liver as a by-product of fat breakdown when blood glucose is low.

It has been theorised that because tumour cells do not seem to have the metabolic flexibility to use ketones for energy, the result of a ketogenic diet would be destabilisation of tumour tissue DNA, reduction of tumour size over time and therefore enhanced survival rates for cancer patients.[14]

### Potential mechanisms for a ketogenic diet in cancer treatment

There are several potential mechanisms that explain why a ketogenic diet can be added as a type of dietary intervention in cancer treatment. The rest of this section outlines a few of them.

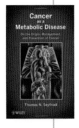

A ketogenic diet may work simply through limiting available glucose to malignant cells. Under the heading 'The dangers of glucose' on pp. 85-6, we saw how Warburg first established the cancer cell's reliance on glucose for energy, a robust hallmark of most tumours.[15] In contrast to our normal cells, data show that cancer cells are unable to effectively generate energy from ketone bodies and rely heavily on glucose.[16] This increased appetite for glucose could result from the fact that most malignant cells have deficient or defective mitochondria, the powerhouses of the cells that create energy.[17] Research carried out by Prof. Thomas Seyfried and his team (prior to publication of *Cancer as a Metabolic Disease: On the Origin, Management and Prevention of Cancer in 2012*) indicates that genomic instability and essentially all hallmarks of cancer, including the Warburg effect, can be linked back to impaired mitochondrial function and therefore energy metabolism.[18] Malignant cells are able to re-programme their glucose metabolism, and thus their energy production, by limiting their energy metabolism largely to glycolysis in the cytoplasm. However, this process is very inefficient for generating energy. Mitochondria can create around twenty times more ATP (the energy currency of the cell) than the process of glycolysis. To compensate for this lower efficiency, cancer cells have developed the ability to up-regulate glucose transporters, notably GLUT1, which significantly increases glucose transport into the cell.[19] Rapidly growing tumour cells typically have glycolytic rates up to 200 times higher than those of their normal tissues of origin.[20]

Due to their faulty mitochondria, cancer cells also depend on glucose to fix free radical damage. Much like our normal cells, cancer cells are under constant attack by free radicals. Since their mitochondria do not function properly, they rely on even more uptake of glucose to counter free radical damage. Limiting this glucose will inhibit their capacity to repair damaged cells.[21] This may also be one of the reasons why restricting glucose through a ketogenic diet may enhance the effects of radio- and chemotherapy.[22]

Like any cell, malignant cells require signalling hormones that tell them to grow and survive. They have receptors, for instance the insulin growth factor receptor (IGF-1R). Insulin growth factor (IGF) can bind to this, as can insulin, which is secreted in our bloodstream in response to carbohydrate consumption. Insulin then activates several pathways that may increase cancer growth and survival.[23] A study in advanced cancer patients carried out in 2012 tested the hypothesis that a carbohydrate-restricted diet will inhibit cancer growth in patients by reducing the secretion and circulating levels of insulin.[24] Minimising the pathways that lead to cancer growth or indeed activating those that limit it, like the AMP-K pathway, is another potential mechanism by which a ketogenic diet can be effective.

## Practical aspects of the ketogenic diet

It seems a reasonable possibility that a ketogenic diet could help to reduce the progression of some types of cancer, although at present the evidence is preliminary. Most of the trials carried out on the ketogenic diet have been animal studies and case-reports, with a few larger randomised, controlled trials currently under way.

The ketogenic diet also has its drawbacks: it is a therapy that requires total compliance and careful monitoring by a trained nutrition professional who is familiar with the required metabolic testing, contra-indicated health conditions and medication. A ketogenic diet for cancer patients cannot be thought of as reduction of macronutrients (carbohydrates, fats or protein). Micronutrients (vitamins, minerals) and anti-cancer nutriceuticals (e.g. curcumin, omega-3 fatty acids, green tea polyphenols) are equally important and their content must be addressed when discussing and evaluating a ketogenic diet.[25] As with any dietary intervention during cancer treatment, a multidisciplinary approach is vital, i.e. looking for synergistic interactions between different therapies that may increase the efficacy of treatment.[26] A low-carbohydrate diet is one of many nutritional and lifestyle interventions that can be used in the management of cancer – certainly a very promising one.

# KETOGENIC PORRIDGE

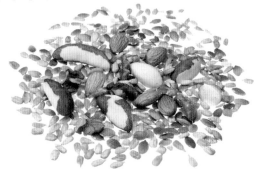

**Serves 2**

**Ingredients**

1/3 cup desiccated coconut

6 whole walnuts, shelled

1 oz ground blanched almonds

2 tbsp pumpkin seeds

1 tbsp whole linseeds
(flaxseeds)

1/2 cup tinned coconut milk

1/2 cup hot water

1 tsp ground cinnamon

1 handful blueberries

**Method**

Put all the ingredients apart from the berries in your food processor. Blend and then put the blueberries on top. You can add sweetener if you like.

# ALMOND COCONUT PANCAKES

**Serves 4** (or 2 and leftovers): whenever I make pancakes, I make at least a double portion and save the rest for snacks, as wraps. Put them in the freezer for another breakfast. It's well worth it!

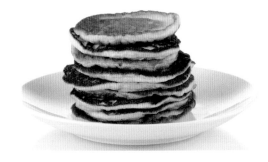

**Ingredients**

1 tsp ground cinnamon

1/2 cup desiccated coconut

1 1/2 cups ground blanched almonds

1/2 tsp baking soda/ bicarbonate of soda

1/4 tsp sea salt

1 cup tinned coconut milk

3 large eggs, organic or free range

2 tbsp (solid) coconut oil

**Method**

1. Sift the dry ingredients and mix together.

2. In a separate bowl, whisk the coconut milk and eggs together.

3. Add the dry ingredients and mix thoroughly.

4. Heat coconut oil in a pan, pour in the batter and cook for 2-3 minutes on each side.

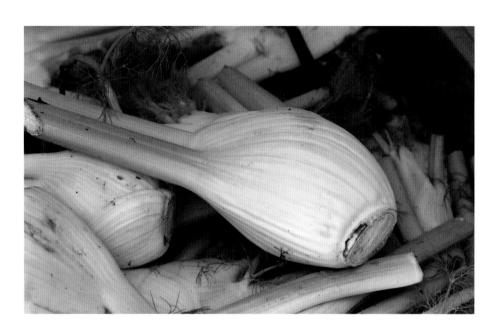

# VENISON STEAK WITH FENNEL

### Serves 4

### Ingredients
4 venison steaks
2 sprigs thyme, fresh
1 tbsp wholegrain mustard
3-4 fennel bulbs, cored
and thinly sliced
1 large onion, sliced
2 cloves garlic, chopped
6 tbsp extra virgin olive oil
2 fl oz dry white wine
A squeeze of lemon juice
4 tbsp (solid) coconut oil

### Method
1. Make a marinade with the thyme and mustard; add salt and pepper to taste (juniper berries are also great). Rub into the venison and refrigerate for at least 30 minutes.

2. In a large frying pan, gently heat the olive oil and fry the onion and garlic, lightly salted, until translucent.

3. Add the fennel slices and cook for 10 minutes, turning occasionally.

4. Add the wine, cover, reduce heat to lowest setting and stew gently for 10 minutes. Season with salt, pepper and the lemon juice.

5. While the fennel is cooking, heat the coconut oil in another pan. When the oil is sizzling, put the venison steaks into the pan, fry at high heat for about 30 seconds on each side until brown. Turn the heat down to low, cover and let cook for 3 minutes. Then turn the venison onto the other side and cook for another 3-4 minutes. Frying time may vary slightly, depending on the thickness of the steak.

### Shiitake mushrooms

Vitamin D deficiency is a major problem in the UK. Low levels of vitamin D are associated with a whole spectrum of diseases, including cancer (see also **Chapter 10**, 'Sunshine and vitamin D'). Boosting your level of vitamin D may help to prevent cancer in several ways, including maintaining healthy cells with normal life spans, discouraging out-of-control cell reproduction, and hindering the formation of new blood vessels for tumours.

Shiitake mushrooms are a good source of vitamin D. Research has shown that outdoor-grown shiitake have seven times more vitamin D than those grown indoors. Mushrooms react to sunlight in the same way as humans and produce a totally natural form of vitamin D. A single 3 ounce serving of outdoor-grown shiitake will provide at least 100 per cent of the recommended daily intake of vitamin D. If you buy dried shiitake, make sure that you find mushrooms that have been dried in the sun, not by some artificial means, in order to gain the benefits of high vitamin D content. Some nutritionists would advise avoidance of all mushrooms, but shiitake have a tradition in the East of being used medicinally and they are a powerful food.

It has also been demonstrated that white button mushrooms exposed to ultraviolet B radiation have dramatically increased levels of vitamin D.

### The importance of water

Water is essential for health. Water is energised as it tumbles through the earth's environmental forces, for example natural vortexes and magnetic fields, and is simultaneously exposed to the sun's energy. During this process, nature adds minerals and oxygen to the water and the result is a natural water, highly structured, mineralised, oxygenated and full of energy and vitality, a kind of water that very few of us are fortunate enough to drink these days.

Living water has a hexagonal molecular structure, which makes it readily absorbable by our cells. Most tap water and bottled water is pentagonal. Research shows that the latter structures are too large for the body to absorb; the body therefore re-structures the water to make it usable, a process that takes up considerable time and energy. In his book *The Water Puzzle and the Hexagonal Key*, the culmination of forty years' work, Dr Mu Shik Jhon concludes that the lack of hexagonal water to drink correlates with disease and lack of vitality.

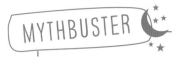

# "IT DOESN'T MATTER WHAT YOU EAT ONCE YOU HAVE CANCER"

This myth has now been thoroughly busted. Sugar and carbs can be converted for energy by cancer cells.[30] Furthermore, your normal cells need top nutritional input to stand a chance of helping you regain health.[31]

In addition to lacking structure, and hence vitality, the tap water that we drink is possibly contaminated with toxins: these include nitrates, herbicides, pesticides, heavy metals, chlorine and fluoride, all of which have a detrimental effect on our health.

Ionised water is made in an ioniser by separating the hydrogen ions (H+) from the hydroxide ions (OH-). Alkaline and antioxidant rich water is made by concentrating the hydroxide ions.

Bottled water is not necessarily of ideal quality because it is affected by storage times and conditions. Even if the water is bottled at source and is rich in particular minerals, the energy of the water will change; if it is packaged in plastic, unhealthy chemicals that mimic oestrogen can leach into the water. If you decide to buy bottled water, choose a natural mineral water; this comes from an underground source and is free of harmful bacteria. Glass bottles are preferable to plastic; if you haven't been able to avoid the latter, don't re-use the bottles as the plastic breaks down more as it ages. Store it away from heat and direct sunlight.

It is essential to drink plenty of water, and it is generally agreed that 2 litres of water per day per adult is the absolute minimum; however if we are ill we should probably drink nearer 3 litres, as water is of paramount importance in assisting our ability to detoxify. So now we are left with the question, what is the best water to drink? You can use the chart available on thecancerrevolution.co.uk, Chapter 5, to decide what you are able to incorporate into your lifestyle to enable the water you drink to be of the greatest benefit to you. Here are three simple recommendations:

- Start the day with a half litre of warm water to which you have added the juice of half a lemon
- Buy a 1 litre glass jug, pop a few quartz crystals in the bottom, keep it with you and drink a full jug of water during both the morning and afternoon; if you are on the move, you can buy some very good non-plastic water bottles
- Have half a litre of warm water each evening infused with nettle, peppermint or rosemary

THE CANCER
REVOLUTION

## Eating problems

### Loss of appetite

The odd day when you have little appetite is not really a problem; but if loss of appetite persists, seek advice to help you work out how you can manage it. Drugs which increase appetite may be considered in some cases. These are a few ideas for a jaded appetite:

- On waking, drink the juice of half a lemon in a half litre of warm water; this helps balance the body
- Try to eat small amounts, often – preferably every two or three hours
- Keep the fridge and cupboard stocked with simple food that you enjoy and is easy to prepare
- Join a box scheme and order a weekly fruit and vegetable box; even when you are not hungry, try to snack on fruit and make vegetable juices
- If you are able, go for a walk to stimulate the appetite
- If possible, share meals with family and friends
- Drink water between meals, not with; drinking at the same time as eating fills you up so that you eat less
- Try some really good nutrient-dense smoothies, which are usually easier to eat than the solids from which they are made

If you are suffering from cachexia, the following additional strategies could be useful:

- If you are hungry at a particular time of the day, make sure you eat at that time, and as much as you want

- Create a space for yourself that is a delight to eat in; a small cloth, a candle and a few flowers make all the difference

- Eat nutritious snacks that are high in calories and protein, e.g. nuts (especially almonds) seeds (especially hemp seed) and eggs

- If the smell or taste of food makes you nauseous, try to enlist someone to prepare your meals; open the window for some fresh air; include more smoothies and salads in your diet

### Pans and utensils

Some pots, pans and cooking utensils are made of materials that have the potential to cause health problems.

Teflon is found in a multitude of everyday objects from frying pans to clothes. Made primarily by DuPont, the 'miracle' coating that stops your food sticking to the pan is a potential health hazard. If it is heated to 260C or above, it begins to break down and to release a number of chemicals, including ammonium perfluorooctanoate (PFOA), which has been linked to cancer. Should you allow the temperature of your pan to reach above 500C, even more hazardous gases are released. An alternative to non-stick pan coatings are cast-iron pans. With proper seasoning and care, food does not naturally stick to this surface. Cast iron has a long history as a safe, sturdy material for cookware, but can add significant amounts of dietary iron to food, especially with acidic foods, which may or may not be nutritionally beneficial. A more recent alternative is Greenpan cookware, which is 100 per cent PFOA-free. They use materials such as ceramic and silicone to provide a smooth, slick surface, which is not quite as non-stick as Teflon, but is without the hazards.

Aluminium is widely used for cookware. Concerns have been raised for many years about exposure to aluminium and links to Alzheimer's Disease: a study from 2000 showed that aluminium in drinking water could lead to a greater risk of Alzheimer's;[32] but organisations working on preventing the disease, for example the UK Alzheimer's Society, say that a relationship between aluminium exposure and the disease has not been demonstrated. Plain aluminium cookware is inexpensive, lightweight and thermally responsive. Aluminium is, however, very reactive to such acidic foods as lemon juice and to such basic ingredients as baking soda. It is definitely best to avoid using these types of ingredient in aluminium pans. Anodised aluminium is made by

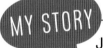

### Jenny Phillips
Nutritionist

*In 2003 I was diagnosed with breast cancer (11 cm, grade 4) and used nutrition alongside conventional treatment to ensure a full recovery and prevent recurrence. My health transformed very quickly, and I am now fitter, healthier and happier than I was a decade ago. I learnt about how biochemistry can be enhanced with foods and supplements, and studied for a degree in Nutritional Medicine. I am now a good food evangelist, and help others to optimise their health naturally.*

placing the material in an acid solution and exposing it to an electric current, creating a layer of aluminium oxide on the surface. Anodising aluminium can eliminate leaching, but some anodised pans contain hazardous chemicals including PFOA in their surface coating. On balance, aluminium is best avoided.

Mixing steel with chromium and nickel produces a corrosion-resistant steel that is both hard-wearing and easy to clean. Stainless steel cookware is considered one of the best and safest choices in cookware.

Bamboo is a non-reactive material with no harmful effects on food. A bamboo steamer is an excellent piece of kitchen equipment for light steaming.

The ubiquitous plastic can have a detrimental effect on your health. But not all plastics are the same, so it is worth understanding the coding system which can be seen on thecancerrevolution.co.uk under Chapter 5.

THE CANCER
REVOLUTION

Bisphenol A (BPA), first synthesised in 1905, was, due to its oestrogenic activity in the body, expected by the pharmaceutical industry to be used as an oestrogen replacement medication. Then when it was tested, it was deemed too dangerous for human medical use and it went on to become a very important chemical in plastic manufacturing.

# CACHEXIA

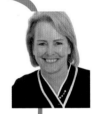

Different types of cancer exhibit different metabolic behaviours: for example, leukaemia cells will metabolise fat instead of sugar as a fuel source.

Weight loss is not normal with cancer, in fact in many instances people gain weight. Some weight loss can occur during treatment which puts the body under strain, often causing changes to your taste-buds and appetite. This usually reverts once treatment stops. Some weight loss may occur naturally as you embark on healthier eating and increase your amount of exercise, and of course that is great. Certain types of cancer, however, can set off a metabolic process known as cachexia, in which the body can break down body weight and muscle at an alarming rate.

The types of cancer in which this can occur are stomach, lung, bowel, pancreatic, ovarian, also head and neck. It can occur in other cancers too, but these are the main ones. It is by no means certain that cachexia will happen, but people with the cancers listed here are more at risk. A sequence of metabolic factors affects the liver and the body's metabolism of protein, setting off a catabolic process. Left untreated, this can be significantly detrimental both to your quality of life and to your ability to get through cancer treatments. With the right advice this can, in my experience, be largely prevented and certainly treated to minimise the effect on the body – the right advice is the key. Cachexia is often dealt with poorly. If you are getting nutrition advice and are nonetheless worried that you may be losing weight rapidly, it is vital that you check out whether the advice you are getting is accurate. Ensure that your practitioner not only knows about cachexia and its physiology, but how to prevent and treat it. If he or she doesn't know or if you are uncertain about this, seek out someone who has experience and knowledge of the subject and can demonstrate that to you.

While not used in the medical field, it can seep into our bodies in a myriad of other ways through plastic containers, wraps, cups, bottles and liners. Constant exposure has been shown to increase cancer rates and to block the ability of chemotherapy to kill breast-cancer cells.[33]

Fatty and acidic foods can break down plastics. Aim to avoid storing food in plastic containers; glass jars and bowls are a far safer option. Detergents can break down plastics, and wear and tear can lead to cracking and toxic leaching. In general, plastics should not be heated, as heating can leach out toxic chemicals. Plastics marked 'microwave safe' are not generally tested for leaching, more likely for durability, so this label is not a guarantee of safety. At this point it is worth considering whether microwaved food is healthy.

Boiling, roasting, baking and grilling all work by transferring heat from a source into the food. The molecules of the food itself don't change, they just get warmer. Microwaves work differently. A microwave oven uses a device called a magnetron tube, which causes an electron beam to oscillate at very high frequencies, producing microwave radiation. Microwave energy alternates between positive and negative polarity billions of times a second, and the same oscillation is induced in the molecules of food, particularly water. In genetic engineering, microwaves are used to weaken molecular structure, to make it easier to insert new genes. Heat is induced from the considerable intermolecular friction. This friction deforms the molecular structure of the food.

After World War II Russian scientists studying the effects of microwaved food found that cancer-causing free radicals were formed within certain trace-mineral molecular formations in plant substances, especially in raw root vegetables. The ingestion of microwaved foods caused a higher percentage of cancerous cells in blood. In addition, due to chemical alterations within food substances, malfunctions occurred in the lymphatic system, causing degeneration of the immune system's capacity to protect itself against cancerous growth.[36]

In 1991 a clinical study undertaken by Dr Hans-Ulrich Hertel at Lausanne University found that people who had eaten microwaved food showed a decrease in the blood level of haemoglobin, which carries oxygen to the cells. White blood cell counts also decreased, reducing immune function.[37]

These and other studies indicate that the effect of microwaving can be to degrade the foods far above the known breakdowns of standard cooking. It is likely that eating microwaved meals can be significantly detrimental to health.[38]

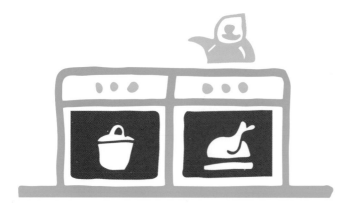

# THE PROBLEM WITH DAIRY

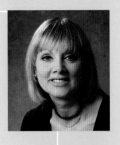

## Prof. Jane Plant

The following is adapted from Jane Plant's book *Your Life in Your Hands*.

When I first came across *The Atlas of Cancer Mortality* in the People's Republic of China, the fact that the statistic for breast-cancer incidence in China was one in 100,000 – as against one in ten here in the West – leapt out at me. Even after careful assessment of all the factors involved, the rates were astonishingly low. The conclusion I drew from the figures is that even if a Western woman were living a Japanese lifestyle in industrialised, irradiated Hiroshima, she would slash her risk of contracting breast cancer by half. Similar conclusions can be drawn for prostate cancer.

The slang name for breast cancer in China translates as 'rich woman's disease'. This is because in China, only the better-off can afford to eat what is termed 'Hong Kong food', a label that can apply to a wide range of luxury items, whether ice cream or chocolate bars, spaghetti or feta cheese.

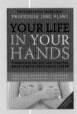

JANE PLANT

In trying to identify specific lifestyle factors that could be contributing to the enormous discrepancy between East and West in terms of cancer incidence, high soya intake is a promising candidate. Soya contains phyto-oestrogens for which there is good evidence of a protective effect.[34] But the 'elephant in the room' turns out to be dairy produce, which was completely excluded from traditional Chinese life. In fact a high proportion of Chinese are lactose-intolerant; and they describe Westerners as smelling of sour milk!

Removing dairy products from your diet is almost as challenging as removing sugar, in that it has found its way into all sorts of products beyond the obvious, including soups, biscuits and cakes. But in my case, the effect of excluding dairy was almost instantaneous and my cancer went into remission quickly. Further investigation revealed data supportive of a link between dairy consumption and the risk of breast cancer stretching back as far as the mid-1990s and earlier.[35]

Probably the most important factor implicated in dairy consumption is hormone intake. Hormones are the chemical messengers that are used to carry information from one part of the body to another. The concentrations of hormones in blood are very small. This is because hormones are so *powerful* that even the tiniest quantities in the bloodstream can have huge effects on the body. Every aspect of breast growth is affected by hormones.

In milk, moreover, other powerful chemical messengers called growth factors, such as epidermal growth factor (EGF), are mixed into this powerful and complex biochemical solution. Milk is uniquely designed to provide for the individual needs of young mammals of the same species. It's not that cow's milk isn't a good food: it is a great food – for baby cows.

And therein lies the source of the problem.

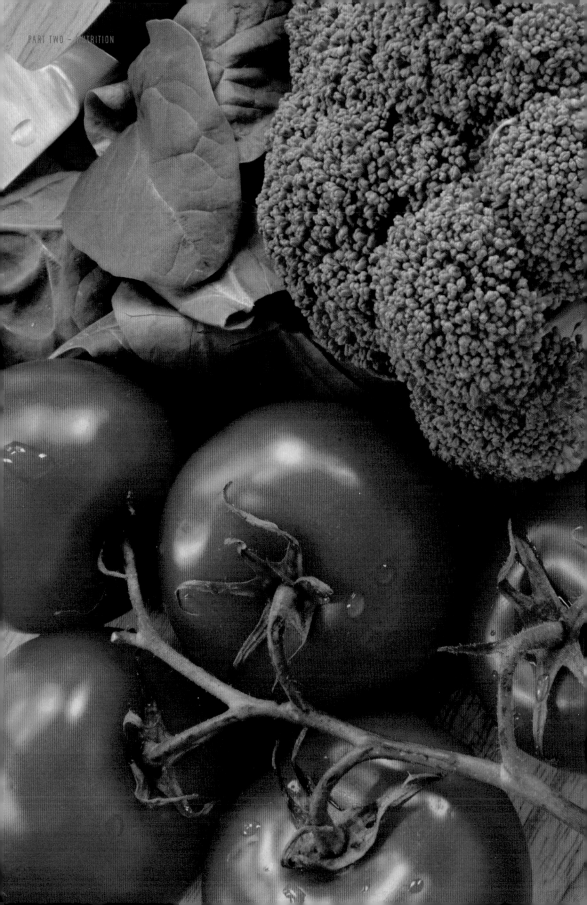

# BROCCOLI IN TOMATO SAUCE WITH GARLIC AND BASIL

Serves 4
Ingredients
2 cloves of garlic, chopped
2 onions, chopped
2 tbsp olive oil
2 1/2lbs tomatoes, chopped
1 1/2 1bs broccoli florets
Large bunch of basil, torn up

Method
1. Cook the garlic and onions in the olive oil, mixed with 4 tbsp of water, until soft.

2. Add the tomatoes and half a pint of vegetable stock.
   Simmer gently for 45 minutes.

3. Blitz in a food processor, then mix in the basil.

4. Steam the broccoli for 2 minutes; do not overcook.

5. Toss the broccoli in the tomato sauce and serve.

# CARROT, ARAME AND CHINESE CABBAGE SALAD

Serves 2
Ingredients
4 oz carrot, grated
1 oz arame, soaked for 20 minutes in
warm water
1/2 Chinese cabbage, finely shredded
1 tbsp hemp oil
1 tbsp olive oil
2 tsp tamari
1 tsp wholegrain mustard
2 tsp sesame seeds

Method
1. Whisk the oils, tamari and wholegrain mustard together in a large bowl.

2. Add the carrot, arame and Chinese cabbage and leave to marinade for
   20 minutes.

3. Divide between 2 bowls; sprinkle over the sesame seeds and serve.

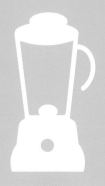

# CHAPTER 6

## CONCENTRATED NUTRITION: JUICING, RAW AND SUPERFOODS

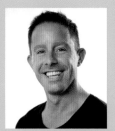

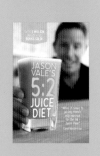

JASON VALE

## JUICING FOR CANCER

### Jason Vale

You cannot talk about holistic methods to prevent and treat cancer without mentioning juicing. And there is simply no way I can cover everything about the topic in this short section alone; 'Juicing for Cancer' could be a book all to itself. The aim here is to provide a little thought-provoking information on this natural holistic approach to cancer in order to highlight the importance of getting the right healing nutrients into the body every day.

The life-giving, nutrient-rich liquid contained within the fibres of all fruits and vegetables have been used to treat and prevent disease for thousands of years. Back then people would literally bash the ingredients in muslin and squeeze the liquid out with their bare hands. It was a long and arduous process, one with which not many would have bothered had there not been good reason for doing so. Luckily, we no longer have to use this long-drawn-out method to extract these therapeutic juices; we are blessed with the technology of the modern world – in the form of a juicer!

It was thanks to Dr Norman Walker (1886-1985) that juicers were introduced to the domestic market and that juicing was shown to benefit those with cancer. His 'Norwalk' juicer was technically the first ever domestic juicer. However, it was – and still is – extremely heavy, very large, complicated to use and very expensive, not really 'domestic' at all. A Norwalk juicer now costs around £1350. It has been succeeded by hundreds, if not thousands, of different types of juicer and you can pick up a juice extractor these days for as little as £15. However, like most things in life, you tend to get what you pay for, and if you have cancer and want to try juicing, a high-speed £15 small feeding tube juicer is not the one to use.

## Choosing a juicer

**Press (£1300 +)** It seems odd, but despite the many years since the Norwalk juicer hit the market, when it comes to working with cancer, many of the top health retreats in the world still insist on using that original model. The Norwalk, unlike conventional juicers, uses a hydraulic-press system. This extracts the maximum amount of juice, while creating very little heat friction. This is important as heat lowers the nutrient content, which is the last thing you want when dealing with cancer. You are looking to retain as close to 100 per cent of the healing 'live' liquid contained within the fruits and vegetables. Having said that, I honestly don't believe you need to use this juicer to get the full benefits of juicing.

**Masticating (£170 +)** The next step down from the hydraulic press, and it's only a small step down, are 'masticating', more commonly known as 'slow' juicers. There are many different types, and these juicers extract almost the same amount as a Norwalk, and also create very little heat friction. Well-designed masticators are easy to clean and can handle leafy vegetables and wheatgrass, although they tend to be bulky and heavy. These are a great choice and there is a wide range for all budgets, with those at the upper end, like the stalwart Champion, built to last for a decade or more. You'll probably need to buy online from a specialist (see **Part Eight, 'Resources'**).

**Centrifugal (£35 +)** This is the most common type of juicer. It works very quickly, but with the speed comes a degree of heat friction and thus a lower quality of juice. It generally doesn't extract as much juice as a masticating juicer, which means that you will spend more on vegetables in the long run and they can be hard to clean. The range available is huge; they can be inexpensive, compact and are readily available on the high street.

However, any juicer is better than no juicer, and any juicer will still enable you to start juicing. The key is to find one that you will use. After all, what's the point of getting a Norwalk or the best 'slow' juicer on the market if you are simply not going to use it? You are better off getting shedloads of slightly inferior juice than none of the very best. If you are making your juice in a really good fast juicer (like the Philips Avance) you need to drink it immediately and, as with any juicer, if you have cancer it is vital to use the best locally grown organic produce whenever possible.

Other important points to note: if you are thinking of juicing wheatgrass, make sure you get a model that is specifically made for the job. Read the reviews to be sure to choose a machine that is really easy to clean; if you don't, it will almost certainly wind up in a cupboard, unused.

## How to juice

If you are using organic ingredients – always the best choice – then there's no need to peel the vegetables or fruit. Simply chop them to fit the feeder tube. There is also no need to remove the core and seeds of apples or pears or the pith of citrus fruits; in fact these possess beneficial compounds of their own, so keep them in.

When juicing ginger or other fresh herbs and spices, put these through the juicer before the other ingredients to obtain maximum juice. You will be using only a little of these, so squeeze out all you can to avoid the juice being lost in the pulp of other ingredients. Harder vegetables such as beetroot will often help push softer ones through a masticating juicer.

## A Wiseman drinks broccoli juice!

In 2003 Ray Wiseman was told he wasn't expected to survive when he was diagnosed with cancer. However, five years later Ray was in the national newspapers after he claimed that his daily glass of broccoli juice had saved his life. Every day his wife Joan would prepare his apple, carrot and broccoli juice. She said: 'We believe my husband's incredible luck is down to broccoli. I hope our experience can help other cancer sufferers.' Scientists from Cancer Research UK even asked for the recipe to study the vegetable's benefits further, so we are making some progress. British scientists at the Institute of Food Research found that men who ate one daily portion had altered patterns of gene activities in their prostates, suggesting that the chemicals in the vegetable might help reduce the risk of prostate cancer. According to a report published in the *British Journal of Cancer* in 2006 natural chemicals found in certain vegetables, such as broccoli, cauliflower and cabbage, can enhance DNA repair in cells, which could help prevent them from becoming cancerous.[1]

## Pomegranate and other juices

Wiseman's example wasn't the first to show how juices have been seen to help prostate cancer significantly. Pomegranate juice has been scientifically tested several times with very positive results. Dr Allan Pantuck, MD, Associate Professor, Department of Urology, David Geffen School of Medicine, UCLA, said: 'We are hoping that pomegranate juice offers a novel strategy for prolonging the doubling time (the time taken for their PSA level, the measure of cancer activity, to double) in men who have been treated for prostate cancer'. They continued: "Pomegranate juice is high in antioxidants, and there is good evidence that inflammation plays an important role in prostate cancer…' Researchers from the Centre for Human Nutrition at the University of Western Ontario, Canada, have found a link between orange and grapefruit juice and the treatment of breast cancer and high cholesterol. Dr Kenneth Carroll, director of the centre, said: 'The implications are potentially enormous because a powerful weapon against breast cancer may be as close as your kitchen.'

There are now hundreds of studies that have shown juicing to be useful in some way as part of a programme of treatment and/or prevention of cancer. What I personally love about juicing is that it meets the first rule of doctoring: 'Do no harm.' No harm can be done by consuming fresh organic broccoli juice and apple juice; and the vital nutrients contained within the 'living' liquid are of paramount importance for strengthening the immune system. All freshly extracted 'live' organic juices are also anti-inflammatory. As virtually all chronic disease is created either by a weak-functioning immune system and/or by inflammation in the body, juicing is one of the best foundational approaches for any disease.

**MY STORY**

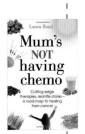

## Gemma Bond
### Ovarian and uterine cancer survivor
(Gemma is the subject of Laura Bond's book *Mum's Not Having Chemo*)

*One of the first things I bought after my diagnosis was a juicer, and most days I make myself a pint of organic, mostly green, vegetable juice. Wheatgrass, kale – and other chlorophyll-filled greens – help flood my cells with oxygen, creating a healthier terrain for my body to thrive in. I chose a low-speed juicer, which I knew would retain the all-important enzymes – essential to healing from cancer. More recently turmeric has been a must in my daily juice; it's now one of the most researched and powerful anti-cancer compounds. While it's not always my favourite beverage of the day, I truly believe in its therapeutic benefits – and it's better than any anti-ageing face cream!*

# ANTI-CANCER JUICE (USE A MASTICATING JUICER FOR BEST RESULTS)

1 apple (organic, preferably
a sour variety)

2 carrots (organic)

1 large broccoli stem or several florets
or a mixture of both
(the idea is to get at least 2oz of juice
from the broccoli)

1 cauliflower (same as above, yielding
around 2oz of juice)

1 medium raw beetroot bulb

2 Brussels sprouts (optional)

1 piece of cucumber, 2 inches

2 sticks of celery

spinach, a handful

kale, a handful (optional)

**To make**
Do not peel anything. Simply juice all in
a masticating or any other type of juicer.
Drink slowly.

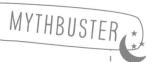

# "YOU CAN'T SUPPORT THE BODY'S PH AND CELLS' ALKALINITY LEVELS"

The body is constantly metabolising its intake and balancing its
pH by itself – true! What you can do is to supply the necessary
nutritional reserves, thus enabling the body to function as well
as possible. An acid diet will drain your reserves of calcium
phosphate salts that the body needs to maintain balance.[2]

## One disease: one solution

The reason I believe juicing to be a perfect natural nutritional therapy for any chronic disease
stems from my fundamental belief that, as far as chronic disease is concerned there is only
one disease. After years of seeing massive changes in people suffering from a huge range of
common chronic conditions, I am convinced that if you remove the toxicity coming into the
bloodstream and replace the nutrient deficiencies, the body is left with the right environment
and has an opportunity to heal. I use the word 'opportunity' here because a lot depends
on the severity of the disease. This is why I also firmly believe that, of course, medical
intervention has its part to play, especially if the disease will kill you before the body can heal
naturally. Deciding what treatments to follow is not easy; many people look closely at what
is available, what makes sense to them, before making a choice. If you do have cancer and
you choose to have chemotherapy or radiation, then I urge you to use juicing in conjunction.
Chemotherapy is not a 'smart bomb'. It cannot kill the bad guys and keep the good guys
alive: it destroys any rapidly dividing cells. The body needs to rebuild itself and this can be
done only with the right nutrition, which is easy to digest and bio-available to the cells.

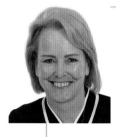

# WHAT TO JUICE

You can use a whole variety of raw vegetables and fruits to make a juice. However, my recommendation is that you use primarily vegetables with just a little fruit to sweeten if necessary. Juices that contain lots of fruit will be very sweet: once the fibre and juice are separated, the sugars (like other nutrients), will be rapidly absorbed. This creates the potential for a rapid rise in blood glucose, which is best avoided.

Certain herbs and spices such as parsley and ginger can also be juiced. They are packed full of powerful phytonutrients and are all valuable for supporting health in various ways.

The following list suggests some of the top vegetables and fruits to use for juicing and pinpoints the reasons why they are so beneficial.

| VEGETABLE/FRUIT | WHY THEY'RE GREAT |
|---|---|
| Apples | This staple fruit yields lots of juice and blends well with most other ingredients. They are rich in vitamin C and a range of other powerful antioxidants. Choose the more sour apples for juicing to keep the sugar content down; good ones include Granny Smith and Bramley. |
| Beetroot | A fair amount of juice can be extracted from beetroots. They are a good source of certain vitamins and minerals, particularly folic acid, manganese and potassium. They are rich in antioxidants and anti-inflammatory compounds as well as nutrients that support liver detoxification. |
| Berries | These yield a moderate amount of juice. All berries are very rich in antioxidant and anti-inflammatory phytonutrients and are a good source of vitamin C. They also contain compounds that help the body to regulate blood glucose levels and slow down ageing processes. |
| Carrots | A good staple for juicing, carrots are full of antioxidants including beta-carotene. Rich in other vitamins and minerals particularly vitamin K, they blend well with many other ingredients. Carrots are high in sugar so caution if you are following a low-glucose diet. |
| Celery | Yielding lots of juice, celery is rich in a range of nutrients, including sodium and potassium. These are important minerals for regulating the body's water balance. Celery is also rich in phytonutrients that help to regulate blood pressure. |

| VEGETABLE/FRUIT | WHY THEY'RE GREAT |
|---|---|
| Dandelion leaves | The small amount of juice that dandelion leaves produce is counterbalanced by the fact that it is very beneficial. The leaves are very rich in minerals including calcium, zinc and iron. They are supportive to the liver and gall bladder and also help to promote optimal digestive function. |
| Ginger | Also yielding little juice, ginger has many benefits for maintaining a healthy system. It is a very warming spice; as juices are generally cooling, the addition of ginger can help to balance the effect on the body. Ginger contains powerful anti-inflammatory compounds, is supportive for digestion and has anti-nausea properties. |
| Lemons/ limes | These citrus fruits produce lots of juice. They are great for livening up any juice and helping to cut through the 'earthy' flavour of some vegetables. A very rich source of vitamin C, they also contain a range of beneficial phytonutrients, many of which are to be found in the pith; therefore include the pith when you juice. Lemons and limes rank among the top most alkalising foods. |
| Parsley | Another herb that yields little juice but is nevertheless very beneficial, parsley is incredibly rich in vitamin K and vitamin C. It is also high in beta-carotene, iron and magnesium and contains a range of other antioxidants and anti-cancer compounds. |
| Salad leaves | These produce a moderate amount of juice. The dark lettuce leaves, watercress and rocket are particularly recommended and are rich in vitamin C, beta-carotene, vitamin K, B vitamins, magnesium and iron. Salad leaves support the digestive system and the liver in particular. |
| Tomatoes | Yielding lots of juice, tomatoes are very rich in vitamin C and other antioxidants including beta-carotene. They also contain lycopene, a phytonutrient with anti-cancer activity. **N.B.**: tomatoes belong to the nightshade family and can cause adverse reactions in some people. |
| Wheatgrass | One of my top juicing vegetables, wheatgrass yields little juice but the juice it produces is very powerful. It is rich in minerals, vitamins and a range of phytonutrients. It is also very rich in chlorophyll, the green pigment found in plants. This mix of nutrients provides the body with a great nutrient boost and also seems to support detoxification and to promote health of the blood. If you are unable to obtain fresh wheatgrass to juice, I recommend purchasing live wheatgrass juice (see **Part Eight, 'Resources'**). |

# WHAT NOT TO JUICE

Not all vegetables and fruit are ideal for juicing. As mentioned above, it's best not to include too much fruit and in particular not the very sweet fruits such as grapes, melon, mango, pineapple and other tropical fruits, thus avoiding a 'spike' in blood glucose levels.

Do not juice if your kidneys are not functioning well. Juicing, particularly of fruits, can give you a large amount of potassium. If your renal function is low you will not clear the potassium from the body and that can be very harmful. If in doubt, check with your doctor. Liver and kidney tests are carried out regularly by doctors when you are having treatment, so the information will be readily available when you want it.

Avoid juicing if you are on blood thinners such as warfarin. Many vegetables contain vitamin K, which if taken in concentrated form can affect the efficacy of warfarin in the body and cause it to work better. This can result in your blood clotting insufficiently.

## When to have your juices

Juices are best consumed as soon as possible after preparation, because the live enzymes are easily destroyed through exposure to oxygen. If you are delayed for any reason, place your juice in an airtight flask and consume within twelve hours.

If possible, have your juice on an empty stomach to allow for maximum absorption of the nutrients. After five to ten minutes follow your juice with some more food – juices make an ideal aperitif. Take the time to enjoy your juice, really savour the experience by sitting in a comfortable chair and allow your body to relax fully. As you drink, absorb the fact that you are being deeply nourished.

## Recovery from illness

Juices make a fantastic aid to recovery from illness. They deliver vital nutrients to support the body in rebuilding tissues, regaining energy, dealing with inflammation, regulating acid/alkaline balance, and boosting immune function. They do all this while putting little strain on the digestive system. As it can be weakened during illness, or sometimes as a result of necessary medical treatments, giving the digestive system a break is important.

## Cleansing the body

Juices provide an easy way to take in nutrients that support the body's detoxification pathways. For this reason juices are a key part of many cleansing programmes. Some of these recommend a large intake of fresh juice every day. Certain types of cleansing regime, however, should take place only with supervision from a nutritionally qualified health professional. On the other hand if you just want to provide your body with a gentle cleanse, a daily juice can be very helpful. Juicing ingredients that are particularly good for cleansing include salad leaves and lemon.

# CANCER-FIGHTING RAINBOW JUICE
RECIPE FROM
DAPHNE LAMBERT

### Ingredients
Half a red pepper
Handful of kale
Bunch of red grapes
Small piece of ginger

1 carrot
Slice of lemon
1 apple

### Method
1. Cut up into pieces that fit your juicer funnel.
2. Juice and drink immediately.

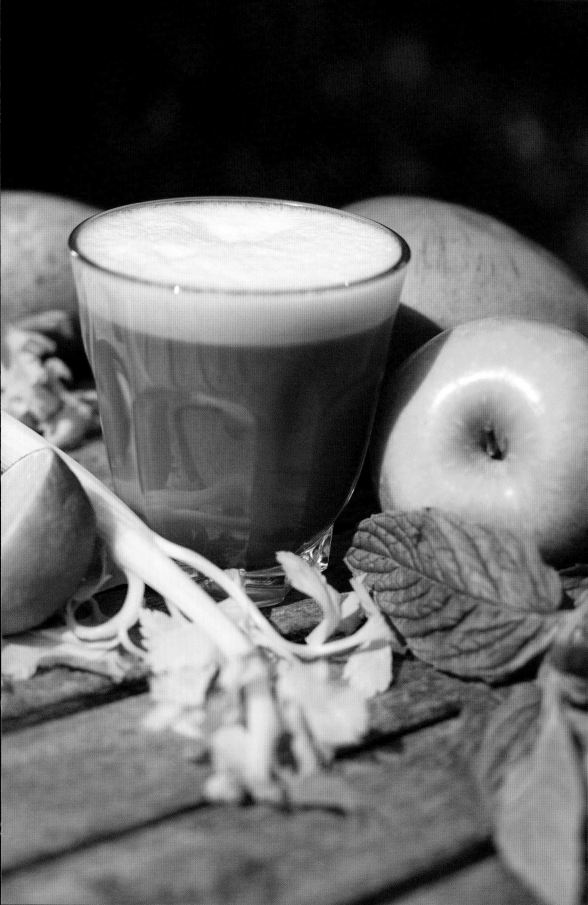

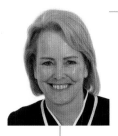

# SMOOTHIES AND BLENDERS

### Juices versus smoothies

People new to juicing and smoothies are often confused about the difference between the two. While each has different properties and uses, both are beneficial to health and wellbeing.

Juicers extract water and nutrients from fruit and vegetables, leaving the fibre behind. As a result they are no longer whole foods and should be used as supplements to the diet. Juicing makes the nutrients much more available to your digestive system, as it doesn't have to break anything down. It is also beneficial for those with sensitive or weakened digestive systems or who cannot tolerate fibre. Nutrients are quickly absorbed, providing a super-fast nutrient infusion to your cells. If there is too much fruit in your juice, however, this can result in blood sugar 'spikes'. Unstable blood sugar can lead to mood swings, energy dips and a risk of insulin resistance. Whether or not to include fruit will depend on your situation and should be discussed with your nutritionist.

Smoothies are fruits and vegetables blended together in the jug to form a smooth, creamy drink, equivalent to a meal. You get the whole fruit, not just the extracted juice of the foods you are blending. The advantage of this is the added fibre, which has numerous benefits. Broken-down fibre is easier to digest than the whole fruit or vegetable. It slows down the digestive process, balances blood sugar and provides a sustained release of nutrients. Fibre also supports detoxification, binding to toxins to help eliminate them. It feeds beneficial bacteria, helping to keep gut flora in balance. Smoothies are very filling and faster to make than juice, so you could enjoy them as a snack or meal replacement. A smoothie uses up less food to make the same amount of liquid, as there is more bulk in the whole fruit. There will therefore be less nutrient quantity per glass, although you do get the added fibre content. On a practical level, smoothies are quick and easy to make as everything goes into the blender and cleaning is easy, which may help you make them more often!

A combination of juices and smoothies in your diet is a great way to reap the many benefits of each. There are certain foods that are difficult to blend smoothly, for example celery, carrots and beetroot, I therefore recommend that they are first juiced, then added to the blender afterwards. Softer vegetables, fruits, herbs and greens are easy to blend. If you have a good blender that can handle ice cubes, it can be nice to add ice to chill your smoothie.

You can also easily add all kinds of nutritious superfoods to your smoothie: try maca powder, chlorella and spirulina, bee pollen, raw cacao powder/nibs, flaxseeds, chia seeds and goji berries. You can use coconut milk or nut milks for a creamy texture and a protein hit; coconut water, which is rich in potassium, can be used instead of water to thin out your smoothie. A good source of extra protein is undenatured whey protein (see 'Foods that may be new to you' on pp. 115, for more details on superfoods).

THE CANCER
REVOLUTION

Caution! Smoothies may not be for you if you have issues with fibre. Many smoothie recipes use lots of fruit which is high in fructose and to be avoided on an anti-cancer regime. Green smoothies made with vegetables can be just as tasty.

(See thecancerrevolution.co.uk, Chapter 6, 'Additional materials', for smoothie recipes).

## Blenders

To make smoothies you will need a blender. There are many on the market from the 'Rolls Royce' of blenders, the Vitamix, to the very cheap varieties. If you intend to use it often (daily or a few times a week), then it is worth spending the most you can afford.

The Vitamix: this is a long-term investment, costing £500 or so. Among its advantages are that it blends everything, including ice and frozen food to a smooth liquid, and that it comes with a five year warranty.

Middle of the range blenders include the Philips HR2162/91 (£50) and the Magimix 11610 (around £160).

Cheaper blenders are plentiful, but don't expect them to last, or your smoothies to be smooth! Buy a cheap model if you want to experiment with smoothie-making before you decide to spend more. One of the better cheaper ones to get you started is the Philips HR2020/50 (£26).

# SMOOTHIE RECIPES
RECIPES FROM
DAPHNE LAMBERT

## Smoothie 1:

### Ingredients
1 dsp flaxseeds
1 oz hemp nuggets
6 fl oz coconut water
4 oz kale
1 pear, quartered and cored
1 tsp spirulina powder

### Method
1. Whizz the flaxseeds in a high-speed blender to crack open.
2. Add the hemp and coconut water and whirl for 30 seconds.
3. Add the remaining ingredients, then whirl again until blended.
4. Pour into a glass and drink at once.

## Smoothie 2:

### Ingredients
1 cucumber, diced
1/2 avocado, peeled and chopped
1 knob ginger, grated
1/2 lemon, juiced
1 tbsp dulse
Large handful green leaves
– chard, spinach and/or kale etc
1 handful broccoli florets

### Method
1. Put everything into a high-speed blender and whizz until smooth.
2. Pour into a glass and drink at once.

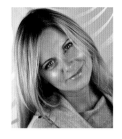

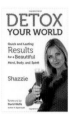

SHAZZIE

# WHAT IS A RAW-FOOD DIET?

## Shazzie

A raw-food diet is the natural diet for all animals on this planet. 99.9 per cent of the world's population follow a raw-food diet, which they've evolved to eat over millions of years. The other percentage, let's call them humans and their companion animals, eat cooked food.[3]

Raw foodism is the oldest diet in the world. For all species on the planet (again excepting humans and the animals they keep), it's the only diet available. It's the ultimate fast food diet – just pick and go!

People on a raw-food diet eat 100 per cent raw, uncooked food. Many people find this a little difficult (often for social reasons) so they choose a 75-99 per cent raw-food diet. Most raw foodists are vegetarian or vegan, but some eat raw fish and meat.

Benefits of a high-raw or all-raw diet include:

• increased energy
• weight loss (if advised)
• disappearance of disease
• happiness – often ecstatic bliss!

Raw foods are cleansing, energy-giving, full of life and help people avoid disease associated with the Standard UK Diet (SUKD) and Standard American Diet (SAD). People who eat a high proportion of raw foods often have a tell-tale glow that can be the envy of all their friends. Raw foodists look to nature to get it right. And it's so simple.

Our meals are based on the following foods:

• fruits, dried, fresh or frozen, especially wild
• vegetables, dried or fresh, especially wild
• seed sprouts (e.g. alfalfa, broccoli, radish, onion, sunflower, quinoa)
• micro greens (e.g. buckwheat, sunflower)
• herbs and spices, fresh and dried, especially out of my garden
• nuts and their butters (e.g. cashew, macadamia, pecan, hazel, walnut, brazil)
• seeds and their butters (e.g. sunflower, sesame, hemp, flax, Salba)
• ancient grains, soaked or ground (e.g. buckwheat, amaranth)
• sea vegetables, often dried (my favourite brand is Clearspring's Japanese variety)
• algae, sometimes frozen, powdered or compressed into tablets (e.g. AFA algae, spirulina, chlorella etc.)
• ecstatic foods ( e.g. cacao, maca, goji berries, Incan berries, wheatgrass, aloe vera, algae)

I sprinkle superfoods onto all our meals, without fail. I usually have between one and three pints of green juice a day, but I don't kick myself if I don't make it for a few days.

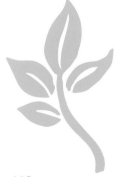

## Will I become deficient in anything if I eat just raw food?

You can be deficient in nutrients on any diet. The SUKD is low in phytonutrients, B12, essential fatty acids, vitamins, minerals, antioxidants and water. The nutrients to watch out for on a raw vegan diet include vitamins B12, D and K2, choline, iron, calcium and essential fatty acids. It is particularly important for pregnant mothers and growing children to have these consciously added to their diets.

Superfoods, hemp protein powder and juiced or blended greens will cover your protein needs when eaten regularly and sufficiently. There is no need to eat animals to get enough protein. I've been a vegan since about 1990 and only ever suspected a protein deficiency when I was eating a high-fruit diet (which I don't recommend). There are also lifelong vegans and raw vegans who are in tip-top health, but you need to take supplementation seriously as it's not natural for us to be 100 per cent vegan.

## How do I start eating raw food?

I've published over 500 raw vegan recipes, so you never need to have the same raw meal twice. I suggest you invest in some books and ebooks that contain good raw-food recipes. It can be exciting to try new things, but guidance in book form is a good choice when going raw, as everything is made differently.

In my experience, the most successful method to adapt to a raw-food diet has been this: change one meal at a time. Become comfortable with that meal before going on to change the next one. For example, you could first alter your breakfast. Make smoothies, eat fruit, make juices, have raw muesli with nut 'mylk'. When you're happy with that, alter your lunch. Make cabbage burritos, lettuce or nori wraps, salads, dehydrated goodies such as burgers or crackers with houmous and guacamole. Top it all with a mix of superfoods such as purple corn extract, Seagreens, Crystal Manna, pink salt, digestive enzymes and spirulina. Then alter your evening meal, dipping into raw recipe books when you have time.

Making your snacks raw could mean fresh or dried fruits, nuts or seeds, raw chocolate or simple vegetable sticks with delicious dips.

If you eat superfoods every day, you will certainly get more minerals and other nutrients that may be missing from a normal raw and cooked diet. Incan berries contain vitamin B12. Goji berries have over 10 per cent protein. Maca has over 10 per cent calcium. These foods are exceptional in their nutritional make-up and we should take advantage of them at every opportunity.

If you're still questioning raw foods, consider the following:

- If you can't eat food raw and unprocessed (like kidney beans and potatoes), ask yourself 'Is this food designed for humans?'
- Watch food as it's cooking: you will see the water disappearing, the colours fading and the textures changing
- Compare how your body feels when you eat raw food compared with when you eat cooked food: which meal makes you more energetic, more alert, happier?; which food sedates you and makes you tired?
- Ask yourself if you're as healthy and happy as you could be; if the answer's 'no', then add superfoods to every meal

## Do I have to go all raw and all vegan?

Most people who start exploring raw food don't eat a 100 per cent raw diet for various reasons. The great news is that you can receive many of the benefits of raw foodism without the dedication that's required to be entirely raw: just eat at least half raw food, in weight, at every meal. Sweet potatoes, buckwheat pasta, steamed vegetables, houmous, wild rice and sprouted breads are all excellent if you choose to eat some cooked food.

There are raw foodists who eat insects, meat, fish, dairy, eggs, honey and other animal products. Raw doesn't mean vegan or vegetarian. If you're not vegan or vegetarian, then eggs are better than animal milk, fish is often better than land meat and bee pollen and honey are good nutritional choices. Take care with raw animal products as they can be loaded with pathogens.

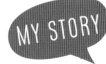

### Perdie
### Cervical cancer, twice

*Having lived with cancer for seven years, raw plant foods, especially greens, which I adore, have given me the energy, clarity, motivation and creativity to create a career I love and live an amazing life. Knowing I am fuelling my body with goodness gives me comfort and allows me and the cancer to co-habit peacefully.*

### Raw-food equipment

To make great raw food easily, you may need a few tools that the average kitchen doesn't boast.

#### Dehydrator
This piece of equipment acts as a low-temperature oven, blowing warm air via a fan over the food. The food then dries out over time to create biscuits, burgers, dried fruits and vegetables, cakes, pizzas, crackers and breads. My favourite brand for a large kitchen is the Excalibur. If you have a smaller kitchen, try the Stockli, as it's more compact, but you can stack as many extra trays as you like.

#### Blender
A high-power blender can make flour out of seeds and grains, and it'll purée everything that you throw into it. That's how we make such smooth soups and patés. I use the Vita-Prep 3, which is a commercial blender. If you don't have a Vita-Prep and there is no liquid in the recipe you're making, then you can use a food processor or hand blender instead (see 'Blenders', p. 111 above).

#### Food processor
I use the Magimix 5000, which has an attachment for making crisps. It has fine and coarse graters as well as several sizes of bowl.

#### Juicer
I don't use my juicer as much as my Vita-Prep, but it's still great for the kitchen. A good masticating juicer will cost a small fortune but it should last a lifetime. My favourite is the Green Power Kempo as it uses magnetic and infrared technology to keep the juice fresher for longer. We also use a citrus juicer, and frequently enjoy freshly squeezed orange juice with some green powder added to it.

#### Sprout bag or nut mylk bag
Probably one of the cheapest and most versatile additions to your kitchen, even a pop sock will do. Use the bag to strain juices, to sprout seeds and to make 'mylks' and 'cheezes' (substitutes for milk and cheese made from non-dairy ingredients).

#### Spirooli, spirali, spiral slicer or spiraliser
These gadgets make 'spaghetti' out of courgettes, squash, mooli and other hard

vegetables. I prefer the spirooli or spirali to the others as it is easier to use and makes slightly wider, less watery, strands.

### Vegetable peeler

This is a standard piece of equipment but I mention it here because it's great for making strips out of vegetables. Use it for slicing the length off a cucumber or courgette, then roll it up with paté for an instant and beautiful treat.

## Foods that may be new to you

You will be familiar with most of the fresh foods that I mention in this chapter. Here's a list of some ingredients that may be new to you. It goes without saying that I use only organically certified or wild food, but I've said it anyway!

### Cacao

Since discovering raw chocolate in Maui in 2003, and co-writing *Naked Chocolate* with David Wolfe in 2005, I've been astonished at how quickly the raw-food revolution has taken off. Cacao is the most nutrient-dense and antioxidant-rich food on the planet. In fact nothing else comes close with a massive 955 ORAC (oxygen radical absorbency capacity – a way of measuring antioxidant capacities) units per gram. Cooked chocolate powder has only 260 ORAC units per gram.

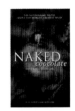

### Goji berries

These berries constitute a real medicinal food and can help you with inflammation, immunity, strength, stamina (in all parts of your body) and hormone function. Just like cacao, they contain chemicals that aid rejuvenation. Gojis berries are known as a fountain of youth.

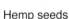

### Maca

The medicinal qualities of this plant are classified as being adaptogenic, meaning that it helps the body to deal with stress and bring bodily functions back to a normal state. For example, it will help raise thyroid function if it's too sluggish, yet it will subdue that function if overactive. Adaptogens help to balance all bodily functions in a similar way.

### Hemp seeds

There are three unique nutritional factors that make hemp one of my favourite ingredients. First, it contains about 35 per cent fats, including omegas 3, 6 and 9. These essential fatty acids come in the ideal ratio for superior human health. Second, it is loaded with trace minerals. Third, it contains the full array of essential amino acids and histidine, meaning it provides a complete protein for children and adults alike.

### Algae and seaweed

Chlorella, though sharing many of its cousins' attributes, has shown a tremendous ability to remove radiation from animals and to help humans detoxify dioxins. Chlorella contains genuine vitamin B12. Spirulina is probably the most familiar of the algae. It is a rich source of essential amino acids. While few clinical trials have been conducted on humans it has been used on animals with some surprising results. People with cancer, or those who have had strokes or suffer from hay fever and brain deterioration, have all benefited from spirulina.[4] All seaweeds have been promoted for weight loss (by stimulating thyroid activity), boosting the immune system, decreasing blood sugar and cholesterol, increasing gastrointestinal tract function, and for decreasing the symptoms of arthritic joint pains.

### Powdered green superfood

I add a touch of one of these to most of our soups and savoury dishes. My two preferred brands are Pure Synergy and Nature's Living Superfood. I also use powdered hemp leaf. If you're organised you can harvest weeds, dehydrate them, powder them and store them for future use.

### He shou wu

Also called Fo Ti, this is an ancient Chinese healing herb particularly favoured by older people and those needing a pick-me-up. The Chinese say it's a 'youth-giving tonic' and can even reverse the greying of hair.

### Mushrooms

With so many varieties at our feet, mushrooms can give us the flavours no other plant-like thing can, but be aware that they often carry other strains of non-beneficial fungi upon them. A thorough rinse in a mild solution of hydrogen peroxide will zap the nasties. There are also many medicinal mushrooms that help improve organ and immune function, such as reishi and shiitake. I advise anyone with cancer to look into the medicinal effects of chaga, as it's known worldwide for helping with this.

### Agave nectar

Agave nectar, or agave syrup, is a popular low-GI sweetener obtained from the cactus-like agave plant of Southern Mexico. Most supermarket varieties have been cooked to death. Make sure yours is raw and pure – you will certainly taste the difference! A word of caution: the reason it is ranked as low-GI is because it has a very high fructose content, even higher than high fructose corn syrup. Fructose will not raise blood sugar, but it can affect liver function and promote obesity.

### Lúcuma

A very popular fruit in Peru and neighbouring countries – in fact it's their favourite ice cream flavour. Rich in antioxidants and vitamin B3, it's a tasty and valuable ingredient. We have it as a powder, and it makes all our sweets really creamy.

### Purple corn

This corn, while almost exactly the same as its yellow brother, contains substantial quantities of antioxidants and other useful phytochemicals. We use it in food as a powder and dark purple extract, also in tea as dried kernels.

### Enzymes

Enzymes are the 'spark of life'. They are biological molecules (proteins) that act as catalysts to help complex reactions occur. Without enzymes our bodies do not properly break down food; and we do not absorb vitamins, minerals and amino acids, which are the basis of health. Vegan digestive enzymes can be sprinkled on food to aid digestion.

### Açaí

This delicious-tasting fruit is packed with antioxidants. Its dark purple skin contains the anthocyanins (antioxidants) that we need to help protect us from our increasingly toxic environment.

### Chia

A South American seed, chia is a rich source of essential fatty acids and is also high in protein, minerals and fibre. It improves bowel function. When ground up, it can be used as a sticky base for dehydrated foods, similar to flax.

## Raw-food recipes

THE CANCER
REVOLUTION

Even with all the ingredients mentioned above, you may be wondering how to make a raw-food meal. I have written down some of my most tried, trusted and loved recipes and hope that you will enjoy experimenting with them. They are on thecancerrevolutio.co.uk, Chapter 6. I also hope that they will encourage you to increase your intake of raw food to that magic 51 per cent a day! Most of these meals have been chosen because the foods within them are known to protect against cancer. Go big on broccoli, chaga mushrooms, raw chocolate and broccoli sprouts. Get your body so vibrant that no disease can survive in there!

**Suppliers:** See Part Eight, 'Resources' for details of specialist suppliers.

# CHEEZY BROCCOLI Serves any number

Comfort food that's healthy - did you know it existed? Well, it does, and it's cheesy, green and delicious. I often double (or even quadruple) this recipe so that I have something spreadable ready for any creamy cheezy whims and for visitors.
Keeps for 5 days when refrigerated in a sealed container.

## Ingredients
3/4 cup broccoli, cut into small florets
4 tsp olive oil
1 tsp apple cider vinegar
3/4 cup raw cashew nuts
1 tbsp nutritional yeast, e.g. Engevita

1/2 cup water for the recipe and additional soaking water
1 tsp ashwaganda extract powder
1 clove garlic, peeled and minced

## Method
1. Soak the nuts in plenty of water overnight, then rinse.

2. Mix the broccoli with the olive oil and apple cider vinegar and set aside.

3. Blend all the other ingredients until very smooth, using a Vita-Prep (or other high-speed blender).

4. Pour the mixture into a shallow container and cover with a dark cloth. Store in a warm dark cupboard for around 8 hours.

# HOLY GUACAMOLE Serves any number

I recommend making double batches of this dish because it will be gone in a flash!
**N.B.**: If you don't serve it immediately, store in the fridge with the avocado stone retained; this will help the lemon juice to slow discolouration. Keeps for 2 days when refrigerated in a sealed container.

## Ingredients
2 avocados, stoned and mashed to your preference (I like it chunkier than normal so the individual
flavours can be savoured and the crunchy bits enjoyed in their own right)
1 red onion
1 small handful of dill (fresh)
or 2 tbsp dried

1 yellow pepper, seeded
2 tomatoes
1 lemon, juiced
1 lime, juiced
3 tsp paprika
1 tsp pink Himalayan salt (or to taste)
1 or 2 spring onions, sliced into small rounds (for garnish)

## Method
1. Scoop the avocado flesh into a medium-sized bowl, discarding the skin.

2. Mince the red onion, tomatoes and pepper and add those to the avocado.

3. Squeeze in the lime and lemon juice.

4. Sprinkle the paprika and salt to taste.

5. Garnish with the spring onions and serve.

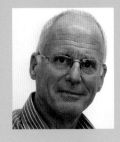

# CHAPTER 7
## SUPPLEMENTS AND NATURAL COMPOUNDS

DR WILLIS

Dr Bernard Willis

Up to 35 per cent of cancers may be due to dietary excesses and deficiencies, especially deficiencies of essential nutrients coupled with excesses of nutrient-poor processed foods.[1]

If you have been diagnosed with cancer and have looked into all the areas outlined in this book, you will probably have embarked on a cancer diet: you may be detoxing, eliminating infections and parasites, practising mind/body therapies and exercising; this chapter focuses on the supplements that can help you to make your body as inhospitable as possible for cancer. Even the most strict anti-cancer diet is unlikely to provide sufficient doses of nutrients to help your body to fight your cancer. So how do you know what to take? You may have consulted Dr Google and been confused by the wealth of information available. There are many natural supplements which can either reduce the side effects of your orthodox therapy or support your body's own defences against cancer. You will certainly need expert advice in order to gain the maximum advantages at every stage, also to avoid wasting money unnecessarily and even to avoid creating additional problems.

Specific nutritional supplements that help to promote normal cell replication and differentiation, boost the body's immunity against abnormal cell growth and reduce DNA damage to cells, are important components in the prevention and management of cancer. When cancer has already begun to grow, it is essential to fight the growth process with specific nutrients that have been shown to inhibit cancer cells and prevent metastasis.

As an integrative medical doctor with thirty years' experience in treating cancer patients holistically, I am confident that an integrative approach, one that incorporates many interdependent factors into a treatment programme of self-help, is essential for all cancer patients hoping for the best outcome.

A good supportive supplement regime will be aiming to achieve for you any of the therapeutic targets outlined on **p. 22** (also detailed on **pp. 39-43** and highlighted with the relevant icons) which are appropriate for the current stage of your programme. Additional targets could include reduction of side effects from standard treatments and anti-fungal action.

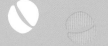

## Nutrition in cancer patients

Cancer itself, or the side effects of cancer treatments, can compromise the nutritional status of cancer patients, often to the state of malnutrition.[2, 3] They often suffer considerable weight loss, a condition known as catabolic wasting or cachexia.[4] The nutritional status of cancer patients can influence many aspects of cancer progression such as treatment tolerance, survival, immune function, cancer growth and spread and especially quality of life.

The list below is not exhaustive, but covers some of the key nutrients that, based on sound research, have been shown to be effective in the prevention and management of cancer. Also, in addition to helping people to fight cancer, these nutrients support overall vitality and have helped many hundreds of my cancer patients.

Please note, the list is not meant to be a menu for all patients, but if you know what treatments with proven benefits are available, then you will be empowered to discuss these therapies with your medical providers and decide which ones would be suitable in your particular set of circumstances. There is no one size that fits all for cancer patients; every treatment programme should be tailored to each individual patient by an expert. It is also important to note that there is a vast number of possible combinations of nutrients, even from the list below. A thorough understanding of potential interactions is essential if the best results are to be achieved.

## How natural products can help in cancer treatments

Natural products have been shown to impede cancer development and progression; they can slow down tumour spread. Many supplements reduce the ability of cancer cells to clump together and grow in size, thus inhibiting angiogenesis, preventing metastasis and boosting the immune system. Many of the following natural supplements have the ability to boost the numbers of a kind of white blood cell called natural killer (NK) cells which, as the name implies, roam through the bloodstream attacking and killing cancer cells.

Cancer is often accompanied by pain, nausea, vomiting, weight loss, fatigue, anxiety and depression, whether as a result of the cancer itself or from the effects of surgery, chemotherapy or radiotherapy.

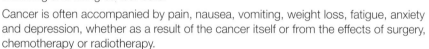

Here are some common symptoms and possible remedies:

- Diarrhoea, neuropathy, heart complications, mucositis can be helped by the amino acid glutamine;[5] there are also many herbal remedies available[6]
- Mucositis, fibrosis, cardiovascular complications can be helped by antioxidants[7]
- Mucositis, anaemia, cardiovascular complications can be helped by melatonin[8]
- Radiation-induced cell damage can be eased by vitamin A[9]
- Neuropathy can be eased by vitamin E[10]
- Nausea and vomiting can be eased by ginger[11]
- Nephrotoxicity (kidney damage) can be helped by silibinin[12]
- Diarrhoea – herbal remedies[13]
- Heart damage can be helped by CoQ10[14]

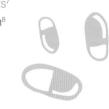

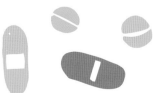

Here is my 'Top Ten' list of supplements/natural compounds for people with cancer, the ones that I have found to be the most helpful for the most people:

01 Vitamin C

02 Curcumin

03 Antioxidants: vitamin A, beta-carotene, vitamin E, selenium

04 Omega-3 fatty acids

05 Coenzyme Q10

06 Medicinal mushrooms

07 Salvestrols

08 Modified citrus pectin (MCP)

09 Iodine

10 Rice bran arabinoxylan compound (RBAC)

## Cancer-fighting nutritional supplements* in common use
(listed alphabetically)

### Alpha lipoic acid (ALA)
This is a wonderful universal antioxidant because of its ability to dissolve in both fat and water. When this acid is in a fat environment, it enhances the effectiveness of other antioxidants. Due to its soluble nature, it can cross the blood brain barrier while many other antioxidants cannot. A major benefit of lipoic acid is that it acts as an 'encourager' and helps to regenerate other antioxidants such as vitamins C and E, coenzyme Q10 (CoQ10) and glutathione, and keeps them in the body longer. It is often added to intravenous infusions of vitamin C. Brain-tumour patients have reported benefit from lipoic acid. High success rates have also been reported in breast, ovarian, prostate, colon and lung cancers. Research has shown good results when used both intravenously and orally in combination with milk thistle, selenium and low dose naltrexone in advanced pancreatic cancer.[15]

### Alpha-tocopherol

As a supplement, this biologically active form of vitamin E, as a supplement, has been shown to reduce levels of vascular endothelial growth factor (VEGF), a tumour-growth factor that helps in the formation of new blood vessels by cancer cells and subsequent tumour invasion of other organs.[16] Blood levels of this cancer-growth factor decreased by 11 per cent in the supplemented group but increased by 10 per cent in the non-supplemented group.[17]

### Amygdalin (laetrile, B17)

Also known as vitamin B17, or laetrile (the synthetic form), this supplement is extracted from apricot kernels and prepared in both tablet and injectable form. The latter is more concentrated and capable of delivering higher doses more quickly than the tablets. Amygdalin is usually recommended at the onset of treatment for patients who are seriously ill. After several weeks or a month, if the patient responds well to treatment, the physician will reduce the dosage and prescribe tablets to replace injections. This therapy is generally used in conjunction with proteolytic enzymes.

* The asterisked items are, in fact, drugs, but used in a way and for a purpose not generally considered within mainstream medicine.

Apricot kernels are taken by many people to prevent cancer.

Please note that laetrile, as a synthetic substance, requires approval to be administered by practitioners in the UK. As this has not been granted, it is not available from practitioners in the UK. Apricot kernels and amygdalin are natural foods and therefore not regulated as medicines.

### Artemisia

An extract from sweet wormwood *Artemisia annua*, this product has been shown to have promising results that were published in the journal *Cancer Letters* (January 2006). Rats were treated with a single dose of a compound known to induce multiple breast cancer. They were then randomly divided into two groups, one group's feed being supplemented with artemisinin. The rats taking artemesinin showed a 40 per cent lower incidence of breast-cancer formation than the control group.[18]

Artemisinin has no known side effects even at high oral doses. It works by reacting with iron molecules in the tissues, forming free radicals that destroy the cells from within. Cancer cells have a greater concentration of iron than normal cells, making artemisinin much more highly toxic to the cancer cells.

### B-complex with folic acid, B6 and B12

These vitamins have multiple properties as nerve and brain enhancers and as co-factors for many other nutrients.

### Beta-carotene

This is a non-toxic form of vitamin A. Beta-carotene can prevent free radicals from damaging a cell's DNA. Such damaged DNA can cause cancer. Hundreds of studies have been conducted on the efficacy of beta-carotene in a cancer setting.[23] Beta-carotene stimulates a molecule that helps the immune system destroy cancer cells.

### Beta-carotene and vitamin A

The supplementation of synthetic vitamin A for twelve months in liver-cancer patients prevented recurrence of the cancer.[24] Vitamin A and its offshoots have been used in the successful treatment of acute promyelocytic leukaemia.[25]

### Boswellia

This is familiarly known as frankincense which comes from Africa, India and the Middle East. It is prepared from resins obtained by tapping *Boswellia carterii* trees. It contains boswellic acids, which have been shown to cause the death of cancer cells, particularly

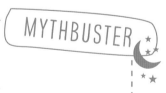

## "SUPPLEMENTS PREVENT CHEMOTHERAPY WORKING"

This is not so much a myth as an over-generalisation. It might be true of some supplements, but some are known to be beneficial.[31] Rather than a blanket ban, what we need is for each person to have a reliably checked programme, specific to his or her treatment.

in brain tumours and leukaemia or colon cancer.[26] A study was published in March 2009 in which the effects of frankincense oil were tested against mutant human bladder cells and compared with normal bladder cells. Results showed that frankincense oil suppressed cell viability in bladder transitional carcinoma cells but not in normal healthy cells. Analysis confirmed that frankincense oil activates genes that are responsible for stopping cell division, suppressing growth of cancer cells, and for the death of bladder-cancer cells. Frankincense oil appears to be capable of distinguishing cancerous from normal bladder cells and suppressing cancer cell health and growth.[27]

### Cimetidine*

Available over the counter, this drug is licensed to treat acid reflux and heartburn. It also possesses anti-cancer activity, inhibiting the ability of cancer cells to adhere to each other on the walls of blood vessels. In 2002 the *British Journal of Cancer* published a study of sixty-four colon cancer patients; they all received standard therapy, some with and some without cimetidine 800 mg daily for a year. The ten-year survival rate for the cimetidine group was 84.6 per cent, while that of the control group was only 49.8 per cent.[28]

### Coenzyme Q10 (CoQ10)

A compound made naturally in the human body, this is used in a process called aerobic respiration, in which oxygen and sugar are converted to energy. CoQ10 enhances antibody synthesis, white blood cell and NK cell activity. It prevents oxidative damage to the cells' DNA. As such, these processes help the mitochondria to generate energy. The body also uses CoQ10 as an antioxidant. It has been shown that CoQ10 helps cancer patients by protecting against heart damage often caused by chemotherapy drugs and their side effects.[29] The use of CoQ10 as a standard conventional treatment for cancer is yet to be established. In animal studies, however, it has shown good results. Inspired by this success, experiments are being conducted in various parts of the world by scientists eager to test its protective powers against heart toxicity in cancer patients treated with the chemotherapy drug doxorubicin.

The first person to pioneer the study of CoQ10 was Dr Karl Folkers (1906-97), Director of the Institute of Medical Research, University of Texas at Austin. In 1994 he chose thirty-two breast-cancer patients, aged between thirty-two and eighty-one. The patients were already at an advanced stage as the cancers had spread to their lymph nodes. Folkers instructed them to follow their conventional treatment and to consume the following nutrients every day for eighteen months:

- 2850 mg of vitamin C
- 2500 IU of vitamin E
- 90,000 IU of beta-carotene
- 387 mcg of selenium (plus secondary vitamins and minerals)
- 1.2 gm of gamma linolenic acid
- 3.5 gm of omega-3 fatty acids
- 90 mg of CoQ10

Two years later, all thirty-two patients were still very much alive and kicking, although four were not expected to survive. Six of them showed partial tumour regression. Under normal condtions, they would not have been expected to live for more than a year. The scientists then decided to increase the prescribed dose of CoQ10 from 90 mg to 390 mg per day in one of the patients, aged fifty-nine and with a family history of breast cancer. Within a month her tumour had spontaneously shrunk. After a second month mammography confirmed that it had disappeared completely – another remarkable success in a very short time, so that the same dose was offered to another patient, this time a woman of seventy-four. A pessimistic lady, she had refused further surgery after learning that her breast cancer had not been eradicated by previous surgery. She was then given daily doses of 390 mg of CoQ10; within two or three months clinical examination showed that her breast tumour was no longer there. Folkers explained that breast-cancer patients have a much lower blood level of CoQ10 than people who are well. As such, breast cancer can be suppressed by taking supplements of CoQ10. Women with low CoQ10 levels have a 38.5 per cent chance of getting breast cancer.[30]

## Curcumin

There are hundreds of studies showing that curcumin, the active ingredient of the spice turmeric, has anti-cancer properties, both preventative and therapeutic.[32] Curcumin works by tracking down cancer cells and altering the regulation of their DNA in order to kill them, at the same time leaving healthy cells and DNA alone so as not to cause harmful side effects. It can slow down the growth of cancers of the prostate, colon and breast.[33, 34, 35]

In one trial of colorectal cancer patients, curcumin in doses of up to 3.6 grams a day reduced inflammation and was not associated with any adverse side effects.[36] Doses of up to 10 grams a day had no adverse effects in humans.[37] It is known to slow the growth of established cancer by reducing the production of growth factors that cancer cells need for angiogenesis.[38, 39] Curcumin is one of the most powerful and promising nutrients that we have for fighting cancer. I recommend that all my cancer patients take it.

## Diindolylmethane (DIM)

Derived from cruciferous vegetables such as cabbage, broccoli and cauliflower, this is of great value in hormone-dependent cancers such as breast and prostate cancer. It helps to ensure that excess oestrogen in the body, which is a prime cause of both breast and prostate cancer, is metabolised via safe and healthy pathways. Patients with these cancers should ensure that they eat at least three portions per week of cruciferous vegetables and consider taking a supplement of DIM.[40]

## Fermented wheatgerm extract

This is a natural compound from a patented process that ferments wheat germ with baker's yeast, which is effective against a wide variety of cancers, including breast, colorectal and skin cancers. It can be used safely during chemotherapy. It was discovered by Dr Máté Hidvégi and is medically approved for cancer therapy in Europe;[19] its use is backed by more than 100 papers which have documented successful clinical results. After its first use in Hungary the mortality rate from cancer began to decline.

Researchers from many parts of the world have found that the supplement:[20]

- helps the body create energy more efficiently from the nutrients we eat
- boosts the body's immune system and strengthens T-cells and macrophages
- helps the body search out and eliminate mutant cells

In 2002 American and Spanish researchers showed that fermented wheatgerm extract has a direct influence on the metabolism of tumour cells, which prevents the cancer cells from reproducing themselves and from carrying out the all-important DNA synthesis. As a result, the tumour does not develop further and the cancer cells die off.[21]

Fermented wheatgerm extract is similar to bread and therefore cannot be taken by gluten-sensitive individuals. It can be taken in conjunction with surgery, chemotherapy and radiotherapy. Prof. Ferenc Jakab, Department Director and Chief Physician at the Uzsoki Street Hospital in Budapest, conducted a trial on 176 patients suffering from colorectal cancer, most of whom were at stages 3 and 4. The average follow-up period was 18.3 months. The trial concluded that, when combined with surgery, radiotherapy or chemotherapy, fermented wheatgerm extract was able to significantly reduce the formation of metastases and to lengthen the lives of those with colorectal cancer.[22]

Fermented wheatgerm extract is taken once a day, in an instant drink mix.

### Garlic

Long known to have anti-cancer properties and the capacity to disrupt the function of cancer-causing agents, garlic is an excellent supplement to boost immune function in cancer patients.[41, 42, 43] It improves the function of NK cells and lymphocyte white cells;[44] it lowers the risk of developing a range of cancers, including those of the stomach, colon, mammary glands, cervix and prostate.[45, 46] Garlic-derived allitridum, taken in combination with selenium, protects against the development of gastric cancer.[47] Various other garlic extracts, including aged garlic extract, allicin and ajoene, are able to help prevent cancer and to offer therapeutic effects.[48]

### Globulin component macrophage activation factor (GcMAF)

The first research on this human protein was published in1993. Since then many papers have appeared showing that GcMAF can reverse cancer by simply activating the immune system. The research was initiated by Dr Nobuto Yamamoto in Philadelphia;[49] hundreds of scientists have followed up this and related projects.[50] While GcMAF has proved effective in the early stages of cancer, in the later stages it is less successful.

How does GcMAF work? In a healthy person it instructs macrophages in our bloodstream to scour our bodies and kill malignancies. But malignant cells like cancer send out an enzyme called nagalase that neutralises the GcMAF. The macrophages therefore never get the message to go into action: while the cancer is suppressing the immune system, the cancer cells are allowed to grow unchecked. To reverse this, GcMAF is made outside the body and is injected once a week for twenty-five weeks in early cancers, fifty or more weeks in late stage (encapsulated tumours require additional treatment).

### Glutathione

This is one of the body's most important antioxidants. It is produced by the body naturally, but can become depleted due to poor nutrition, high levels of toxins or radiation as well as stress and some medications. While acting to clear out toxins such as heavy metals, it is normally recycled by the body, unless the toxic load becomes too great, at which point levels start to become depleted. Furthermore, glutathione regulates the nitric-oxide cycle, which plays a vital role in the immune system and is involved in DNA synthesis and repair. Glutathione levels can be increased by eating cruciferous vegetables or by exercising, but in chronic conditions, supplementing is needed to restore balance.

### Grape-seed extract

Research has shown that grape seeds contain anti-cancer chemicals that act on breast, colorectal and prostate cancers, also on leukaemia as well as head- and neck-cancer cells. The extract creates conditions that are unfavourable for cancer cells to grow. It does this both by damaging the DNA of cancer cells and by disrupting the pathways that allow cancer cells to repair.

A report published in the *Cancer Letters* journal, research carried out by the University of Colorado (CU) Cancer Center, showed that grape-seed extract is effective in inhibiting the growth of colorectal cancer cells.[51] The breakthrough news is that the more aggressive the colorectal cancer cells are, the more grape-seed extract inhibits their growth and survival. This is done without harming healthy cells, which means healing can take place without suffering the adverse side effects of chemotherapy and radiation.

Grape-seed oil can be added to salads, and grape-seed extract can be bought in capsules. Standardised grape-seed extracts that contain at least 40 to 80 per cent pro-anthocyanidins have the best therapeutic effect.[52]

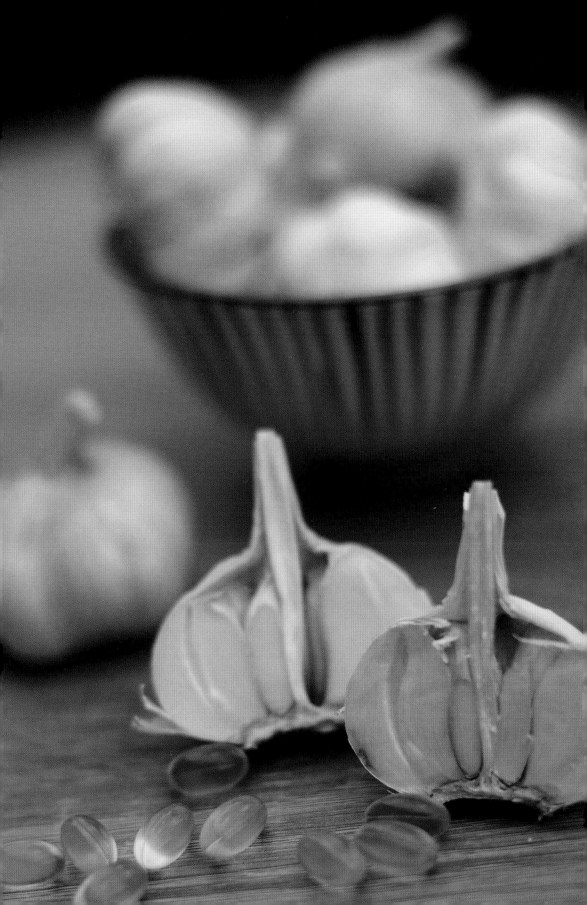

### Graviola

Derived from the seeds, leaves, bark and stem of the South American plant *Annona muricata*, this has marked potential for killing cancer cells; it is especially effective against prostate and pancreatic cancers and works well against lung cancer. Much of the activity of graviola is due to phytochemicals called annonaceous acetogenins. In 1997 Purdue University (Lafayette, Indiana), where most of the research has been done, published promising news that several of the annonaceous acetogenins 'not only are effective in killing tumours that have proven resistant to anti-cancer agents, but also seem to have a special affinity for such resistant cells.'[53]

Another study showed that six acetogenins (four known and two newly discovered) exhibited significant activity in cytotoxic tests against two human hepatoma cell lines.[54] As a review in the *Skaggs Scientific Report* of 1997-8 states: 'Annonaceous acetogenins [...] have remarkable cytotoxic, anti-tumor, anti-malarial, immunosuppressive, pesticidal, and anti-feedant (inhibiting normal feeding) activities'.[55]

Graviola is very safe and has few side effects. The dose for effectively killing cancer cells is much lower than that which would damage healthy human cells. It is probable that graviola will benefit more than colon cancer alone; it now seems that it is worth considering for all cancers, particularly prostate cancer.

### Green tea

The ingredients in green tea are believed to be beneficial in the treatment of cancer. Catechins and theaflavins, compounds found in green and black teas, have anti-cancer properties.[56] Clinical trials have shown that consuming five or more cups of green tea a day may help to reduce the risk of recurrence in those who have survived breast cancer.[57] Consumption of green tea also significantly improves the survival of women with ovarian cancer and reduces the risk of developing cancers of the lung, breast and prostate.[58, 59, 60]

Green tea has been a favourite of Asian people for centuries and has become a popular cancer remedy throughout the West. The active ingredient is a chemical compound epigallocatechin gallate (EGCG), which has a marked ability to scavenge free radicals. EGCG in green tea has long been known to have properties that can prevent cancer.[61] EGCG also inhibits angiogenesis.[62]

### Herbal anti-inflammatory supplements

Out of several proprietory formulations available, the one I use contains ten different herbs. According to the Sloan Kettering website, preliminary studies in 2007 suggest that its ingredients not only have anti-inflammatory properties but also can reduce the growth of cancer cells and prevent them from forming new blood vessels.[63]

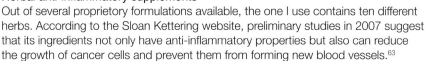

This compound inhibits the proliferation of oral cancer, pancreatic cancer and melanoma cells in the laboratory. In animal trials, it has been shown to inhibit the growth of both hormone-sensitive and hormone-insensitive prostate cancer, and to reduce prostate specific antigen (PSA) markers.[64] It may potentiate the cancer-killing effects of certain chemotherapy drugs, including gemcitabine, taxol, doxorubicin and bicalutamide. The individual components of this supplement have anti-inflammatory and possible anti-carcinogenic properties. In various preclinical studies, it has been shown to suppress the expression of certain genes involved in the inflammatory response and in cancer progression.[65] In other preclinical studies, it has demonstrated anti-cancer activity on its own, and the capacity to be combined with hormonal and chemotherapy agents for improved cancer suppression.[66]

Herbal anti-inflammatories of this type are generally well tolerated.

## Herbs

Echinacea, ginseng and astragalus are among the herbs that can strengthen the immune system and may be beneficial to cancer patients.[67] Red ginseng boosts the immune system of those with gastric cancer who are undergoing chemotherapy after surgery.[68] Five years after diagnosis, those who had taken red ginseng had significantly higher overall survival (76 per cent) than non-supplementing subjects (39 per cent).[69] Astragalus has been shown to increase the number of white blood cells, which can be very important after chemotherapy.

## Inositol (IP-6)

This is a natural plant chemical found in rice bran. Clinical trials have shown that it is a non-toxic compound that can slow down the rate of cell growth, increase NK cells, normalise cell physiology, increase tumour-suppressor gene activity and inhibit inflammation.[70] It is a naturally occurring carbohydrate found in whole grains, wheat germ, dried beans, rice, nuts and seeds.

In 1998 Dr Abdulkalam Shamsuddin, Professor of Pathology at the University of Maryland School of Medicine, theorised that IP-6 could stop the growth of liver cancer, so he conducted two studies published in *Anticancer Research*.[71] In the first of these, he treated human liver-cancer cells with IP-6 and found that it slowed down cancer-cell growth partially in some cells and completely in others, depending on the dosage. In the second study, one group of mice received human liver-cancer cells that had been pre-treated with the compound, while another group received untreated cells. 71 per cent of the mice with untreated cells developed tumours. No tumours were found in the mice with the pre-treated cells. He concluded that IP-6 makes cancer cells behave like normal cells. Although IP-6 inhibits the ability of cancerous cells to colonise, it doesn't affect normal cells.[72]

IP-6 can be taken as a supplement, preferably one that also contains magnesium and calcium. IP-6 binds to those minerals, making it easier to absorb.

## Iodine

It has been shown to kill breast-cancer cells without damaging normal cells.[73] Researchers in India and Mexico have made encouraging progress in this area. In June 2006, a group from the Sanjay Ghandi Institute of Medical Sciences in Lucknow found that iodine is cytotoxic to several lines of human breast cancer cell.

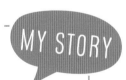

### Alan Hancock
Prostate cancer survivor

*After being diagnosed in 2006 (at the age of 71) with prostate cancer that was too aggressive to be operated on, I was told by the oncology nurse that I would need hormone tablets, hormone injections and radiotherapy every day for six weeks.*

*I read about the Pfeifer Protocol and decided I would try that instead. The protocol involved taking four different supplements: a powerful natural immune booster, micro-nutrients, vitamins and herbs.*

*I also changed my diet, cutting out all processed foods, red meat and dairy products. In a few months my PSA dropped dramatically and I have now had a PSA reading below zero for years. I now only take a very small maintenance dose of the protocol.*

When iodine was applied to human blood cells (monocytes), it inhibited growth and proliferation, but it didn't kill the cells.[74] Later the same year (December) the group in Mexico tested the effect of iodine on the MCF-7 form of human breast-cancer cells. They found that iodine (but not iodide), along with an iodinated fatty acid, inhibited the MCF-7 cancer cells while also establishing that the iodine neither harmed nor inhibited fibroblasts (a normal type of human connective tissue cell that helps to support breast tissue and other tissues throughout the body). Other technical details led the researchers to suggest that iodine may become active against cancer cells when it is bound to certain lipids or proteins that are normally present in the breasts.[75]

These research reports give new hope and an added tool for breast-cancer patients. The evidence is not yet conclusive, but we need not wait for academic and scientific certainty. If you have breast cancer and are undergoing regular treatment, adding iodine to your supplements is likely to increase your odds of a favourable outcome – and it is very safe. Numerous studies have proved that iodine (and its iodide form) are among the safest of all the elements.[76]

Please note that, even though iodine is generally safe, some individuals are sensitive to iodine and/or iodide. There have been anecdotal reports of iodide causing autoimmune thyroiditis, hyperthyroidism and hypothyroidism. Too much iodine in a few individuals has caused iodism, an acne-like rash accompanied by a runny nose and a bad taste, all of which go away when the dosage is reduced or eliminated. Nevertheless, iodine is well worth considering if you have breast cancer.

### L-carnitine

Using the amino acid L-carnitine as a supplement can reduce stress and fatigue, both of which are often either a symptom of the cancer or a side effect of treatment.[77] Giving L-carnitine during chemotherapy with doxorubicin has been proposed as an adjuvant therapy since1985.[78]

### Lipoic acid palladium complex (LAPd)

This compound contains various minerals, vitamins and amino acids such as lipoic acid, palladium, B12 and other B-complex vitamins. It is a nutritional supplement that is considered to be a non-toxic alternative to chemotherapy. Because it is said to be capable of crossing the blood brain barrier, this product is generally used in the treatment of brain tumours, but it is said also to be effective against cancerous growths in the lung, ovaries and breast. The indications are that it boosts the immune system, reduces pain and helps people to regain energy and appetite. It is considered a powerful antioxidant that can turn the toxins released by cancer into energy. According to its proponents, the compound attacks cancerous cells and protects DNA and RNA. They contend that the lipoic acid component allows the various minerals, vitamins, and amino acids to be easily absorbed into the system where they can kill cancerous cells.[79] LAPd also repairs cancer cells that have been abnormally altered. In 1994 in Canada, the oncologist Dr Rudy Falk used LAPd with a group of his cancer patients. He reported that when it was used in conjunction with chemotherapy, patients experienced such benefits as lessened pain, improved appetite, weight gain and revitalised energy.[80]

### Low-dose naltrexone (LDN)*

Our natural opiate chemicals, endorphins, make us feel happy, relaxed and boost our immune systems. We all have the ability to try to resist cancer by increasing or modulating what are called our opioid receptors. As LDN is a powerful antagonist of opioids, it blocks opioid receptors, preventing signals from getting through. Another action is stimulating certain immune-system cells that tend to kill cancer cells, including T-cells and NK cells. For treating drug or alcohol addiction it is used in much higher doses than those used for cancer.

LDN is also used in the treatment of certain immune-related disorders, including HIV/AIDS, multiple sclerosis, Parkinson's disease, cancer, fibromyalgia and in autoimmune diseases such as rheumatoid arthritis or ankylosing spondylitis, Crohn's disease, ulcerative colitis, Hashimoto's thyroiditis and central nervous system disorders. LDN is believed to increase your body's production of met-enkephalin and endorphins (your natural opioids), hence improving your immune function.

Dr Burton M. Berkson, of the Integrative Medical Center of New Mexico in Las Cruces, has published two studies on intravenous LDN coupled with alpha lipoic acid (ALA) for the treatment of cancer.[81] The first, on the reversal of pancreatic cancer, was published in 2006, and the other, on the reversal of B cell lymphomas, came out in 2007. Both sets of results were promising. LDN is taken at bedtime, which blocks your opioid receptors for a few hours in the middle of the night. LDN can be prescribed by your doctor, and should be prepared by a reliable compounding pharmacy.

LDN

For further details of past and current research, see the LDN website.

### Lycopene
Abundant in tomatoes and tomato-based products, this caritenoid can protect against cancers of the prostate, colon, pancreas, ovaries, breast and bladder.[82, 83, 84, 85, 86, 87] It is a powerful antioxidant that has been shown to slow the growth of both prostate and breast cancer.[88]

### Medicinal mushrooms
Having been known to be useful in treating cancer and other immune-deficiency diseases for thousands of years, mushrooms are now confirmed to have particular properties that enhancie immune function and the production of T-cells. Mushrooms contain a polysaccharide compound called beta-glucan, which has shown strong anti-tumour activity in many animal studies.[89]

In patients suffering from gynaecological cancers, mushroom extracts increased the activity of NK cells.[90] A study of eight patients with various cancers revealed that a combination of maitake mushroom MD-fraction and whole maitake powder resulted in a good response in 23 of 36 cancer patients. Symptom improvement and regression of cancer was shown in 69 per cent of those with breast cancer, 63 per cent of those with lung cancer, and 58 per cent of those with liver cancer. In patients with leukaemia, stomach or brain cancer, the study found a much smaller response, less than 10 to 20 per cent improvement.[91]

The mushroom coriolus contains a substance called PSK, which has often been shown to increase NK cell activity. In one study 225 patients with lung cancer received radiotherapy with or without PSK. Results showed that more than three times as many patients taking PSK were alive after five years, compared with those not taking PSK. In a study of colon cancer, published in the British Journal of Cancer in 2004, the five-year survival rate was 75 per cent in the PSK group, compared with only 46 per cent in the control group.[92]

If you have cancer, beneficial mushrooms include coriolus, cordyceps, reishi, maitake, agaricus, phellinus and umbellatus. Some formulae contain all of these.

### Melatonin
The sleep hormone melatonin, produced at night by the pineal gland, has anti-cancer effects.[93] The use of melatonin (20 mg a night) during chemotherapy improves survival as well as quality of life in lung-cancer patients.[94] Melatonin also reduces the growth of prostate- and breast-cancer cells.[95]

Blind people, who generally have high melatonin levels, have lower rates of cancer.[96]

Most cancer patients have low levels of melatonin.[97] Melatonin supplements improve immune function in patients suffering from a variety of cancers, including gastric, renal, prostate and bladder cancers, without any apparent adverse effects.[98]

Numerous studies have established melatonin to be one of the most effective natural anti-cancer treatments in existence. It inhibits the growth and proliferation of cancer cells; it stimulates the immune system and increases the cancer-killing activity of macrophages, monocytes, NK cells and T-helper cells (which, as their name suggests, contribute to the activation of T-cells), all of which are involved in destroying cancer cells; it induces apoptosis; it stops new tumour blood-vessel growth, and prevents harmful forms of oestrogen from stimulating cancer-cell growth. Its effects have proven to be superior to those of many chemotherapeutic drugs. As an antioxidant, melatonin reduces inflammation, a condition that enables cancer cells to survive, and it scavenges free radicals so that they don't damage normal cells. In one 1996 clinical trial, patients with glioblastoma, a type of brain cancer, were given either radiation and melatonin or radiation alone. Twenty-three per cent of the patients who took the melatonin were alive after a year, while those who had received only radiation had all died.[99] Similarly, in another study in Italy, patients with non-small cell lung cancers who had failed chemotherapy were given melatonin. They were compared with other patients with non-small cell lung cancers who weren't given melatonin. A year later, 26 per cent of the patients who had taken melatonin were still alive, whereas none of the non-melatonin group had survived.[100]

Studies have also revealed melatonin to be more effective for treating pancreatic and lung cancers than a drug commonly used to treat those two types of cancers.[101]

### Milk thistle

Silymarin, the active ingredient in the herb milk thistle, has shown anti-cancer potential properties against prostate-cancer cells and may be one of the resources for treating prostate cancer.[102] Used in combination with ALA and LDN, silymarin has proved to be useful in the treatment of pancreatic cancer.[103]

### Mistletoe extract

A fermented preparation of the European mistletoe (*Viscum album*), which grows on deciduous trees, is widely used to treat cancer throughout Europe, especially at integrative clinics. There is much research to show that this extract benefits the immune response by increasing NK cells and enhancing the function of white blood cells. Mistletoe extract is now recognised in Germany and Switzerland – and to some extent in the UK – as a medicine. It is calculated that 60 per cent of all cancer treatments in central Europe include mistletoe, often in conjunction with chemotherapy or radiotherapy.

Studies have shown that mistletoe extract reduces tumour size and prolongs lives. Patients with cancers of the cervix, ovaries, breast, stomach, colon and lung should consider using this herb. It can also be beneficial for cancers of the bone marrow, connective tissue, lymphomas, sarcomas and leukaemias. A study involving over 10,000 cancer patients published in 2001 showed that patients who were given mistletoe lived 40 per cent longer than those in the control group.[104] It is generally well tolerated with few side effects.[105]

Please note that patients on anti-depressant drugs should not take this herb.

### Modified citrus pectin (MCP)

This natural substance is high on my list of essential cancer supplements. Derived from the pith of citrus fruit and then modified through an enzymatic process to meet specific molecular chain and weight characteristics, MCP directly attacks cancer by binding to galectin-3 molecules ('sticky' surface molecules that promote angiogenesis and metastasis) and blocking them. As a result the cancer cells can't spread and grow. 2009 research showed that MCP also blocks the growth of primary tumours and prevents the formation of new blood vessels that would feed the tumour. Further advances have introduced an even more potent form of this compound and have demonstrated compelling results among late-stage cancer patients.[106]

### Omega-3 fatty acids

Omega 3 helps to prevent cancer metastasising to other parts of the body. It is also a powerful anti-inflammatory agent and can help to prevent the weight loss in advanced cancer patients, known as catabolic wasting or cachexia (see also 'Cachexia', p.97, in **Chapter 5, 'Diet as the foundation of good health', p.97**). Fish oil contains a high level of omega-3 fatty acids that help to stop the spread of cancer by reducing angiogenesis. It counterbalances the effects of omega-6 fatty acids' production of inflammatory chemicals. This is because omega-3 and omega-6 fatty acids compete for cell receptors in the cell membrane. Omega-6

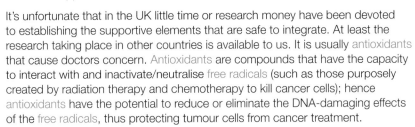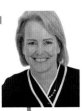

# TAKING SUPPLEMENTS ALONGSIDE ORTHODOX TREATMENTS

There is much confusion about which supplements are beneficial to take during chemotherapy and radiotherapy, or alongside other drugs. There is a lack of uniform policy and response on this from the medical profession, which adds to the confusion. Some hospitals offer a pharmacy-checking system to clarify their recommendations; others put a blanket ban on all supplements, which is obviously less time-consuming for them; and some express no concern over your choice of supplements.

It's unfortunate that in the UK little time or research money have been devoted to establishing the supportive elements that are safe to integrate. At least the research taking place in other countries is available to us. It is usually antioxidants that cause doctors concern. Antioxidants are compounds that have the capacity to interact with and inactivate/neutralise free radicals (such as those purposely created by radiation therapy and chemotherapy to kill cancer cells); hence antioxidants have the potential to reduce or eliminate the DNA-damaging effects of the free radicals, thus protecting tumour cells from cancer treatment.

Relatively little research on the effect of antioxidants on treatments has been published. Some compounds such as turmeric, which is classified as an antioxidant, have been shown in many studies to improve the efficacy of chemotherapy. What is also being revealed is that the whole action of antioxidants may indeed have been incorrectly identified. There is further concern about herbal medicines causing interactions, but a reputable herbalist will know what is safe to use. International databases currently list all known interactions for clinicians to use.

Ideally, if your hospital has an established pharmacy system for checking for potential interactions, you and your practitioner can work together to establish what is acceptable to your oncologist. If he or she puts a blanket ban on taking supplements, try to establish if that is because they don't have any knowledge or avenues for checking interactions. They may be willing to work with your practitioner in exploring his or her specialist knowledge to help compile a support programme.

fatty acids cause weakening of the immune system, suppression of cytokines, reduction in T-cell proliferation as well as inhibition of white cells and NK cells responsible for controlling cancer growth. Furthermore, omega-6 fatty acids support angiogenesis in many cancers, and therefore encourage the growth of cancer cells. Conversely, fish oil prevents cancer cells from attaching to healthy tissues. It also slows down the rate of tumour attachment in the lymph nodes. It is a useful adjunct during chemotherapy as well as radiotherapy. Human studies confirm that fish oil increases the efficacy of chemotherapy drugs such as mitomycin, cisplatin and vincristine, because it enhances their cytotoxicity. Breast-cancer patients with high fat-tissue levels of omega-3 fatty acids respond better to chemotherapy. In short, omega 3 prevents cancer from spreading with or without chemotherapy.[107]

### Proteolytic enzymes

Digestive enzymes, specifically pancreatic enzymes, can be used to induce two effects: first, to expose the cancer cell by removing its fibrin coating, thereby making it an easier target for the immune system; and second, to reduce the adhesiveness of cancer cells, so making it more difficult for them to stick together and form a larger mass.

One of the available brands is a patented complex of digestive enzymes that includes bromelain (from pineapple) and papain (from papaya), which can digest proteins and other molecules, safely and effectively. Most tumours and cancer cells are covered by a sticky resistant coating, which keeps them safe from immune cells and to some extent even protects them from chemotherapy. This complex can dissolve away this protective coating, leaving the cancer cell vulnerable to attack by the body's immune system. It can also enhance the effects of chemotherapy because the chemotherapeutic agent will be more likely to penetrate the cancer cells.

In 1987 Dr Nicholas Gonzalez set up a private practice with Dr Linda Isaacs in New York. They achieved excellent results using high doses of proteolytic enzymes and dietary manipulation in many types of cancer, including late stage pancreatic cancer.[108] I usually advise all cancer sufferers to take an enzyme complex as I am impressed with the results achieved by Dr Gonzalez.

### Pine bark extract

This antioxidant, which is obtained from the French maritime pine tree, is excellent for those patients undergoing chemotherapy or radiotherapy. Research has shown that it can significantly reduce nausea, vomiting and diarrhoea.[109]

### Quercetin

This special flavonoid, present in onions and apples, destroys cancer cells while leaving normal cells intact. Quercetin can enhance the effect of chemotherapy agents such as cisplatin and adriamycin, as well as tamoxifen and also radiotherapy. It acts to prevent the spread of cancer by stimulating our immune system in a similar way to medicinal mushrooms, that is, by increasing the number of NK cells. It also alters the DNA and genes in tumour cells and increases apoptosis. Quercetin slows down the growth of oestrogen positive and oestrogen negative cancer cells.[110]

### Resveratrol and salvestrols

These are found in more than seventy species of plants, including mulberries, peanuts and particularly in grapes. Salvestrols, of which resveratrol is the best known, serve as defensive molecules that act against fungus in grapes and other crops. They are found in abundance in crops that are not treated with artificial fungicides. Fresh grape skin contains about 50 to 100 micrograms of resveratrol, while red wine concentrations range from 1.5 to 3 milligrams per litre. Salvestrols are strong antioxidants that stop the enzymes necessary for cancer growth. A clinical study from the Hematology/Oncology Division of the Department of Medicine at the Josephine Ford Cancer Institute, Michigan in 2000 showed that cells in an HL60 human leukaemia cell line exposed to resveratrol were destroyed.[111] This flavonoid also prevents the development of pre-cancerous lesions in mouse mammary glands treated with a carcinogen in culture. Additionally, it inhibits other tumour growths in mice. At the time of writing, no toxic side effects have been reported. In the UK new salvestrols have been isolated from certain fruits and vegetables by scientists in Leicester. Their research on these supplements for treating people with cancer is very impressive and exciting. It has become clear to me that salvestrols should be high on the list of possible supplements for every cancer patient.[112]

### Rice bran arabinoxylan compound (RBAC)

This is a product that I have found very useful in cancer treatment; it is one of my 'Top Ten', see p. 120. A very safe natural food supplement made from rice bran, it has been clinically proven to boost failing immune systems.

RBAC has been shown to increase NK cell activity by as much as 300 per cent in just two weeks, while the acivity of T-cells and B-cells (both of which are involved in making

# LIPOSOMAL VITAMINS

First described in 1961, liposomes are an increasingly popular way to administer both drugs and supplements. Some chemotherapies are now available in this form. A liposome is a tiny bubble, made out of the same material as a cell membrane. The liposomes are absorbed by melting into the human cell, since they have an outer layer that is made from the same phospholipids as the cell membrane. With all oral treatments there is variability as to how much is absorbed and how much is destroyed or malabsorbed by the individual's gastrointestinal tract. Most nutrients and drugs are molecules that are too large to be absorbed. The most common way in which food is absorbed is by nutritional molecules being broken down to a size where they can slip between the stomach and intestinal cell walls, thus entering the bloodstream. The liver and other organs then re-assemble the molecules. Liposomal preparations have the advantage of directly entering the cell. In 2010 it was shown that stress can influence absorption; low vitamin D levels in winter can also be a factor, hence the potential for variables is high.[114]

Vitamin C is now available in liposomal form. An oral dose, the size of which has always been limited by the tolerance level of the gut, results in a far higher absorption than was previously possible. This makes it either a viable alternative for those unable to obtain intravenous treatment or a useful additional treatment. Do not attempt to take other oral forms of vitamin C in high doses as it will adversely affect the gut. The vitamin itself should never be viewed as a direct replacement for chemotherapy. Recent indications are that, whereas it is a good recovery strategy, its effects are short-lived, and it therefore should not be relied on exclusively.[115]

antibodies) is increased by 200 and 150 per cent respectively. It has proved to have anti-inflammatory effects and antioxidant scavenging activity, as well as the capacity to improve glucose tolerance, to enhance pancreatic and liver function, to reduce the adverse effects of chemotherapy, and to improve general quality of life. RBAC has been shown to be completely non-toxic, even in extremely high doses. It is also safe for children and infants (intake scaled down by body weight). Much of the scientific and clinical research on this supplement has taken place in Japan, the USA and Europe, and has been published in peer-reviewed journals. RBAC's immune-enhancing effects are apparent in just a few days, and it takes only a few weeks for the immune-boosting effect to reach 90 per cent of its peak. It is not a drug, a synthetic chemical or genetically modified and can be taken long-term.[113]

### Selenium

This essential mineral is a powerful antioxidant that protects cells from the damaging effects of oxygen free radicals. Certain studies have indicated that selenium reduces the risk of cancer by helping to destroy free radicals; in so doing, it protects cell membranes.[116] Other studies show that the use of selenium reduces unpleasant side effects such as nausea and vomiting as well as headache during chemotherapy.[117] Cancer patients often lack selenium. Supplementation of selenium works synergistically with vitamin E in combating cancer.[118]

### Skullcap (Scutellaria baicalensis)

This herb has been extensively researched and shown to have pronounced anti-cancer properties. Chinese skullcap is a member of the mint family and grows in China and Russia. It is a rich source of over thirty-five flavonoids, the most important one being baicalein, which is being studied for its anti-cancer, anti-inflammatory, antiviral, antibacterial and anti-allergy effects. Capable of slowing or even stopping the replication of various human cancer cells, it appears to be able to block the growth of cancer cells, to induce cell death and to prevent metastasis. It is also a powerful antioxidant.

Baicalein inhibits the enzyme which converts testosterone to dihydrotestosterone (DHT). This beneficial action makes it potentially useful for the treatment of testosterone-dependent disorders, including prostate enlargement and prostate cancer. In a 2000 study performed by researchers from the University of California at San Francisco and the Memorial Sloan Kettering Cancer Center in New York, baicalein was administered to prostate-cancer patients with metastasis to other organs which had failed to respond to the usual conventional treatments. Baicalein demonstrated reversal of their condition with significant reduction of PSA levels and improvement in survival time in a large proportion of patients. Studies following men with prostate cancer for up to four years have also shown that this herbal extract reduces prostate-specific antigen (PSA) levels and improves survival.[119]

### Sodium bicarbonate

This chemical compound is commonly known as baking soda. Moving the body from acidity to mild alkalinity is one of the crucial strategies for making your body hostile to cancer cells (see 'pH balance', p. 39, under 'Therapeutic targets', p. 38 in Chapter 1, 'Taking an integrative approach'). Sodium bicarbonate, given orally or transdermally (through the skin) in a bath, can be a useful alkalyser.

### Soy

It contains an active ingredient called genistein, which has been shown to prevent cancer cells that have persisted after surgery from invading new organs and spreading.[120] This potential to arrest the spread of cancer is linked to genistein's ability to reduce production of the growth factor VEGF, a necessary substance for cancer spread and invasion.[121]

## Vitamin C

Rose hips, apples, oranges and other citrus fruits are all rich in vitamin C, which is a beneficial supplement for those with cancer. It is a potent water-soluble antioxidant. While most animals synthesise their own vitamin C, humans do not.

Vitamin C is an excellent antioxidant. It fights cancer by:

- stimulating the production of white blood cells, primarily neutrophils, which attack foreign antigens such as bacteria and viruses
- repairing cell damage from free oxygen radicals
- strengthening the terrain around the tumour and inhibiting the spread of cancer
- destroying cancer-causing viruses through its stimulation of the activity of the white blood cells
- correcting the vitamin-C deficiency common in cancer patients
- stimulating and stabilising the formation of collagen (the 'glue' that holds tissue together)
- elimination of cancer toxins

- increasing hydrogen peroxide and free radical generation in the cancer cell under a high iron environment. Hydrogen peroxide kills cancer cells as they lack an enzyme called catalase that normally functions to remove hydrogen peroxide[122]

In 2013 doctors at the University of Iowa Carver College of Medicine conducted a study in which 50 to 125 grams of vitamin C were infused into patients with pancreatic cancer once a week on a weekly cycle ('intravenous' or 'IV' treatment). The standard chemotherapy drug for pancreatic cancer was also administered on a weekly cycle as usual. The average treatment duration was six months (range: 60 to 556 days) during which patients lost an average of only 11 pounds, which is much less than would usually be expected. Side effects of the IV treatment included diarrhoea and dry mouth, but these symptoms were generally mild. Apart from increasing survival to 12 months, the IV vitamin-C therapy also increased progression-free survival to 26 weeks (12.7 weeks have been reported in other trials). The researchers did not report on overall tumour-size development, except for one patient who experienced a dramatic nine-fold reduction in the size of the primary tumour after four months of treatment.[123]

Vitamin C is helpful for most cancer patients, preferably by IV infusion, but if the expense is a problem, oral liposomal vitamin C in large doses, up to 16,000 mg daily, can be taken as part of a supervised programme with other synergistic supplements (see the 'Liposomal **vitamins**', **p. 133** above). Vitamin C in high doses is toxic to cancer cells and can also improve the potential success of chemotherapy. It is an often quoted myth that vitamin C can reduce the effectiveness of chemotherapy, but there is much research to disprove that premise.[124]

## Vitamin D3 (as cholecalciferol)

Cancer patients invariably have low levels of vitamin D, a fat soluble vitamin that occurs in several forms. It promotes normal cell differentiation and is an excellent immune booster. 90 per cent of our vitamin D is manufactured from sunlight and the incidence of cancer is higher in the northern hemisphere than in the south. Natural vitamin D from sunshine lasts longer in the body than vitamin D from a supplement. Ten minutes of exposure to the sun at mid-day, without sunscreen, should be mandatory for all cancer patients.[125] I would advise everybody with cancer to have their blood level of vitamin D measured, and if low they should take a vitamin D supplement (see **Chapter 10, 'Sunshine and vitamin D'**).

### Vitamin E (mixed tocopherols)

A key nutrient needed for combating the effects of cancer, vitamin E strengthens the immune system and is an important fat-soluble antioxidant. Research is being done on the use of vitamin E together with chemotherapy and radiotherapy. Positive indications from studies on vitamin E include the following:

- Vitamin E succinate has been shown to convert highly malignant melanoma cells in vitro (isolated under laboratory conditions) into normal cells after a few days contact[126]
- Brain-cancer cells can be affected by vitamin E succinate[127]
- In ovarian and cervical cancer, vitamin E can slow down the activity of cancer cells without affecting normal cells[128]
- In radiotherapy, vitamin E succinate can help to destroy cancer cells and protect normal cells[129]
- Tamoxifen can be more effective against breast cancer when combined with vitamin E[130]
- Animal studies indicate that vitamin E may have activity against colon cancer and melanoma[131]

### Vitamin K3

The addition of vitamin K3 to vitamin C in cancer therapy can substantially increase the cytotoxic properties of vitamin C. By exerting an oxidant effect on cancer cells, hydrogen peroxide is released in the cells; unlike healthy cells, cancer cells do not have the enzymes to metabolise hydrogen peroxide and are therefore vulnerable. Many Integrative Oncology practitioners give an infusion of IV vitamin K3 after an IV vitamin-C infusion for its additive effect.[132]

# SUMMARY

This formidable but not exhaustive list above is intended to empower you with the knowledge you need to make a start in building your own anti-cancer programme with your practitioner. I am certain that you will soon begin to feel the benefits inherent in a carefully considered supplement regime. The supplements that are appropriate for you will depend to some extent on the type of cancer you have and what stage it has reached; other personal health factors are of course equally relevant. Again, I want to underline the importance of consulting an experienced integrative doctor or specialised nutritionist who will have the depth of knowledge and experience needed to help you to decide your best way forward in making your body a hostile environment for cancer.

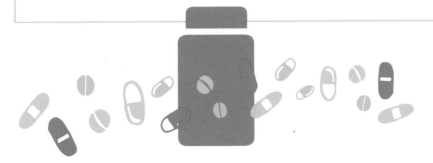

# CASE REPORTS

I follow with two cases illustrating how supplements can contribute to an integrative programme:

A sixty-two-year-old white man was diagnosed with organ-confined prostate cancer in November 2010 with a Gleason score of 5 (2 + 3); there is a simple description of the Gleason scoring system on the Prostate Cancer UK website. He was initially treated elsewhere with monthly leuprolide therapy. Prostate-specific antigen (PSA – the standard marker for assessing prostate-cancer progression), first recorded as 1 in April 2010, increased to 27 in July 2011. Treatment was deferred as the patient had no symptoms. Scans of his bones, abdomen and pelvis showed no spread. In September 2011 blood appeared in his urine and transurethral resection (surgical tissue removal) of the prostate was performed. Pathological examination of the removed tissue revealed adenocarcinoma of the prostate, Gleason score 8 (4 + 4 ).

PC UK

The patient declined further hospital treatment and came to my Optimal Wellness Centre in Auckland, New Zealand. PSA was 18.8, with still no sign that the disease had spread locally. However, a bone scan showed skeletal metastases.

He began an 80 per cent raw-food diet, particularly eliminating dairy products. In March 2012 he began intravenous infusions of vitamins C and K3 with glutathione, alpha lipoic acid and bicarbonate of soda in gradually increasing doses. He began supplementing with liposomal vitamin C, lycopene, melatonin, curcumin, DIM, quercetin, iodine and modified citrus pectin. In June 2012 his PSA had decreased to 13.6, and to 8.1 by October 2012, then stabilised to between 3 and 8. A repeat bone scan in January 2013 demonstrated improvement of bony metastases and he continued to have weekly infusions. At his last follow-up in April 2013 he was asymptomatic.

In October 2010 a seventy-three-year-old New Zealand farmer was diagnosed with widespread non-Hodgkin's lymphoma. Biopsies and CT scans showed that he had cancer in all the lymph nodes from his chest up. He was treated with chemotherapy for eight months, resulting in a remission. In July 2011 he began losing weight (30 lbs). He returned to his oncologist and a CT scan at that time showed recurrence. He had further chemotherapy in September 2011. In December 2011, with no change in the cancer, his immune system was so depressed that he developed a case of shingles and the chemotherapy was stopped.

I first saw this gentleman in March 2012. He was given infusions of vitamins C and K twice a week. In addition he undertook a plant-based diet with the occasional portion of fish. He was given a wide range of supplements, including curcumin, green tea extract, quercetin and artemisinin. Three months after beginning vitamin-C therapy, a CT scan showed a reduction in the lymph nodes. Another CT scan in February 2013 showed that the lymph nodes were clear and his oncologist declared him to be in complete remission.

# PART THREE

## FURTHER LIFESTYLE
# FACTORS

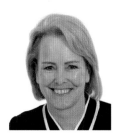

# INTRODUCTION TO PART THREE

Patricia Peat

Along with nutrition (covered in Part Two), the lifestyle factors investigated in this part of *The Cancer Revolution* probably represent the most important ways in which each of us can personally influence our wellbeing and our ability to meet the challenges of cancer. Understanding of the massive impact that an exercise programme or meditation, for example, can have on wellbeing and survival is growing exponentially. You simply cannot afford to ignore any of these avenues to health.

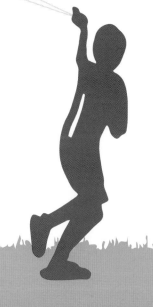

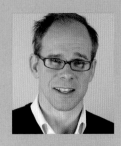

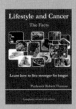

CANCERNET

# CHAPTER 8

# THE BENEFITS OF PHYSICAL ACTIVITY AFTER DIAGNOSIS

## Prof. Robert Thomas

Most of us realise – whether we do anything about it or not – that regular exercise and a healthy lifestyle reduce our risks of developing many serious diseases, including cancer. What is less well known is that, after a diagnosis of cancer, exercise can bring enormous benefits, not only to reduce the side effects of treatment and improve physical and psychological wellbeing, but also to increase the chances of long-lasting remission and cure. In many cases, the magnitude of these benefits is on a par with that provided by chemotherapy, yet mainstream oncology units have been slow to offer exercise guidance and support for their patients.

This chapter reviews the evidence from published clinical studies and describes the underlying mechanism of how exercise fights cancer. It also makes tried and tested suggestions on how, when and how often to exercise.

### Evidence that physical activity improves wellbeing after cancer

Through a combination of earlier detection and enhanced treatments, the chance of surviving cancer has significantly improved during the last two or three decades. For example, the average chance of living five years from diagnosis for a woman with breast cancer when I first became a consultant in 1990 was just 54 per cent; by 2012 it had become 84 per cent.[1] To achieve this and similar successes in other types of cancer, however, patients usually have to endure complex and arduous therapies, often involving acute or long-term side effects, that can considerably diminish their quality of life.

Fortunately, well-conducted clinical studies have demonstrated a significant benefit for exercise and that it can play a major role in reducing the severity of many of these adverse effects. A meta-analysis of thirty-four randomised trials, published in the *British Medical Journal* in 2012, showed that patients who took exercise after cancer experienced improvements in terms of fatigue, mood, anxiety, depression, muscle power, hand grip, exercise capacity and quality of life.[2] Other trials have shown that regular exercise during and after cancer treatments reduces the serious risk of blood clots, which affects up to 15 per cent of cases, and in some can be life-threatening.[3] The evidence for the benefits of exercise spans the common cancer types and has been demonstrated following a range of treatments including surgery, radiotherapy, chemotherapy, hormone treatment and even the newer biological therapies. I now go on to describe some specific programmes and clinical studies addressing some of the common symptoms that often plague those who have survived cancer.

## Cancer-related fatigue (CRF)

Fatigue has overtaken nausea and pain as the most distressing symptom experienced by cancer patients both during and after cancer treatments. It is reported by 60-96 per cent of patients during chemotherapy, following radiotherapy or after surgery.[4] CRF can have a profound effect on the whole person, physically, emotionally and mentally, and can persist for months or even years following completion of treatment.[5] It is also reported in up to 40 per cent of patients taking long-term treatments such as hormone or biological therapies.[6]

The first step to treating CRF is to correct, if possible, medical conditions that can aggravate it – anaemia, medication, electrolyte imbalance, liver failure, steroid withdrawal, depression, nocturia (the need to get up in the night to urinate), night sweats and pruritis (the desire to scratch).[7] Drugs such as opiates, antihistamines, anti-sickness medication and sedatives can also worsen the condition.

The self-help strategy most extensively investigated for CRF is exercise. There have been two meta-analyses addressing the use of exercise to combat CRF. The first showed a modest benefit. The second subdivided the data into two main exercise strategies:

- Home-based programmes, involving patients being advised to exercise, unsupervised, in their own homes
- Referring patients to a supervised exercise programme, including a combination of aerobic exercises (e.g. running or rowing) and resistance exercises (e.g. weight lifting)

The studies involving supervised aerobic exercise programmes showed a statistically significant improvement; the degree of improvement was also better than that of the home-based programmes.[8]

## Weight gain and body composition

Weight gain during and after adjuvant chemotherapy is becoming an ever-increasing concern. Nearly half of women with breast cancer, for example, report significant weight gain, often at a time in their lives when losing it is difficult. In men, a study of 440 prostate-cancer survivors reported that more than half were overweight or obese.[9] For individuals with bowel cancer, a trial showed that a third of these patients were overweight after chemotherapy, and that a third were obese or very obese.[10] There are several reasons for this. Some patients are concerned about undue weight loss, perhaps as a result of outdated and misleading information, and they tend to overeat; others with fatigue and nausea stop exercising. Certain drugs, including steroids and hormone therapies such as Tamoxifen (for breast cancer) or Zoladex (for prostate cancer), can also promote weight gain. Numerous reviews and meta-analyses of published medical literature have demonstrated that individuals who gain weight after cancer treatments have poorer survival rates and increased chances of complications.[11] Fortunately, supervised exercise programmes have been shown to reduce weight problems and to be significantly beneficial for body constitution and fitness, including lean mass indices, bone mineral density, heart and lung function, muscle strength and walking distance.[12]

## Psychological wellbeing

Being diagnosed with cancer is of course a stressful experience and requires a high level of emotional and social readjustment. While many people accept a cancer diagnosis reasonably well, psychological distress is consistently reported in over a quarter of patients.[13] Still, psychological wellbeing, including mood status, depression and anxiety, is under-diagnosed in up to half of cases.[14] As well as being distressing for the patients and their carers, depression may have a physical impact. Cohort studies (those examining a selected group of similar patients) have suggested that people with lung and breast cancer who are also depressed, for example, have reduced survival compared with those who are psychologically healthy.[15] A number of observational studies (those with no control group of patients for comparison) among people undergoing chemotherapy, radiotherapy, hormone and other therapies, have demonstrated reduced levels of depression and anxiety as well as improved quality of life, mood, happiness and self-esteem for those on an exercise programme, especially when group activities are involved.[16]

## Overall quality of life

Regular exercise has been shown to improve quality of life at all stages of illness and for several different types of cancer. For example, in a study involving 1966 patients with colorectal cancer, those achieving at least 150 minutes of physical activity per week had an 18 per cent higher Quality of Life (QoL) score than those who reported no physical activity.[17] Another study showed similar benefits in relation to exercise in a randomised trial of breast-cancer survivors who had completed surgery, radiotherapy or chemotherapy; it also demonstrated that change in peak oxygen consumption (a measure of physical fitness) correlated with change in overall QoL.[18] Another randomised trial compared supervised resistance exercise versus a similar group of 135 men with prostate cancer and not involved in exercise who were scheduled to receive hormone therapy for at least three months. There was a significant improvement in QoL in the exercise group and a significant decline in the comparison group.[19]

## Bone health (osteoporosis)

Pre-menopausal women who have had breast-cancer treatment are at increased risk for osteoporosis and fracture due to reduced levels of oestrogen brought on by a premature menopause; this can be caused by chemotherapy, surgery or hormones. Men who receive hormone-deprivation therapy for prostate cancer also have an increased risk of developing osteoporosis.[20] Post-menopausal women are at a higher risk if they receive aromatase inhibitors such as Arimidex.[21] Osteoporosis, its precursor osteopenia and increased rates of fracture have also been noted in those who have survived many other types of cancer, including testicular, thyroid, gastrointestinal and that of the central nervous system as well as non-Hodgkin's lymphoma and various haematological (blood) malignant diseases.[22] Medical conditions associated with a higher risk of osteopenia include thyroid disorders and prolonged warfarin or corticosteroid intake. Lifestyle factors that increase the risk factors for developing osteoporosis include a low intake of calcium, a low-protein diet, lack of physical activity, smoking and excessive alcohol intake.[23] A number of well-conducted retrospective and randomised studies have identified exercise as an intervention to reduce the risk of bone mineral loss, which is a common factor in all the conditions listed above.[24]

## Summary

- Regular light exercise reduces cancer-related fatigue
- Too much intense exercise can make fatigue worse
- Supervised exercise regimens have the best results for reducing fatigue
- Exercise programmes improve psychological wellbeing
- Group and socially interactive programmes have the best results for improving mood and anxiety levels
- Regular exercise reduces the risk of blood clots during chemotherapy
- Regular exercise during cancer treatments helps prevent weight gain
- Regular exercise helps individuals lose weight after cancer treatments
- The best weight-control programmes combine exercise with a healthy calorie-reducing diet
- Weight-bearing exercise is best to prevent bone loss
- Non-weight-bearing exercise nevertheless also helps to prevent bone loss
- Exercise has to be sustained for several months before any benefits are noticeable

## What type and how much exercise do we need?

In terms of improved wellbeing and reducing side effects of cancer treatment, the best results appear to involve programmes that combine of aerobic and anaerobic exercise, particularly within a social group. Studies have demonstrated benefits in those who practise gym, Medical Qigong and Tai Chi Chuan or those who dance in such styles as Celtic, American, Jazz, Afro-Cuban, Reggae, Middle Eastern and Cajun. The precise amount of exercise has to be determined on an individual basis: the choice of limit depends on such factors as pre-treatment ability, current disability caused by the cancer itself, surgery, radiotherapy or chemotherapy and how much time there is before the next major treatment. Exercise programmes supervised by trained professionals can offer significant advantages. They can design a bespoke regimen that starts slowly and gradually builds up to an acceptable and enjoyable pace. They can help motivate the individual to continue exercising, whether on a short- or long-term basis. They can judge the optimal exercise levels to reduce fatigue, not to aggravate it.

In terms of exercise to reduce the chances of a cancer relapse, most of the cohort studies (studies of a selected group of similar patients) suggest moderate exercise for around two and a half to three hours a week for those with breast cancer, while men had less risk of dying from prostate cancer if they walked for four or more hours per week. In addition, compared with men who walked for less than an hour and a half at an easy walking pace, those who walked for that amount of time (or longer) at a normal to very brisk pace halved the risk of death from all causes. More vigorous activity, and longer duration of activity, was associated with significant further reductions in risk.[25] In a separate study of 1455 men with prostate cancer, researchers found that walking at a pace of at least three miles per hour for three hours or more per week halved the risk of relapse compared with men who walked the same amount, but slower.[26]

## CONCLUDING REMARKS

There is little doubt now that maintaining regular exercise not only reduces the risk of illness, but can also have a significant effect on your recovery. Even during treatment, efforts made to exercise regularly affect energy levels and can accelerate recovery. Many GPs are now able to 'prescribe' sessions at exercise classes, gyms and with personal trainers – do ask your doctor about this. After treatment, exercise will get you well and keep you well. It is all absolutely worth the investment of time and effort.

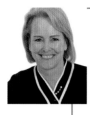

# EXERCISE, OXYGEN AND HORMONES

## OXYGEN AND EXERCISE

Exercise has a direct beneficial effect on the oxygen levels in the body and the environment in which our cells exist. But as with everything in integrative programmes, balance is important: it is possible to overdo things. Ordinary levels of exercise produce free radicals. Intense exercise produces more, which may overwhelm the body, leading to oxidative stress and damage to the very cells you are trying to support.

We have an anabolic/catabolic balance (between constructive and destructive metabolism) in our bodies, the two processes working together to produce a healthy energy level. Catabolism acts as the energy provider and anabolism helps the body draw on that energy for healthy cells. Exercise which is too intense will upset the balance and deplete the cells. So remember to exercise regularly and well, but not to push your body too far.

## OTHER WAYS TO INCREASE OXYGEN LEVELS

The virtues of increasing your oxygen levels are extolled throughout this book. Exercise is clearly vital in this process, but for those of you in a very debilitated condition, not a viable option in the short term. So what else can you do to get more oxygen into your system?

### Hyperbaric oxygen therapy (HBOT)

This therapy involves breathing 100% oxygen in a chamber under pressure (greater than 1 atmosphere, the normal air pressure in which we function every day). Regular air contains 21% oxygen. HBOT has been recommended for a variety of diseases, including multiple sclerosis.

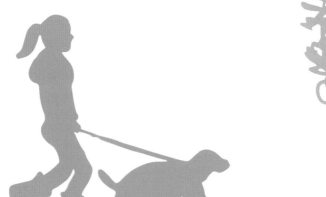
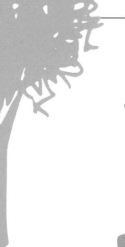

When oxygen is delivered under pressure, the red blood cells carry the maximum amount of oxygen possible. Under these conditions, more oxygen moves into the plasma, where it is carried to the body areas that have decreased blood flow. Some of the many benefits of increased oxygen levels are outlined above (see 'Oxygenation', pp. 40-41 in the 'Therapeutic targets' section of **Chapter 1**, **'Taking an integrative approach'**). Additionally, oxygen improves white blood cells' ability to kill bacteria, and can increase the action of certain antibiotics.

Hyperbaric oxygen chambers can be found in many centres for treating multiple sclerosis, where they are available at a reasonable cost (see **Part Eight, 'Resources'**).

### Oxygen concentrator

There are many models of oxygen concentrator available, the portable ones being easiest for use at home. The machine extracts oxygen from the air, giving up to a 95% concentration (see **Part Eight, 'Resources'**). Some will find the cost prohibitive as good quality machines are several hundred pounds or more. I recommend that they be used only under the supervision of a qualified practitioner.

### Oxygen therapies

Integrative doctors often offer specialised treatments to increase oxygen levels throughout the body, or in some instances, specifically within a tumour. Ozone therapy is one example. Talk to your practitioner if you are interested in pursuing any such approaches.

# HORMONES AND EXERCISE

If you have one of the many cancers influenced by hormones, exercise can be key to how quickly and well you recover, as it is vitally important in hormone regulation. Our bodies need to methylate hormones to ensure that toxic elements don't remain in the body to sustain the growth of cancer cells. Taking regular exercise will help to ensure that your body is capable of reducing potentially harmful hormone levels naturally and healthily.

## MYTHBUSTER

# "OXYGEN CAUSES CANCER CELLS TO GROW"

On the contrary, oxygen actually helps treatments to work better. New understanding is that low levels of oxygen may be the reason that cancer spreads.[27]

# EXERCISING AT HOME OR LOCALLY

## Patricia Peat

A resounding message in this book is the importance of exercise. Suggestions about finding the best forms are offered throughout this chapter. Here I focus on how to achieve regular exercise if symptoms and side effects have depleted your energies and reduced your capacity. Any amount of exercise is good, no matter how little. If you are unwell and become less mobile, within forty-eight hours your muscles will start to break down – so unfair if you have made an effort to develop them. Our lymphatic system slows down and becomes more stagnant, and the process of removing toxins from the body becomes less efficient. All the studies show that resting does nothing to relieve treatment-related fatigue, but exercise does.

Aim to achieve whatever you can manage and the next day aim to extend your goals. If going for a walk, try to make it a brisk and longer one, paying attention to making your body work. If you are in pain, consider cycling or a home bike if this is comfortable. Swimming is excellent for the lymphatics, and the sense of being weightless in water often means that this is the one form of exercise that is unlikely to lead to discomfort. Some people are understandably not keen on the chemicals in swimming pools. If so, have a swim and then rub down afterwards with sodium bicarbonate on a cloth in the shower. The benefits will far outweigh any detriment.

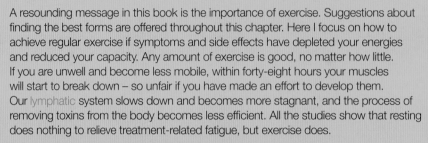

At home there are several easy ways of increasing your exercise regime: rebounders (mini trampolines), for example, are very effective; even if you manage only gentle bouncing, you will be moving the lymph, developing muscle and pushing oxygen round the body more effectively than resting. Walking up and down the stairs a few times every day, increasing duration and speed, is incredibly effective.

Yoga and Pilates (the latter named after its inventor Joseph Pilates,1883-1967) can be gentle ways of getting your muscles moving. Learning to extend and control your breath is both relaxing and invigorating. Deep breathing techniques used in practices such as qigong have proved beneficial for people with cancer (see also **Chapter 3 'Who's who in Integrative Medicine', p. 63, Chapter 3**, for more about qigong).[28]

If you can't get out to a class regularly, there are many DVDs or online videos you can use at home. Try one of the exercise consoles such as Wii or Xbox, for which there are a wide range of fun-based activities that will get you on your feet and moving. There are many dance-based programmes, also great fun – and you can look as daft as you like.

If you are feeling very immobile, after surgery for example, there are small oscillating plates available. You can stand or sit on a Reviber, while the machine tones your muscles. Another device that can be a great help with regaining mobility and improving circulation is the Chi Machine; while you lie down and relax, with your ankles resting on the machine, it creates a gentle, undulating motion throughout your body.

Think about your protein intake and consider glutamine supplementation to enable the building of muscle fibres. Always drink lots of water. You don't have to start running marathons or sign up for Ironman, but you do need to make an effort to take some exercise every day. Invest a little time slot here and there in your daily programme, put them all together and get into the habit of exercising regularly. Before you know it, you have contributed to keeping cancer at bay and made yourself feel good into the bargain. As a cancer 'treatment', exercise surely ranks as one of the most appealing.

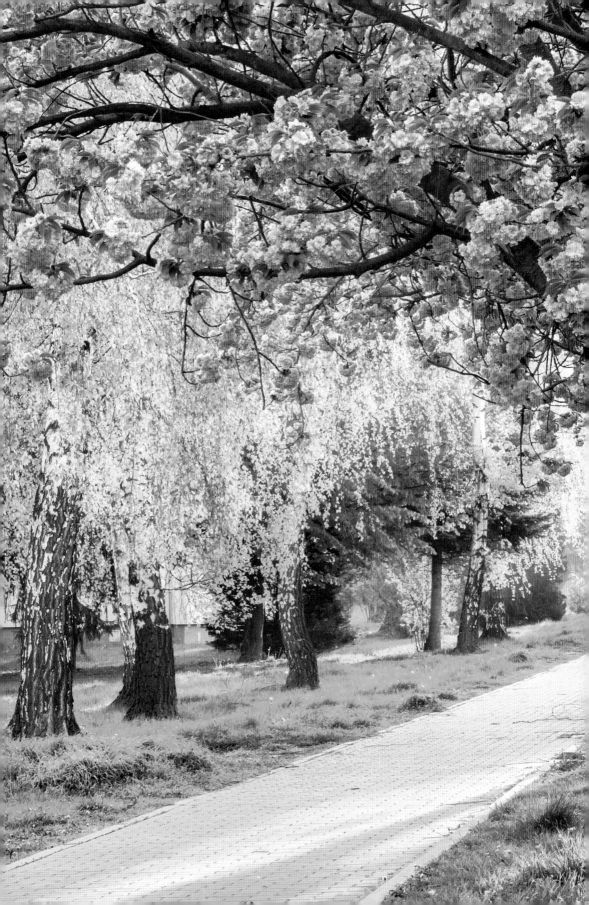

# YOGA EXERCISES FOR YOU TO TRY

Barbara Gallani

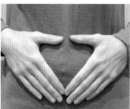 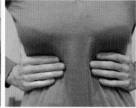 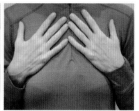

*Pranayama*: use your breathwork to feel calm and grounded

This Sanskrit word means 'extension of breath', which is a central component of yoga practice. As you learn to use your breath, you will begin to feel calm and grounded.

These instructions will guide you through Dirga Pranayama (or three-part breathing), an exercise that you can do either lying on your back or sitting comfortably on the floor, on a cushion or on a chair:

- Close your eyes and observe your natural in-breath and out-breath
- Place your hands on your lower belly and feel the movement of your abdomen under the palms of your hands, with every in-breath and out-breath; continue for at least two minutes
- Now move your hands to the lower ribs, so that your thumbs are hooked around the side of your torso; feel the expansion of the ribcage with every in-breath, but still keep the lower belly soft; continue for at least two minutes
- Next move your hands to the sternum, just below the collarbones; as you breathe in, feel the upper chest lifting and the tops of the lungs filling with air; keep the rest of the body soft and the breath natural, without forcing the air in or out; continue for at least two minutes
- If an area is affected by physical and associated emotional distress, for example as a result of surgery, the muscles tend to tense, and scars or adhesions can also restrict movement; aim to use the breath to bring some movement gently into the affected areas; try to build space with every in-breath, and to maintain the space during each out-breath
- Bring your arms along your body
- Open your eyes

*Namaste**

* This ancient Sanskrit greeting remains in common use in India and Nepal. Rough translations include 'From my heart to yours' or 'The spirit within me salutes the spirit in you'.

## Bird's Breath

In yoga practice a sequence of consecutive poses combining breath and movement is called Vinyasa. One of my favourite sequences, which is intended to bring movement and flexibility to the spine and shoulders, is the Bird's Breath.

Sit tall and comfortably, either on the floor, on a cushion or on a chair. Then:

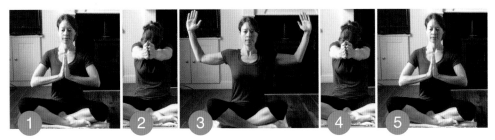

1. Bring the hands into prayer position at the heart and breathe in

2. As you breathe out, bring the chin to the chest, extend the arms forward, keeping the palms of the hands pressed against each other and curve the spine, pushing your navel back

3. As you breathe in, lift the head and open the chest, bringing the arms into cactus-arms pose

4. As you breathe out, bring the chin to the chest, extend the arms forward, keeping the palms of the hands pressed against each other and curve the spine, pushing your navel backwards (as before)

5. As you breathe in, lift the head and bring the hands into prayer position at the chest

Repeat the sequence four or five times.

*Namaste**

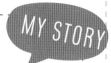

## Susie
### Breast-cancer survivor

*The thought of exercising after the cancer operation and while having radiotherapy was daunting. I was guided by Prof. Rob Thomas' simple advice in his book* Lifestyle and Cancer: The Facts, *to take things very easy and only progress in small steps, when I felt I could. It was tough to start with, but got a little easier, and following the advice and tips, I was comforted by Rob's book.*

*Exercise gave me a new focus, and Rob's advice gave me a structure to follow. The psychological benefits of having somewhere to go, and a focus on exercising were as important, if not more so, than the exercise itself. I have progressed to having exercise as a lifestyle choice thanks to the information provided in the book. Thanks Prof. Rob!*

# Balance Exercises

Lizzy Davis

Always warm up for at least five to ten minutes before beginning these exercises, preparing your body for movement and helping to prevent injury. Try a brisk walk, a gentle dance around the living-room to your favourite piece of music or even some seated marching. All of the following can be practised at home.

## Simple mobilisation exercises

Really try to connect the breath to the movement, inhaling through the nose and exhaling through the mouth. Imagine you are blowing bubbles. Soften the shoulders to begin.

### Shoulder rolls

• Inhale as you lift the shoulders up towards the ears and roll them back down again on the exhale; repeat this three times

• Reverse the direction; repeat this three times

### Shoulder shrugs

• Inhale as you hug the shoulders up towards the ears and release them back down again on the exhale; repeat this three times

### Neck stretches

• Inhale deeply and exhale as you lower the chin towards the chest; inhale to lift the head back up again

• Exhale to tilt the left ear towards the left shoulder, inhale to return to centre

• Exhale to tilt the right ear towards the right shoulder; inhale to return to centre

• Exhale to float the chin over the left shoulder; inhale to return to centre

• Exhale to float the chin over the right shoulder; inhale to return to centre

• Exhale to lower the chin towards the chest; inhale to lift the head back to centre

• Repeat the sequence

## Equilibrium

As children, we respond naturally to anything that challenges our equilibrium. As we age, however, we give less and less thought to the importance of balance, and our sensory receptors become less sensitive. This means that the brain receives less information about the body's position. Balance can often deteriorate as a result of failing eyesight, surgery, loss or change of sensation caused by cancer treatments, restricted range of movement or diminished muscle strength. A fall, or merely feeling anxious about the possibility of falling, may encourage you to withdraw from daily activities, which can then affect your quality of life.

Balance training can help to strengthen your legs and wake up your reflexes, while also improving control, co-ordination, gait and posture as well as enhancing body awareness. Spending just five to ten minutes each day on the following four exercises can make a significant difference.

• Repeat each balance exercise three to five times, once or twice a day

• Use a chair/wall for support if balance is poor to begin with

• As you progress, try incorporating exercises into your daily routine – while standing at the sink, watching TV, in the park, talking on the phone

## Standing/seated side stretch

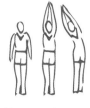

- Begin with arms by your sides; relax the shoulders away from the ears and look ahead
- Pull your abdominal muscles in and up; keep the hips even
- Turn the left palm towards the ceiling; inhale as you slowly raise it up and over the head
- Turn the palm towards the floor; exhale as you lower the arm back down with control
- Repeat on the right side
- Focus on pressing your shoulders down and keeping them level; your neck and back are forced to compensate for uneven shoulders; this affects your spine and compromises balance
- If shoulder range of motion is poor, place fingertips on the shoulder and raise the elbow towards the ceiling

## Single leg stance

This exercise helps to strengthen the hip of the standing leg and improves balance and stability. Breathe deeply throughout:

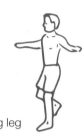

- Look straight ahead and pull the abdominal muscles in and up; keep the hips even and try not to sink into the hip of the leg you are standing on
- Stand with your weight evenly distributed across both feet
- Lift one foot slightly off the ground, shifting your weight over to the supporting leg
- Try to maintain balance for five to twenty seconds before lowering the leg
- Hold onto a stable surface for support or place arms across the chest
- Repeat on the other side

## Heel raise

This exercise will strengthen your legs, hence also stabilising your foundation. Breathe deeply throughout:

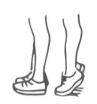

- Stand with your feet hip-width apart and your weight evenly distributed
- Try to think of your feet as the four corners of a room
- Lift your heels so that you are standing on the balls of your feet
- As you slowly lift, try to hold this position and balance for a moment; then bring your heels back down to the floor with control
- Ensure that the ankles are firm and don't roll inwards or outwards
- To develop this exercise, try lifting your arms up over your head as you lift the heels; then slowly lower the arms and heels together

## Leg circles

This exercise encourages you to shift your body constantly, relocating your centre of gravity. Keep the body upright, shoulders relaxed and even, pull the abdominals in and up. Breathe deeply throughout:

- Hold onto a chair for support and stand with feet together to the left of the chair; place your right hand on your hip for added support
- Extend your right foot in front of you and point it, so that the toes are touching the floor
- Slowly trace a circle on the floor by taking your foot to the right, then around to the back, bringing the feet together again in the starting position; repeat this four to six times
- Repeat this with the left leg
- To progress this exercise, try lifting the foot off the floor

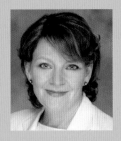

# CHAPTER 9
## MANAGING STRESS

Dr Rosy Daniel

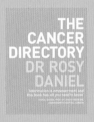

HEALTH
CREATION

## THE IMPORTANCE OF EMOTIONAL SUPPORT

Despite the early controversy and battles fought to promote understanding of the emotional and self-help needs of people with cancer, there is now hardly any cancer centre, hospice or support group in the UK that does not offer some level of emotional, spiritual or complementary therapy to help you through whatever problems you are facing. Indeed, we are now well advanced in the development of 'survivorship programmes' based on helping those who have survived cancer and its treatment to deal positively with the changes that cancer has created in their work, finances, relationships, wellbeing and mental health.

There are, however, a huge ideological differences when it comes to the ethos underpinning these services and in the beliefs held by those running them. And these differences are of major significance to those using them. Critically, professionals and support workers within the integrative health movement believe that working with emotions and the interacting state of mind and body can activate our immunity and self-healing, promoting physical recovery and improvement of our chances of survival. By contrast, many emotional cancer-support services are targeted towards the emotionally based goals of learning how to develop our coping skills, how to accept and improve our current quality of life, and when the time comes, perhaps even how to have a good quality of dying. This difference is like night and day to those confronted with the limited power of modern medicine to cure cancer. It is healing work at the powerful interface of body, mind and spirit which has motivated every single day of my twenty-five year career as an Integrative Medicine Cancer Consultant, guiding people to get the best of all worlds, orthodox and complementary, while crucially activating self-healing, health-promoting beliefs, behaviours and lifestyles.

What was started entirely intuitively by Penny Brohn and her support team at the Bristol Cancer Help Centre in 1980 (renamed Penny Brohn Cancer Care in 2006) has now been proven by mind-body science, and the evidence for the role of mind in quality of life and survival is now so strong that in my opinion it is completely unethical for psycho-spiritual care not to be provided routinely for everyone who is diagnosed with cancer. This chapter discusses the discoveries made since the 1990s and also explains how that research can help you find the resources and therapies you need.

PENNY
BROHN

But first, let's take a step back and acknowledge, before anything else, that there are emotional needs and stresses that *everyone* who is diagnosed with cancer has in common. Given that you are reading this, there is a good chance that you or someone close to you has been newly diagnosed and is experiencing the shock, fear and uncertainty that diagnosis brings with it. If that is so, my heart goes out to you, and I now offer the following facts that have the power to provide you with comfort.

# TEN VITAL FACTS FOR YOU TO KNOW AND COMMIT TO MEMORY

**01** Cancer is a two-way process; it can grow but it can also shrink or go into remission

**02** People have recovered from every single kind of cancer and are living to tell the tale

**03** A healthy body has detection and repair mechanisms for cancer cells; the integrative healthcare approach works to repair and boost these natural anti-cancer mechanisms within the body

**04** Apart from orthodox medicine, there are many factors over which you have primary control and that can positively affect your health and wellbeing

**05** Your personal response to your cancer can make a huge difference to both your quality of life and survival

**06** You are a unique individual; average medical statistics cannot be applied to individuals

**07** Your conventional treatment is only one component of your approach to fighting cancer

**08** You do not have to rely entirely on the effectiveness of medical treatment alone to 'cure' you of cancer; give up the passive patient role and join forces with your doctors, getting as proactive as possible in recovering your health

**09** It is you, not your medical team, who is in overall charge of your situation; your doctors are there to serve you and it is your wishes, not theirs, that really matter

**10** Astonishingly, many people who have embarked on the self-healing approach to cancer have landed up saying that they are actually grateful for their illness because they have come to feel much happier, healthier and more alive than ever before

Keep re-reading these facts until the message sinks in. I suggest that you copy them onto a card or phone to carry with you at all times.

You can then read them again whenever you feel the need.

Go forward in the knowledge that:

- You are a very powerful person in your anti-cancer team
- There is a great deal of help available to strengthen, support and guide you in your treatment and self-help programme
- It is possible to stabilise and live with cancer; it is equally possible to go into remission altogether
- A cancer diagnosis can start a profound and exciting journey of healing and self-development, giving you the push and permission to change what may have been making you ill or unhappy for years
- This book is here to help you understand and discover every type of help that is available; it has been written to empower you in both your fight against cancer and your personal healing journey

## Facing the demons

It is very important for you to identify and change any negative beliefs that you have about cancer, so that you don't risk buying into these beliefs and giving up before you even start. This chapter goes on to show that what we believe can have an extremely strong bearing on the outcomes of our chosen treatments.

So straight away I must protect you from taking on board and succumbing to negative programming, whether this is based on your own beliefs about cancer, your family's beliefs or society's collective fear. It is also vital that you do not take to heart statistics from your consultant about average survival times with your particular kind of cancer. These are generally based on results of outdated medical treatments that were recommended to people who were not proactive in their own defence. Average survival rates will mask the results of people who have done extremely well and are still living happily in total remission. Please remember that statistics connot be applied to individuals. The course of your illness and recovery is unique to you. There are over two hundres types of cancer and the way each one develops is different in everyone who has it. Challenge and change your negative beliefs by re-reading the ten facts on the previous page. People really have survived with every single kind of cancer, even reversing and surviving late stage cancers. There is no reason why it should not be you who has a remarkable recovery and goes on to be living proof of these facts.

## Understanding your emotional needs and how to meet them

While I was Medical Director at Bristol Cancer Help Centre (1993-9), we ran a research project with the help of the Bristol Oncology Centre and Warwick University's Department of Sociology. Fifty-four people with cancer and their carers in four major UK cities were asked about the emotional journey they had experienced through the diagnosis and treatment of cancer. These were not people who had come to Bristol, but a group made up of those who responded to an invitation from their medical team to participate in this qualitative research.

The range of emotions and feelings that these people had experienced was immense: fear, confusion, anger, despair, terror, isolation, confusion and bewilderment; in some cases there was elation and even relief to have an excuse to stop and take a complete break from the pressures of life. Coping strategies ranged from taking full control in finding information and engaging with the best medicine, through exploring therapies and self-help systems, to having none at all. The resources that they found varied greatly, with some finding full-spectrum holistic support, while others had never found or been offered any support whatsoever. The emotional outcomes therefore ranged from being positively transformative at one end of the scale to remaining in unpleasant anxious preoccupation or helplessness at the other. Clearly this was very far from equitable and it pointed to a huge gap in the provision of emotional care. Furthermore, it underlined that some people were natural fighters who would go out and find every possible type of resource, while others were much weaker in their own defence.

The resulting piece of work *Meeting the Needs of People with Cancer for Support and Self-Management*, quoting from those consulted, could be summarised as follows:[1]

- Our emotional needs are as great if not greater than our physical needs when diagnosed with cancer, and we need emotional support services to be provided routinely alongside our medical care

- We need complementary therapies and psychological, spiritual and emotional support services alongside our medical services to help us cope better with our mental, physical and spiritual symptoms; it is urgent that equitable access is provided to these services throughout the UK, and not just to the lucky few whose hospitals provide services themselves or information about how to access support services in the community

- We need to be cared for by healthcare professionals with excellent communication skills, people who will listen to and respect our needs and healthcare values

- Our need to find alternative ways to fight for our lives must be taken seriously and supported by our healthcare professionals in the light of the often limited power of medicine to cure us

- We need an unbiased link worker to help us understand our state, needs and healthcare values and to inform us about the full range of support and self-help services that exist

The really helpful outcome of this work was that we were able to identify the points of greatest vulnerability encountered along the cancer journey; studying the emotional needs that everyone had encountered helped us to define our 'ten key needs'. We also heard about the range of resources that people consulted to meet these needs and what strategies were found to be the most useful. These are summarised in the table on the following pages so that you can quickly identify your current stage and immediately check that you are doing all you can to get appropriate support.

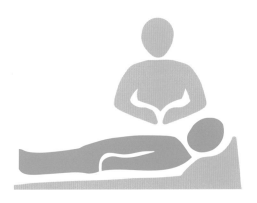

# MEETING THE TEN KEY EMOTIONAL NEEDS

## MEETING YOUR EMOTIONAL NEEDS

| VULNERABLE TIME | THE TEN KEY NEEDS | |
|---|---|---|
| 1 Facing getting tested for possible cancer | Support to get a clear diagnosis (especially if you are too frightened to face going to the doctor) | You may need to:<br>• Get a friend to go through the process with you<br>• Talk to a counsellor to help you work through your fears and resistance to seeking medical help<br>• Get a hypnotherapist to help you deal with any phobias you have<br>• Talk to an integrative doctor or your GP to help you evaluate the seriousness of your situation, and to form a strategy to get the help you need |
| 2 Waiting for and going to get test results | Support to face getting the diagnosis | While waiting for test results, do you need:<br>• A talk with your GP to find out more about what you might expect to hear?<br>• A talk with your practice nurse, health visitor, social worker or the practice counsellor?<br>• A talk with your consultant or the hospital support team?<br>• A talk with a counsellor?<br>• To confide in a friend or family member?<br>• To tell colleagues at work and arrange to be excused from normal work duties?<br>• To take time off work?<br>• To cancel social events?<br>• To speed up results if you have been waiting for over a week by telephoning your GP, the practice nurse, the consultant's secretary or the pathology department at the hospital where your tests were done?<br><br>And when you go to get your results:<br>• Do you want to go alone or with a supporter?<br>• Is there someone who can be at the end of a phone to support you or stay with you overnight if the news is bad?<br>• Is this arrangement confirmed?<br>• Will you ask the clinic staff beforehand if there are any support staff in the hospital to help you if the news is bad, such as a counsellor, psychologist, chaplain, social worker or volunteer, specialist nurses or complementary therapists? |

| 3 | Receiving a diagnosis (or re-diagnosis) | Help with reaction to the shock and upset of diagnosis, with emphasis on taking time, not making important decisions while in shock, allowing for the effects of shock in home and work life | Take really good care of yourself and be sure to:<br>• Make allowances for the degree of shock you are in<br>• Take your time to go through your emotional reaction before trying to make important decisions<br>• Adjust your own and others' expectations of what you will be able to do while you are in shock<br>• Realise that the full range of emotions being experienced is normal<br>• Seek immediate help in the community from your GP, the surgery counsellor if there is one, the practice nurse, practice health visitor or social worker, Macmillan or Marie Curie nurses or relevant spiritual advisers<br>• Seek help at work from the occupational health and/or human resource team<br>• Think carefully about what you are going to tell to whom, who will deliver the news to others and who will provide the support for the close ones in your circle, those who may also be shocked and upset |
|---|---|---|---|
| 4 | Feeling isolated and frightened after diagnosis | Help to set up the appropriate emotional support network | Set up an appropriate emotional support network, especially if you live alone' by:<br>• Getting a counsellor[2]<br>• Joining a community support group, whether general, holistic, relating to gender, race, religion, type of illness or disability<br>• Thinking about creating a personal support group (see Appendix 3, 'When Do You Need a Practitioner?')<br>• Finding a cancer buddy who has been through what you are experiencing<br>• Communicating your state and needs well to your carers, family, friends and colleagues |
| 5 | Facing and making the right treatment decision for you | The need to find high-quality information in order to make an informed decision and appropriate support and guidance to make an authentic one | Get all the information to make a treatment decision from all relevant sources before agreeing to treatment:<br>• For orthodox medicine, from your consultant, GP, second opinion specialists in national and international centres of excellence for your type of cancer, Macmillan Cancer Options, Cancer Research UK<br>• For Integrative Medicine, from Integrative Medicine Consultants, Yes to Life, Cancer Options<br>• For alternative medicines, from specialist alternative medicine doctors, centres and information services, Yes to Life, Cancer Options |

157

# MEETING THE TEN KEY EMOTIONAL NEEDS

| VULNERABLE TIME | THE TEN KEY NEEDS | MEETING YOUR EMOTIONAL NEEDS |
|---|---|---|
| 5 continued | | Find help to clarify your own wishes in the light of conflicting advice and differing healthcare values: |
| | | • Good sources of help are Integrative Medicine consultants, who aim to form a bridge between orthodox and alternative medicine, enabling patients to get the best of both worlds |
| | | • GPs (who can be supportive, but generally know little about holistic possibilities) |
| | | • The Cancer Options Team offers a service to find out about all the medical frontier treatments and new research findings for your type of cancer |
| | | • Yes to Life supports patients in building their own integrative treatment programme |
| | | Never forget that the key and final authority is you; you will know somewhere inside what is right for you; you may just need to be given the necessary space, time and support to tune in to this knowing; you will then find the courage to follow your convictions |
| 6 Preparing for treatment | Making the appropriate psychological preparations pre-treatment | Make appropriate preparations for treatment by: |
| | | Preparing mentally |
| | | • Develop a strong belief in your treatment and visualise it healing you (you may find my CD 'Cope Positively with the Symptoms and Treatment of Cancer' useful at this point |
| | | • Reduce fear and anxiety levels through Emotional Freedom Technique (EFT), hypnosis, relaxation therapy, relaxation/meditation exercises, counselling, massage and healing |
| | | • Get all the information about how the treatment will be, so that you are in control |
| | | Preparing physically |
| | | • Read Part Two of *The Cancer Revolution*; consider adopting my Eat Right plan or Tough Times plan to optimise your nutrition; if time, do two or three days detox |
| | | • Take recommended vitamin and mineral supplements |
| | | • Cut out smoking and drinking if possible |
| | | • Build your energy levels with healing and other energy medicine |
| | | • Rest well |
| | | • Take appropriate exercise (examples available on the Stretch and Breathe tracks of my 'Cope Positively' CD) |
| | | • Drink plenty of good water (see 'The importance of water' p. 94) |

Preparing practically
- Prepare the family and all your support team
- Delegate your major work and social responsibilities
- Organise shopping, cooking and cleaning or delegate to others
- Make your home feel clean, comfortable and calm for your return from treatment

| 7 | Facing treatment and getting the best possible treatment outcomes | Making the appropriate psychological preparations going through treatment and after treatment |
|---|---|---|

Going through treatment:
- Research the likely side effects of treatment and be prepared with all the complementary remedies or therapies that have been pre-identified to help you
- Know how you will access support when you are in hospital
- Based on the advice of your practitioners, organise an appropriate amount of time off work
- Tell the medical team if you are having adverse reactions, either physically or emotionally
- If it is too much, ask the team to stop treatment until you are able to cope

When in hospital:
- If you are to be an in-patient, arrange for good food and drink to be brought to you e.g. soups, home-made juices, salads, fruit, good water
- Bring your supplements and an iPod or portable CD player, relaxation recordings and your favourite music
- Think about arranging for a healer, masseur or reflexologist to visit you in hospital

Recovery from surgery:
- Make adequate convalescent plans in advance; choose physiotherapy, yoga, massage, osteopathy or craniosacral therapy as required.

Recovery from radiotherapy:
- Be aware that the flare reaction and energy depletion can continue for up to six weeks
- Convalesce properly, as recommended by your practitioners
- Get good energy therapy and do a detox programme

Recovery from chemotherapy:
- Do a detox programme
- Take build-up drinks, supplements and immune stimulants to get your weight and your immune system back to normal
- Convalesce properly, as recommended by your practitioners, taking the time you need off work to recover fully before taking up full duties again

# MEETING THE TEN KEY EMOTIONAL NEEDS

| VULNERABLE TIME | THE TEN KEY NEEDS | MEETING YOUR EMOTIONAL NEEDS |
|---|---|---|
| 8 Facing the changes and losses that treatment may bring | Help to think about adaptations you may need to make to your lifestyle and self-image – in both the short and long term – due to the illness and its treatment | It is important that you:<br><br>• Prepare yourself emotionally, preferably before any loss occurs (e.g. of any organ or of hair); you can do this by honouring the way you have been until now through enjoying your own ritual, photographs and portraits or remembering playful adventures<br>• Take time to process feelings; grieve your loss and come to accept and love the new you<br>• Find support groups that deal specifically with the issue you are now confronting. For example, there are groups for people with intestinal stomas, facial disfigurement, lymphoedema, loss of limbs and many other conditions<br>• Find ways to deal with these changes creatively through beauticians, stylists, prosthetic specialists, wig makers<br>• Find support to explore new ways of expressing yourself physically and sexually if your mobility and sexuality have been affected |
| 9 Facing the end of treatment | Coping when the medical support system goes; help with planning the route to recovery and rekindling hope and motivation | Embarking positively on a proactive self-healing and prevention strategy:<br><br>• Adopt a 'survivorship programme' such as the Living Well programme of Penny Brohn Cancer Care or mentorship through the Health Creation Programme<br>• Think about your 'coping style' – having 'fighting spirit' conveys a significant survival advantage compared with stoicism, anxious preoccupation and helplessness; it is important to get psychological support to move into fighting spirit if you are not naturally a fighter<br>• Build in lots of extra support, especially if you live alone<br>• Think about the circumstances in which you got ill and whether you can make healthy changes in your lifestyle going forward<br>• Think about the message of illness<br>• Become clear whether there is any secondary gain in being ill (e.g. attracting attention) that can be diverted into safer, healthier activites<br>• Work at understanding the causes of cancer; remember that a healthy body fends off cancer so that you can maximally support your body to prevent recurrence<br>• Take charge of your health and wellbeing, moving from passive patient to proactive self-healing |

- Let go of your dependency on the medical model alone to prevent recurrence
- Improve your immune function by working with the mind-body connection
- Determine the areas of vulnerability in your own health, state and lifestyle and (if necessary) get the coaching/mentorship support you need to change
- Enjoy a nutritious, healthy diet to nourish, cleanse and defend your body
- Lift your energy at all levels – body, mind and spirit – to re-power your body's fighting force
- Use the power of the mind to visualise yourself healed
- Eliminate excessive stress and over-activity
- Engage in that which excites and fulfils you in life
- Nourish your spirit with beauty, love and a form of spiritual communion that works for you, whether through healing energies and/or prayer

| 10 | Facing your worst fears | Looking directly at your beliefs and fears about death and dying (whether that happens soon or much later) will help you to achieve peace of mind and clarity about your needs and wishes | Working with a mentor or spiritual advisor, you could:<br>• Go through your emotional reaction to confronting your mortality<br>• Look at the big questions about the meaning of life and death for you and what unfinished business you may have to take care of before the end of your life<br>• Prepare yourself emotionally, practically and spiritually for the end of your life, however far away that might be, so that you are not living in fear<br>• Create an advance directive for your carers so that your wishes will be known and respected |

Wherever you are on this emotional journey, help is at hand to meet your needs and get you back into a calm, positive and well-supported place. In **Part Eight**, 'Resources', at the end of the book you will be able to locate all the best support resources. Remember, if things are tough, it is usually because you don't have enough support. Do not struggle on your own, bottling up your feelings and trying to keep everything going as normal. 'Normal' is where you got ill. Learning to express your feelings, share your vulnerability and crucially become able to receive help will not only improve your coping skills but become a vital part of the change needed for you to recover your health and flourish in life.

## How work with the mind-body connection affects health and survival

While Penny and her therapy team at the Bristol Cancer Help Centre felt convinced that our personal reaction to cancer can make all the difference to our survival, the first evidence for this came in the mid-1980s from Dr Steven Greer at the Royal Marsden Hospital in London. He had witnessed how those with natural fighting spirit tended to do very much better than those who collapsed into anxiety and helplessness. In fact, his first seminal study showed that at the five-year point, there was a staggering 60 per cent difference in survival between those found by his team in the first week of diagnosis to display fighting spirit, i.e. those with a positive belief that they could influence the outcome of their illness, and those who did not.[3] In later studies he was not able to repeat the positive finding for those with fighting spirit, but he repeatedly found that those who were depressed and anxious fared worse than those who were coping well. Critically, for those who do not have fighting spirit naturally, he was then able to demonstrate that with Cognitive Behavioural Therapy (CBT), his patients could significantly improve their coping style and self-belief with commensurate improvement in outcomes.

Since Greer's early work, there have been a number of studies that show both that up to half of all people with cancer are depressed, and also, worryingly, that the depressed are at greater risk with cancer.[4, 3] In other words, the same illness has a different prognosis according to the mental state of the person. These facts alone mean that the provision of positive psychological support and the learning of good coping strategies to beat depression are not just a 'nice to have' comfort for those with cancer, but a vital therapeutic intervention which may well be as potent as the medical treatment. Positive evidence of improved rates of survival was also shown in those attending support groups.[5]

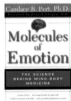

Next, there was a great breakthrough in understanding with the advent of the new science of psychoneuroimmunology (PNI), during the 1990s, pioneered by Dr Candace Pert (1948-2013) and colleagues in *Molecules of Emotion*, which gives definitive proof that our emotions profoundly affect our body chemistry, immune systems and the functioning of all body tissues. This science shows that communication within the body is not just coming to and from our brains but that all of our cells make and receive messages via 'informational substances' known as neuropeptides. If we are sad, depressed, stressed and emotionally repressed, our tissue functioning also becomes depressed. Most critically in cancer, this means that cells lose their innate protection mechanisms and also that our immune function depletes, resulting in there being fewer white bloods cells that are less aggressive in nature and with a lower number of the all important natural killer (NK) cells that can detect and kill cancer cells.

It is vital to realise that our emotions and moods are not the cause of cancer. The disease forms in tissues that are inflamed by either carcinogenic chemicals, infections or radiation, which cause gene mutation. We are all exposed to these factors to some degree. Gene mutation is more common in tissues that are older, acidic, low in oxygen and high in sugar, all of which can promote the growth of infective agents, including fungus in the body. Resulting gene mutations can be corrected if we have the right levels of protective vegetable plant nutrients and oxygen in our system, and they can be avoided altogether if our body-mind chemistry is right. Beyond that, we are further protected by an abnormal cell-suicide system called 'apoptosis' which destroys abnormal cells if the right genes are switched on in our cells. If that fails to happen, our immune T-cells should be able to detect and destroy cancer cells if they form. If our immune cells are in poor condition, whether because we are exhausted, sad, dispirited and/or full of the stress chemicals adrenaline and cortisol, our bodies are 'off guard' and disease states can develop. But this can be reversed through good integrative healthcare and self-help. There is no place whatsoever for any sense of guilt or blame, just a big window of hope opening, allowing us to listen to the message that our bodies are giving us, and to restore healthy balance in all aspects of our lives.

Controversy has raged for decades about whether stress can make us vulnerable to cancer and heart disease; some people appear to be more able than others to tolerate high levels of stress without getting ill. In 1978, however, Dr Suzanne Kobasa of the City University New York discovered that those who are prone to suffering ill-effects from stress are likely to have a 'learned helplessness' response to difficulties, rather than what she called 'personality hardiness' and a tendency to thrive on challenge. It has also been shown that if we have developed certain psychological skills, we will be at less risk than those who are stressed and without any power to control their situation.[6]

Happily, there are many ways that we can take charge of our emotional state, and it has now been proven that even if our self-belief and fighting spirit is low, with the right balance of counselling, mentorship, cognitive behavioural therapy (CBT), hypnosis and/or loving support, we can change our underlying beliefs and coping styles, thus developing the mindset and associated blood chemistry that goes with being a fighter and a survivor.

Furthermore, even when therapy and support is not available we can change our own body chemistry through practising various self-help techniques, including relaxation, breathwork, meditation and visualisation. This is called auto-regulation, in which individuals achieve mastery over the state of their bodies through deliberate practices. In 1972, Candace Pert and colleagues finally identified the opiate receptor, laying the basis for the subsequent discovery of endorphins, the body's natural form of morphine neuro-peptide that is produced when we feel happy, loving and satisfied. Since then, not only has mindfulness meditation been shown to reverse depression and anxiety but being able to visualise blood counts improving and chemotherapy curing us is known to have measurable physical benefits. Furthermore, Prof. Walker showed that people having chemotherapy who were taught to imagine it curing them had over 17 per cent better survival rates thirteen years later, more than doubling the benefit of the chemotherapy, which conferred a 15 per cent benefit.[7]

The next breakthrough in our understanding has come from the science of epigenetics (a term coined in 1942 for the study of external or environmental factors that turn genes on and off). Throughout the 1980s and 90s, Dr Dean Ornish began to open the door to an even deeper understanding of the power of the mind to heal the body, and in 2005, Bruce Lipton's seminal book *The Biology of Belief* described how our predominant states of mind affect the expression of our genes. Dr Ornish provided evidence of this through his GEMINAL study, published in 2013, which examined a group of men with prostate cancer who were engaged in emotional support groups, yoga, relaxation, low-fat diet and daily exercise. Within only twelve weeks on this lifestyle programme, the men displayed dramatic changes in their cells; as key oncogenes became protectively regulated, oncogenes promoting cancer were down-regulated and those suppressing cancer were up-regulated, resulting in measurable drops in the tumour-marker PSA levels.[8] Ornish later stated that these results are just as dependent on the emotional support and improvement in mental state as on improvements in fitness and nutrition.[9]

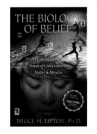

Thus we can see that support, emotional healing and the development of positive states of mind and spirit are far more important than simply making us feel better. They help create the climate within the body in which all of our healing mechanisms activate, and this can provide the crucial step to take us into remission from cancer.

Certainly in all my work since the early 1990s, which has focused on self-healing in my clients, I would say that it is almost always when people re-ignite their passion for life and raise their spiritual and mental energy that great recoveries occur. And usually the catalyst for this is love – a huge love of life and everything that is precious, a love that is re-ignited when life is threatened. But the big healing happens when the shift is made towards a great love of ourselves, changing any tendency to overwork, stress, neglect and abandon ourselves into a newly respectful way of caring for ourselves. Of the countless people I know who have recovered from cancer, all have said that they needed to learn the magic word 'No' and to begin to put themselves at the very top of the list of people about whom they care.

## Staying true to yourself on your self-healing journey

As we reach the end of this chapter, I am sure that you will realise that taking the path in which you believe is the most powerful thing that you can do to gain control of your situation. Placebo studies have repeatedly confirmed that when we believe in our medicines and healers, they help us in a way that is far stronger than the power of the medicine and practitioner alone. It is therefore essential that we listen to our own intuition about what is right for us, that we stay absolutely true to what we know we need. In the first flurry of fear and panic that can be overwhelming when we are newly diagnosed, it is easy to get swept along and accede to the wishes of others. But this is your life, your body and your decision. Do not allow yourself to be rushed, bullied or emotionally blackmailed into treatments that you do not want. Surround yourself with those who enable you to hear your own highest truth and who will support you to stick to it. Your doctors are there to serve you and not the other way around. If you choose a path that is not the one that that they have suggested, that is your decision and they must honour and support it. Similarly, if family members would do things differently themselves, again you must politely tell them that you appreciate their concern, but that the best way they can support you is by lovingly encouraging you to be absolutely true to yourself. The role of a good Integrative Medicine consultant is to explain to you all your choices – medical, complementary, psycho-spiritual and self-help – and then support you to create the very best and most powerful programme for you.

## Summary

This chapter explores the emotional needs of people diagnosed with cancer and offers advice on how we can meet these needs to:

- Understand and process what is happening to us
- Strengthen our ability to cope
- Build our personal support team
- Develop positive beliefs and healthy hope to sustain our fighting spirit
- Deepen our loving relationships and ability to communicate our needs, wishes and desires

We have learned that work with our mind-body-spirit connection improves not only our peace of mind and quality of life, but also enhances our health and survival.

We have understood that if we embark on a self-healing journey and tensions arise in relation to our medical team, family and friends, we must learn to:

- Listen to and follow our authentic truth
- Allow others to have their say while making them aware that ultimately all decisions about our health, wellbeing, quality of life are ours; and have to be based upon our own truth

We have learned that scientific research has now established, beyond doubt, that the mind-body connection is one of the most powerful tools in supporting recovery of the body.

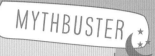

# "INTEGRATIVE MEDICINE PRACTITIONERS RAISE 'FALSE HOPE' IN PATIENTS WITH A POOR PROGNOSIS"

Many patients complain of being given a 'realistic' prognosis by their oncologist, based on statistics. The effect of this is often to destroy their 'reasonable' hope. Statistics cannot 'realistically' be applied to individuals, and proactive patients can strongly influence their chances. Good practitioners know how to work skillfully with people at each stage of illness, setting realistic expectations and goals. Even at later stages, integrative approaches can help with quality of life, but that is a world away from promises of easy cures. People, and particularly families, can often place unrealistic expectations on integrative therapies when standard care has failed, for which the practitioners are blamed. A good relationship is based on an acknowledgement and clear view of the situation and of what may be achieved.

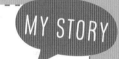

## Kathy Wickam
Breast-cancer survivor

*In June 2011, aged 69, I had a mastectomy and lymph nodes removed. I decided to decline further treatment and follow a natural path, as I had a strong belief in the power of self-healing and natural medicine. I contacted Dr Rosy Daniel for a consultation, and we quickly worked out that I needed emotional healing. So she referred me to an Emotional Freedom Technique practitioner who is also a spiritual healer.*

*Throughout my life I had felt really unvalued and unloved, and unaccepted for who I was. I was carrying a lot of anger from childhood abandonment. But over time I came to develop a strong self-love, having experienced unconditional higher love during the healing sessions. This also had a direct effect on me physically and, without a shadow of doubt, on my immune system too.*

*As well as attending to my emotional healing, I have fully embraced a healthier diet, supplements, natural chemotherapy, acupuncture, shiatsu, yoga, and enjoy lots of lovely fresh air and fun. I have to say that I have never felt so well, happy and alive, and surrounded by so much love from my family and friends. I am still on my journey to full health, but what an amazing journey this is, full of miracles and learning to live fully each moment, every day.*

# CHAPTER 10

## SUNSHINE AND VITAMIN D

### Dr Damien Downing

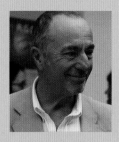

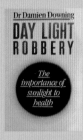

DR DAMIEN
DOWNING

Vitamin D is the nutrient that is single-handedly establishing the case for the vital role of the correct nutritional elements for recovery and survival in cancer. As typically found in Integrative Medicine, this proves to be true not only of cancer but also of many chronic diseases. Vitamin-D deficiency is linked with development of Parkinson's disease, multiple sclerosis, heart disease, muscle weakness in the elderly and many other chronic conditions.

Researchers are now discovering the many elements that regulate cell function. The role of vitamin D is complex: with cancer, a key function is apparently to control inflammation in the body; its regulation of calcium and phosphorous is also attracting research. We have long cast envious glances at some of our European neighbours and their lower levels of cancer, attributing it to a healthier diet. While that is undoubtedly true, it may well be that their greater exposure to sunshine may also be a leading factor (all too often, those of us in the UK can settle for only two weeks of sunshine per year). What is certain is that having inadequate vitamin-D levels increases our risks of developing many types of cancer, and that supplementing vitamin D reduces those risks and increases our chances of recovery.

Some basic facts about vitamin D:

- If you are deficient in vitamin D, you are four times more likely to develop cancer than if you are not
- Vitamin D is only a 'vitamin' because we do not get enough of it from sunlight
- Most people throughout the world are deficient in vitamin D
- Even in Australia and the Arabian Gulf, lifestyles and the use of sunscreens mean that most people are deficient

Almost everybody is deficient in vitamin D. Unless you have just returned from a summer holiday on a sunny beach, you too are very likely to be deficient in this crucial nutrient, which, as already noted above, is only a vitamin (i.e. needing to be obtained from food) because we do not get enough sunlight to enable us to manufacture it in our skin. In the UK, the government's advisory committee on these matters, the Scientific Advisory Committee on Nutrition, still sets the threshold for deficiency ridiculously low at 25 nmol/l (nanomoles per litre is the standard measurement used to quantify the level of vitamin D in the blood); see Illustration 1.

To put this in context: even using this ultra-low benchmark, 15 per cent of all adults are deficient, rising to 30 per cent in those over sixty-five and, curiously, 25 per cent in those aged between nineteen and twenty-four.[1] In the USA, over 50 per cent of adults are below their official deficiency level, and this seems to hold true for the entire world.[2] Using a higher, but still not optimal threshold of 75 nmol/l, a London-based informal study of results from a nutritional testing service found that 95 per cent of users were deficient in vitamin D.[3] It is not known how many of them were cancer sufferers.

Illustration 2 shows that it takes about 4000 IU of vitamin-D supplements to bring the serum level to around 100 nmol/l. Above that point, further increases have progressively less impact as the body's feedback mechanisms cut in. Responses vary considerably, however, from one individual to another, which has led the campaigning group D*Action to recommend taking 6000 IU per day to ensure a serum level over 100. Compare this with the 20,000 IU that a healthy young adult will manufacture on exposing most of his/her skin to mid-day summer sun for twenty minutes, even in the UK. The vitamin-D yield will be half that for older people, but note that they are not advised to expose themselves for longer if this could lead to a risk of sunburn.

It is important to note that people of Asian or African origin have higher levels of the pigment melatonin in their skin, which delays both vitamin-D production and burning, so they can and should extend their exposure time by a factor of two (Asians) or three (Africans). Given this, it is no surprise that Reinhold Vieth's challenge to the biomedical community, to demonstrate an instance of vitamin-D toxicity at doses less than 10,000 IU per day, remains unanswered.[4]

The very few cases of vitamin-D toxicity that have occurred are in fact all at over 100,000 IU per day.

* See table of skin types on p.169

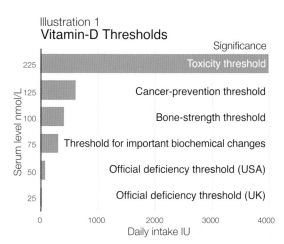

Illustration 1
**Vitamin-D Thresholds**

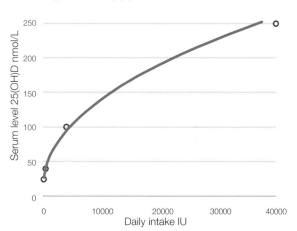

Illustration 2
**Vitamin-D Blood** Serum Levels

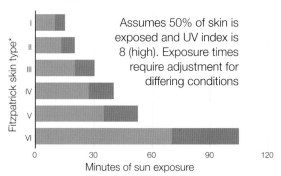

Illustration 3
**Recommended exposure for different skin types**

Assumes 50% of skin is exposed and UV index is 8 (high). Exposure times require adjustment for differing conditions

In evolutionary terms, this makes sense – humanity developed in the tropics, without any clothes, and worked outdoors. Electric light is now available in most places and some of us may go outside for only minutes or even seconds a day, when moving between the front door and the car, or the train station and the office. This was clearly shown in a study done in 1983 in San Diego, one of the sunniest cities in the USA.[5] Sunlight deprivation has been happening, and getting worse, for at least a century – not long enough for our bodies to adapt, but long enough for the effects to be passed down from generation to generation. And passed down it is: mothers who are low in vitamin D suffer more complications and need more Caesarean sections than others; their offspring are less healthy and at greater risk of diabetes and atherosclerosis as they age. A 2011 study showed that it is safe and effective to give pregnant women 4000 IU of vitamin D a day.[6]

Another study from 2007 even suggests that vitamin D may slow down the ageing process, because higher vitamin-D levels were associated with greater telomere length (telomeres are the repeating endpieces on chromosomes that are shortened by one every time the cell replicates). The difference in telomere length between the lowest and highest vitamin-D levels was estimated to translate to five years of life.[7]

It is also likely that there are benefits other than increased production of vitamin D to be obtained from sunlight. Research since the early 20th century suggests that ultraviolet (UV) may kill tuberculosis organisms by oxidative damage – nothing to do with vitamin D. This may also be so for a number of other skin diseases which sunlight is known to help, including eczema, psoriasis, vitiligo and scleroderma. Sunlight's mood-elevating effects may have as much to do with beta-endorphin release as with vitamin D. And UV light hitting the skin produces nitric oxide, which is the subject of intense research interest for its widening of blood vessels (vasodilation), immune boosting, regulation of the nervous system (neuromodulation) and other effects.

It would probably be easier to list the mechanisms that are not relevant to vitamin D's anti-cancer effect than those that are. Leaving aside the important issue of the 'Warburg effect' (see 'The dangers of glucose', pp 85-6, in Chapter 5, 'Diet as the foundation of good health', p.85) – cancer cells' impaired ability to use oxygen to generate energy – such cells exhibit several behaviours that are clearly different from healthy cells, and clearly necessary for a cancer to thrive:

- Uncontrolled proliferation – the normal processes that inhibit growth are absent

- Loss of differentiation – healthy cells grow to be clearly identifiable as one specific type, e.g. liver cells

- Enhanced angiogenesis – generally a healthy process for growth and wound healing; a growing tumour uses angiogenesis to increase its blood supply by invading adjacent tissue with microscopic blood vessels

- Loss of apoptosis – healthy cells have an allotted cycle at the end of which they self-destruct

In both laboratory and animal studies, vitamin D has demonstrated a beneficial impact on all these behaviours. The most recent review of laboratory research available at the time of writing states that it 'is a potent anti-cancer agent, affecting cancer cells in cultures and tumour progression in animal models by a variety of mechanisms, including but not limited to [the above]'. A study of post-menopausal women carried out in 2007 concluded that vitamin-D usage could reduce risk by as much as 77 per cent.[8]

As a result of this and other studies clearly showing reduction in cancer risk from vitamin D, a number of treatment centres in the USA now recommend 5000 IU per day to those diagnosed with cancer. It is perhaps unsurprising that there are no published intervention trials using vitamin D alone in the treatment of cancer. There was a wave of interest in using vitamin D, mainly in conjunction with, for instance, chemotherapy, that peaked in 2011 and has receded since. Despite this, it is hard to find a reason not to take a substantial dose – 10,000 IU per day for instance – when one has been given a cancer diagnosis.

# STRATEGIES FOR GETTING MORE VITAMIN D FROM SUNLIGHT

Patricia Peat

Have a 'vitamin D thought' every day!
Make a great contribution to your health by making vitamin D your daily habit. Remind yourself on your calendar, a post-it note on the fridge, anywhere that will get you to assess your vitamin-D intake every day. Ask yourself regularly: 'How am I getting my vitamin D today?' 'Will I be outside for longer than half an hour?' If not, schedule some outdoor time:

- walk the dog
- go for a bike ride or roller-skating
- walk instead of taking the bus or tube
- sit outside to enjoy hot or cold drinks, also for lunch and/or dinner
- join an exercise group that uses the park instead of the gym
- get a regular outdoor sport; you could choose tennis, football, cricket, bowls, rowing, rambling or anything that appeals to you

Above all, expose your skin to the sun as often as possible. Uncover your arms and legs whenever you can. Try wearing layers to make this easy.

Make every day your 'vitamin D thought' day!

| FITZPATRICK SKIN TYPE | SKIN COLOUR | SKIN CHARACTERISTICS |
|---|---|---|
| I | White - very fair; red or blond hair; blue eyes; freckles | Always burns, never tans |
| II | White - fair; red or blond hair; blue, hazel or green eyes | Usually burns, tans with difficulty |
| III | Cream white - fair; any eye or hair colour; very common | Sometimes mildly burns, gradually tans |
| IV | Brown; typical Mediterranean Caucasian skin | Rarely burns, tans with ease |
| V | Dark brown - mid-eastern skin types | Very rarely burns, tans very easily |
| VI | Black | Never burns, tans very easily |

# PART FOUR

## AVOIDING OR REDUCING
# TOXINS

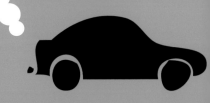

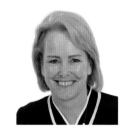

# INTRODUCTION TO PART FOUR

Patricia Peat

It is a well-accepted fact that we now live in a toxic environment and also that toxins are one of the key drivers of cancer. What is specific to Integrative Medicine is the importance of both reducing exposure to toxins and removing accumulated toxins from your body in order to allow your overloaded immune system to recover its full functioning.

This part of the book explores all the ways in which you might be exposing yourself to toxins, suggesting strategies to avoid or reduce exposure and approaches to detoxing your body.

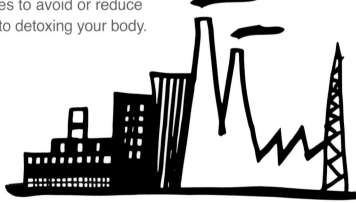

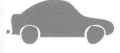

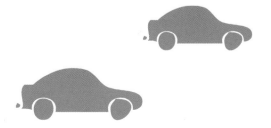

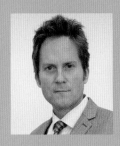

# CHAPTER 11

# ENVIRONMENTAL TOXINS

Robert Verkerk

ANH

## ADAPTING - OR NOT - TO THE INDUSTRIAL CHEMICAL AGE

There is no doubt that our bodies are armed with a series of extraordinary mechanisms for dealing with toxins, whether these are produced internally (endogenous toxins) or externally (exogenous toxins). The latter, particularly those that are foreign to human metabolism ('xenobiotics' – derived from the Greek *xenos,* meaning foreign, and *bios,* life), are the most likely type to overwhelm our innate capacity for detoxification (or, more correctly, 'biotransformation').

The liver is the organ most commonly associated with biotransformation, supporting a complex, phased system that enzymatically oxidises a wide range of chemicals (Phase I), then binds or conjugates the breakdown products (Phase II) and finally excretes them (Phase III). This biotransformation system, however, with the liver as its central powerhouse, is far from the only one in the body that is capable of coping with our toxin load.

In a healthy body, antioxidants, many of which are derived from foods, are capable of 'quenching' potentially damaging, short-lived, highly reactive atoms or molecules referred to as 'free radicals' (also known as 'reactive oxygen species' or ROS). Free radicals, which are a by-product of metabolism and can be produced in greater quantities by the harsh Phase I oxidation reactions or by intense physical activity, can damage cell membranes and DNA, and have been associated with an increased risk of cancer.[1] Antioxidants present in the bloodstream, other body fluids and in interstitial (between cells) spaces, protect cell membranes from damage. Free radicals are frequently produced in greater amounts in bodies suffering an excessive toxin burden.[2]

But there are further armaments available to guard ourselves against harmful chemicals. The immune system is also involved with highly complex responses to substances that the body deems foreign. As scientific knowledge of the interconnectedness of the various bodily systems expands, it has become clear that the immune system does not react in isolation from other systems. The immune and nervous systems – sometimes described as the 'super-systems' of the body – work closely together, and have immense capacity, when functioning optimally, to protect us from biological or chemical substances that have the potential to inflict harm.[3] Working in a co-ordinated fashion, they not only alter the function of internal metabolic pathways, they can alter our behaviour and emotional state. The science of these 'super-systems' is referred to as psychoneuroimmunoendocrinology, more commonly abbreviated to psychoneuroimmunology or PNI.[4]

We must recognise that the sheer sophistication of these complex networks and pathways within our bodies has not adapted to cope with the onslaught of synthetic, environmental chemicals to which most of us are now exposed every day. Quite simply, not enough time – in evolutionary terms – has elapsed for our bodies to adapt adequately to the 20,000 – 30,000 or more industrial chemicals now in common circulation.[5] In Europe alone, there are around 100,000 'existing substances' listed on the European Inventory of Existing Commercial Chemical Substances (EINECS); the European Commission states that these '[account] for about 99% of the chemicals' volume on the [EU] market', while only around a quarter of these are widely used. The vast majority of such industrial chemicals have come into circulation since World War II and the boom in the chemical industry that has resulted a cluster of chemical and pharmaceutical companies becoming among the largest corporations on the planet.[6] The biotransformation systems with which our bodies are gifted, supremely sophisticated as they are, have co-evolved over millennia with the natural world around us, and of course with our primate ancestors before us. It cannot be contested that nature contains a huge variety of toxins; in the main, however, we are admirably capable of handling those to which we are commonly exposed through natural diets and through clean, unadulterated water and air.

## THERE ARE TWO MAIN FACTORS THAT AFFECT OUR ABILITY TO TOLERATE THE ENVIRONMENTAL TOXINS TO WHICH WE ARE NOW EXPOSED.

The first is toxic load or burden. While a large and continually growing body of evidence demonstrates that individual chemicals or substances can cause or predispose the body to cancer, it appears that in many cases it is the overall chemical load or burden for an individual that is likely to be more important.[7] The body of evidence on single chemicals (see thecancerrevolution.co.uk, Tables 1 and 2, Chapter 11) has developed largely because it is easier to study chemicals in isolation than it is as mixtures. For many years, toxicologists thought that the toxicity of a xenobiotic would always increase with dosage (i.e. the dose makes the poison); later research on particular chemicals, however, notably xenoestrogens found in plastics, cosmetics, food and drink containers suggests otherwise (see thecancerrevolution.co.uk, Table 2, Chapter 11). In the case of these endocrine-disrupting chemicals, the dose is not always proportionate to the response, with minuscule doses – at or even below the limit of detection – sometimes yielding large, adverse effects.[8]

THE CANCER
REVOLUTION

The second is known as compromised biotransformation.The response or tolerance of an individual to a given chemical burden varies considerably, in part because of genetic differences between individuals. This has led to a significant rise in environment-associated disabling conditions, including multiple chemical sensitivity (MCS), fibromyalgia, chronic fatigue syndrome (CFS), electric hypersensitivity and amalgam disease.[9] As a result, a given threshold of safety determined by a government regulator based on average populations may well lead to adverse effects in a highly susceptible one. Among the reasons for less tolerance or increased sensitivity, even hypersensitivity, is an individual's history of chemical exposure and one or more compromised biotransformation pathways. These are the pathways through which the body chemically alters nutrients, chemicals and toxins. Reasons for compromise include a deficiency of particular nutrients needed to enhance biotransformation and genetic defects (polymorphisms) that compromise the rate or effectiveness of detoxification. Polymorphisms, which affect the body's ability to produce specific detoxification enzymes, are common even in healthy populations.[10] People's varying ability to detoxify caffeine or paracetamol is a good example of this. Another probably relevant factor is that some chemicals, including specific pesticides and drugs, may be made more, rather than less, toxic through the body's attempt to biotransform them.[11]

Cancer risk, and an individual's predisposition to cancer when exposed to particular environmental chemicals, have been found in recent studies to be affected by:

- the function of DNA and gene-repair systems in the body
- the function of our cell division (cycle) and apoptosis systems
- folate metabolising enzymes
- vitamin/hormone receptors

## Product types or groups associated with carcinogenic potential

Based on the existing scientific literature, it is possible to identify a few types of exposure that are more likely to be associated with increased risk of cancer. Population-based studies would suggest that it is also important to bear in mind the duration of exposure to carcinogens (the longer, the greater the risk) and the age at which the body has been exposed (exposures in early life probably confer greater risks than in late adulthood).

Accordingly, long-term, chronic (regularly repeated) exposure to the following is likely to present an increased risk of development of particular types of cancer (in alphabetic order):

- air pollution
- alcohol consumption
- benzene and other industrial solvents
- certain pharmaceutical drugs and hormonal treatments
- chlorination by-products in drinking and washing water
- chronic infection by various viruses or bacteria
- diets rich in red meat
- diets rich in refined carbohydrates
- dry-cleaning chemicals
- excessive exposure to the sun
- high-temperature cooked foods

- inadequate intake of unprocessed fruits and vegetables
- industrial or domestic 'heavy-duty' cleaning products
- ionising radiation exposure (X-rays, CT scans, mammograms, occupational or accidental nuclear-radiation exposure)
- metal fumes
- moulds in food
- nitrates in municipal or groundwater drinking-water supplies
- occupational exposure to paints, pesticides or other industrial chemicals
- oestrogens or oestrogen-mimics in drinking water or medications

- overweight and obesity
- pesticide residues in food
- petroleum-based products (applied to the skin)
- petroleum-derived combustion products (inhaled)
- physical inactivity
- plasticisers (chemicals e.g. xenoestrogens like bisphenol A that soften plastics)

- preserved meats and foods (containing nitrite or nitrate preservatives)
- tobacco (smoking, second-hand smoke, chewing)

There are countless other chemical types, such as food additives, which undergo assessment by government regulators and which are not currently classified as carcinogens. For example, interactions in soft drinks and preserved fruits or vegetables are not necessarily observed between the 'approved' preservative sodium benzoate and vitamin C, either added or naturally occurring. The reaction produces small amounts of benzene, rated as a Group I 'proven' carcinogen by the IARC (see thecancerrevolution.co.uk, Table 2, Chapter 11, in 'Additional materials'). Since the discovery of this problem in the USA in 2005, testing has shown that a large proportion of soft drinks (carbonated and fruit juices, e.g. cranberry) contain detectable levels of benzene, and many contain levels above the US level set by the Environmental Protection Agency (EPA) for drinking water.[12] But, as is the case with so many levels set by governments, the thresholds are based on limited data and are somewhat arbitrary. Accordingly, the carcinogenic risk to an individual will depend on many factors, including his or her genetic and physiological predisposition, the amount and frequency of consumption and the effectiveness of their biotransformation processes.

THE CANCER
REVOLUTION

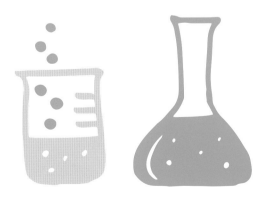

## Routes of exposure

We can absorb environmental toxins in three main ways:

- **By mouth (oral exposure).** This might be in the food we eat (e.g. food additives, contaminants, micro-organisms, pesticide residues) or via pharmaceuticals, herbal products or food supplements.

- **Through our skin or eyes (dermal exposure).** Skin and the surface of our eyes are far from impermeable barriers. Vast numbers of chemicals are absorbed readily into our bloodstream. Generally those with a low molecular weight and high affinity to fats or oils (fat-soluble) are more likely to be readily absorbed than those of both high molecular weight and water solubility.

- **Through our breathing (inhalation exposure).** The inhaled chemical can be a gas (e.g. solvents from paints, carbon monoxide from poorly serviced boilers, fluorine released from non-stick coated cookware); it might be adsorbed on the surface of dust particles (e.g. domestic pesticides, chemicals in the workplace); or the toxin could be a fine particulate or in the form of tiny mist droplets that can be inhaled directly (soot, asbestos, exhaust fumes, pesticide spray drift).

## Where in our environment might we be exposed?

THE CANCER
REVOLUTION

A detailed list can be accessed on the Cancer Revolution website (see thecancerrevolution.co.uk, Table 2, Chapter 11), under the following categories:

- foodstuffs
- drinking water
- skin exposure

- dentistry
- air
- occupational exposure

## Strategies for coping with environmental toxins

### Reducing or avoiding exposure

The most important way of modifying risk to environmental toxins is to avoid, or at least reduce, exposure to them.[13] Reduction or avoidance strategies include:

- Avoid processed foods; consume whole foods, home-prepared for freshness and to avoid nutrient loss, where possible

- Consume organically certified or guaranteed pesticide-free produce; this is especially important when consuming fatty foods (e.g. dairy produce, vegetable oils, fatty meats) that tend to accumulate pesticides, veterinary drugs and Persistent Organic Pollutants (POPs)[14]

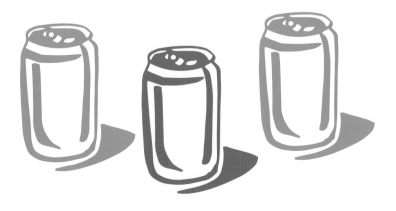

- Reduce or eliminate personal-care products that contain harmful ingredients (e.g. phthalates, parabens, polyethylene glycol (PEG), propylene glycol)[15]

- Eliminate or avoid excessive exposure to petrochemicals, agrochemicals and other sources of environmental toxin, e.g. garden chemicals, dry cleaning, car exhaust, second-hand smoke

- Reduce or eliminate the use of toxic household cleaners (use low-toxicity, environmentally-friendly versions; wear gloves to avoid skin contact)

- Avoid unfiltered, municipal tap water; the only two systems that remove xenoestrogens employ reverse osmosis or distillation, although it is advised to re-mineralise water (to at least pH 7.5) with a suitable mineral source before drinking

- HEPA/ULPA filters and ionisers can be helpful in reducing dust, moulds, volatile organic compounds and other sources of indoor air pollution

- Avoid high-temperature cooking, such as frying and deep frying

- Avoid using non-stick-treated pans, which may release fluorine gas during high-temperature cooking

- Do not drink water or drinks from plastic bottles, unless they are guaranteed to be BPA-free; use glass bottles

- Avoid storing food in plastic containers or covering food in plastic wrapping, unless it is guaranteed to be BPA-free; use glass or earthenware for food storage

- Clean and monitor gas-heating systems for release of carbon monoxide

- Houseplants throughout the home (including bedrooms) will help filter the air and increase oxygen concentration

- Air dry-cleaned clothes in well-ventilated space before wearing or storing

- Use solvent-free or low-solvent paints if decorating

- Avoid inhaling heavy traffic fumes, especially when exercising heavily (e.g. running, cycling); a respirator will reduce inhalation exposure to some toxins, but filters should be changed regularly

- Understand all sources of possible workplace exposure and take action to avoid or minimise; in some cases it may be helpful to engage a relevant trades union for assistance

- Use a carbon filter on baths or showers (and replace regularly according to manufacturers' specifications); otherwise reduce their length of use

- Avoid chlorinated swimming-pools; preferably dip in seawater or ozone-treated pools

- Prospective mothers should ensure that they have minimised exposure to environmental toxins six to twelve months before planning to get pregnant; minimise exposure to xenobiotics throughout breastfeeding[16]

- Avoid taking antacids, paracetamol or other common over-the-counter medications and seek support for natural/non-drug alternatives

- Remove allergens and dust from your home as much as possible

- Minimise exposure to electromagnetic radiation (EMR) from mobile phones by ensuring that time spent with handset near head or body is minimised; do not carry phone on your person; do not sleep with phone near your bedside if left on; use 'airtube' headset to reduce proximity of phone to head/body when talking

- If working on a computer, ensure screens and main computer are at least 30 cm from your body. Use a separate wired keyboard and low-radiation screen if your main computer is a laptop

- Do not use cordless telephones, as most base stations emit EMR equivalent to a transmission mast 250 m away; use corded phones for landlines
- Avoid watching television for more than one or two hours a day; sit more than 3 m away from the TV set when watching
- Do not use microwave ovens
- Avoid excessive exposure to sun; avoid burning (see **Chapter 10, 'Sunshine and vitamin D'**)
- Avoid any exposure to X-rays other than that regarded as medically essential (see **Appendix 2, 'Understanding scans'**)
- Reduce heavy metal exposure (e.g. predatory and river fish, water, lead paint and thimerosal-containing products)

Addressing this long list in detail represents a formidable task for most people. Try to prioritise the items in the list in accordance with the exposure risk associated with your own lifestyle and environment. Once you have identified the highest risks along with some of the most easily achievable reductions, you can adjust your priorities accordingly.

## Supporting the body's detoxification capacity

There is a large body of research, as well as decades of clinical experience, supporting nutritional approaches to enhancing biotransformation processes in the body.[17, 18]

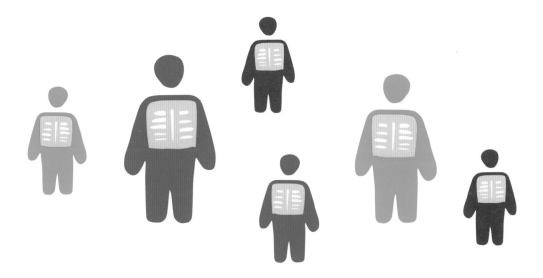

## Improve elimination of toxins

- Have one or two bowel movements a day
- Drink six to eight glasses of water a day or about 2 litres
- Sweat regularly – whether as a result of exercise, steam baths or saunas; infrared saunas are often particularly beneficial
- Regular exercise, yoga, or lymphatic massage can improve lymph flow thus helping to flush toxins out of your tissues into your circulation and contributing to detoxification
- Increase fibre intake (to around 30 g a day)
- Eat lots of beans, whole grains, vegetables, fruits, nuts and seeds
- Taking probiotics such as *Lactobacillus* and *Bifidobacterium* species helps to normalise gut flora and reduce endotoxins (produced by imbalances in gut bacteria)

## Foods and phytochemicals that enhance detoxification

- Try to eat at least one cup of cruciferous vegetables (cabbage, broccoli, collards, kale, Brussels sprouts) a day
- Eat a few cloves of garlic every day or take a garlic supplement
- Decaffeinated green tea can be a healthy way to start your day
- Fresh vegetable juices, including mixtures of carrot, celery, cilantro, beets, parsley and ginger are delicious and beneficial
- Try prepared herbal detoxification teas containing a mixture of burdock root, dandelion root, ginger root, liquorice root, sarsaparilla root, cardamon seed, cinnamon bark and other herbs
- Eat high-quality, sulphur-containing proteins, e.g. eggs and whey protein, as well as garlic, and onions
- Consume citrus peels, caraway and dill oil (which contain limonene)
- Consume bioflavonoids in grapes, berries and citrus fruits
- To help liver detoxification, improve the flow of bile and increase urine flow, consume dandelion greens
- To increase the flow of urine and aid in detoxification, eat celery
- Consume fresh coriander, which may help eliminate heavy metals
- Rosemary, which contains carnosol, is a potent booster of detoxification enzymes
- Curcuminoids (turmeric, used in curry) have powerful antioxidant and anti-inflammatory action
- Burdock root is a good aid in detoxification
- So is the chlorophyll in dark green leafy vegetables and in wheatgrass
- Take pycnogenol (found in grape seeds) in supplement form for support of detoxification and circulation

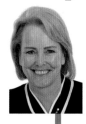

# THE LIVER AND DETOXIFICATION

Four major organs are involved in eliminating toxins from the body – the liver, the intestinal tract, the kidneys and the skin. The liver works to detoxify harmful substances, whether they are produced internally through normal processes such as energy production or through one of the many external sources outlined in this chapter.

The liver plays many vital roles: it acts on nutrients to break them down and to build up body tissue; it stores nutrients; and it produces special red blood cells that scour the bloodstream for harmful micro-organisms, while also producing glycogen, a long-term energy source. The liver regulates hormone levels and it breaks down fat-soluble toxins to make them water soluble, so that they can be excreted.

The detoxification processes in the liver are broken down into Phase I (oxidation) and Phase II (conjugation). In Phase I, a group of enzymes work to neutralise toxins, which they can achieve with some unwanted chemicals. Others, however, have to be converted to an intermediate form that requires Phase II to complete the detoxification process. Curiously, the intermediate forms tend to be more chemically active than the original toxins, highlighting the importance of well-functioning Phase II processes, without which the intermediate toxins can be a significant hazard, even carcinogenic.

These processes themselves produce unwanted by-products in the form of free radicals. If the liver is overloaded with toxins, then the build-up of these free radicals can damage liver cells. However, this type of damage can in turn be limited by antioxidants such as natural carotenoids and vitamins C and E. Conversely, a shortage of antioxidants combined with a high level of toxins can potentially lead to malignancy.

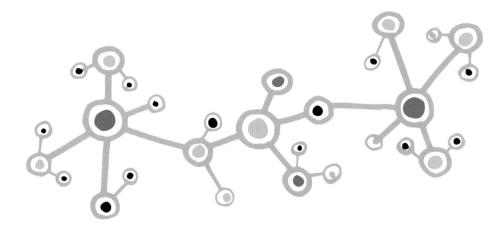

# IN CONCLUSION

Physically, it is a matter of fact that we are what we eat, drink, breathe and absorb – other than what we eliminate. Excessive loads of xenobiotics have been shown to contribute to a wide range of health conditions in humans, particularly in the ways they affect the immune, endocrine, neurological and skeletal systems. Concerns about the adverse effects that environmental toxins continue to have on health and wellbeing are still increasing. Given their sheer number and their ubiquitous nature, there is an urgent need for further research on the safety of so many, and, in evolutionary terms, the shortage of time for genetic adaptation.

Although data remain limited, it is clear from the extensive work done on smokers and asbestos workers that the risks of exposures to mixtures of chemicals, as occurs in the real world, can be synergistic and 'more than additive'.[19]

It has been demonstrated that chronic exposure to toxins may augment pathological processes, accelerate ageing and create self-amplifying intolerance; it may also play a significant role in triggering or amplifying cancer and other chronic disease, along with neurological conditions such as Alzheimer's and Parkinson's diseases.[20] Accordingly, all efforts should be made to minimise exposure to xenobiotics, this being especially important for those with compromised health, so as to avoid diverting valuable resources (e.g. energy, nutrients) required for biotransformation processes.

Seeking the support of a suitably qualified and experienced healthcare professional who specialises in Ecological Medicine, Functional Medicine, Integrative Medicine or related disciplines can be of enormous value. Such a clinician could help you to identify genetic susceptibilities (including polymorphisms), important sources of past or current environmental toxin exposure, and help you to develop suitable diet and lifestyle-based protocols to optimise the effectiveness of biotransformation pathways.

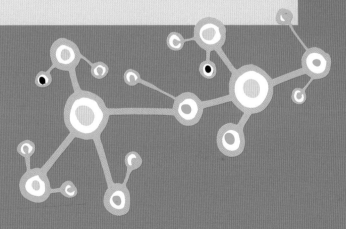

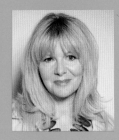

# CHAPTER 12

# TOXINS IN THE HOME

Janey Lee Grace

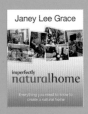

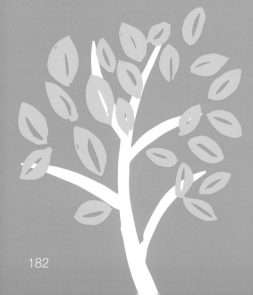

IMPERFECTLY
NATURAL

It is a worrying fact that many of us are exposed to more pollution in our own homes than when we're outdoors.[1] Toxic chemicals are present in building materials, floorings, furnishings, cleaning and personal-care products, clothing and food products – sometimes all on top of smoke, air fresheners and the effects of electromagnetic fields (EMFs).

Cleaning is an everyday activity. How you clean and care for your home is very much connected with your wellness and your ability to maintain a healthy immune system. The air quality in our homes often contains far higher concentrations of toxic chemicals in a confined space than a busy street corner does.

Where possible, planting trees around our home is about all we can do to reduce the effects of traffic and airborne pollution; few of us are likely to be able to stretch to a purpose-built eco home. We can certainly, however, make sustainable healthy choices in our personal-care products and in what we use to clean and refresh our personal space. How you choose to clean your home can play a big part in reducing your toxic load. Fortunately there are many natural substitutes for commercial, conventional cleaning and air-freshening products.

## What's wrong with conventional detergents and air fresheners?

The answer to that is: just about everything. They are unsustainable, many are petrochemical-based (and petrol is a non-renewable resource, harmful to the environment), they contaminate rivers and seas, many contain chemicals that are creating strong superbugs and an unbalanced ecosystem. They also contribute to ill-health. Many cleaning agents contain carcinogens and/or hormone-disrupting chemicals; these can cause respiratory problems, lowered immunity and low-level fatigue. Laundry products can also be a skin irritant and lead to allergies. By contrast, however, a wealth of great plant-based substitutes for toxic products is available for cleaning our homes and clothes.

Studies have shown that women who work in the home have a 55 per cent increased risk of getting cancer.[2] Research also shows that women suffer from headaches due to VOCs (volatile organic compounds, which will also aggravate respiratory conditions such as asthma); artificial fragrances which can be hormone disrupting and can even cause depression.[3] (The word 'Parfum' or 'fragrance' in the ingredients list of a product can mean that up to 100 different synthetic chemicals have been used to create that aroma.). VOCs are found in a host of household products, including paints, aerosol sprays, cleansers, disinfectants, air fresheners and dry-cleaned clothing. Plastics can also give off a toxic formaldehyde gas, as can soft furnishings, new mattresses and even new suitcases.

Of course one might hope that the safety data are reliable and that standards are in place to ensure that any commercially available products are safe to use, but the issue is not with any one bottle of washing-up liquid, carpet cleaner, window spray or even shampoo and conditioner. Most of us have an inordinate number of different containers under our kitchen sinks and in our bathroom cabinets. There are approximately 100,000 different synthetic chemicals approved for industrial use; it is impossible (and not economically worthwhile) even to begin to ascertain what happens when these chemicals interact in limitless possible combinations. Because of the affordability and huge choice available, we can end up swimming in a toxic soup. In her book *Cleaning Yourself to Death*, Pat Thomas, former editor of the *Ecologist* magazine, wrote: 'To test even the commonest 1000 of these chemicals in combination would require at least 166 million different experiments. Even if scientists worked around the clock it is estimated that such data would take 100 years to compile'. We actually need far fewer of these products than we think. You can easily make your own DIY-cleaning concoctions and room sprays. If you do choose to buy, you can opt for one of the more natural eco brands, which use plant-based surfactants which are much kinder to the environment and our skin. And of course, don't forget that houseplants can also enhance the air quality in your home.

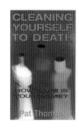

## Do-it-yourself cleaning

For general cleaning, microfibre cloths are a truly wonderful invention. Some are specifically designed to be used without detergents: they trap bacteria within them, which are then killed by nano-particulate silver, either within the cloth or when they get tossed into the washing machine. Other staples of a DIY-cleaning kit include lemons, vinegar and good old bicarbonate of soda, which is brilliant for neutralising smells. You probably already know about using vinegar and newspaper for cleaning windows. Many of the DIY cleaning ideas that follow are similarly 'old school'.

### Vinegar
Mixed with bicarbonate of soda, vinegar makes a really strong fizzing solution, excellent for cleaning and unblocking drains. Vinegar on its own will help to prevent limescale in the toilet bowl; for removing limescale around taps, soak a cotton-wool pad in it, pop a plastic bag around the tap and leave for a couple of hours before washing off. You can mix it with lemon juice and water to clean surfaces and floors and to descale kettles.

### Lemons
These should be kept to the bitter end, because a used lemon will shine a ceramic sink beautifully. You can add salt to half a lemon with the flesh all used up and use it as a scouring mitt. A tiny bit of lemon peel in the cutlery tray of the dishwasher works a treat too.

### Bicarbonate of soda
There are countless uses for this wonder product. To mention only a few: it neutralises odours (simply leave some in a carton or jar), cleans plastics and removes stains from mugs and coffee pots (as a paste with a bit of water); and it also polishes chrome. As already mentioned, mixed with vinegar it can be used to clean toilets and drains; wiped on the inside of your oven, it can be left overnight as a cleaning agent; and if you want to refresh a carpet, shake bicarbonate of soda over it and then vacuum it up. It can even be used as a dry shampoo and a toothpaste.

### Essential oils
It is worth investing in some essential oils. Tea-tree oil *(Melaleuca aternifolia)* is antibacterial and can be used to clean the toilet seat or anywhere that you feel might need some extra germ-killing help; try mixing oils such as lavender, lemon and citronella.

### Air fresheners
The obvious way of keeping the air in your home fresh is often overlooked nowadays – open the windows. Many people live in sealed units with triple glazing, keep their radiators on full and wonder why they can't shake off infections. My advice is to open your windows wide, especially when you clean the house. No-one need ever again buy air freshener. Many oncologists in breast-cancer units are telling their patients to avoid both aerosols and the 'scary' plug-in types. Artificial fragrance merely masks an odour; it is far better to get to the root of the problem and deal with it. If you must buy an air freshener, choose one of the natural room sprays with essential oils as fragrance. A far cheaper opton is to use a plant sprayer, half-filled with water and two or three drops of essential oil added. Lemon, lavender and geranium work well, as does eucalyptus or tea tree for a more antiseptic whiff. You can add a drop of vodka or a few drops of vinegar as a preservative.

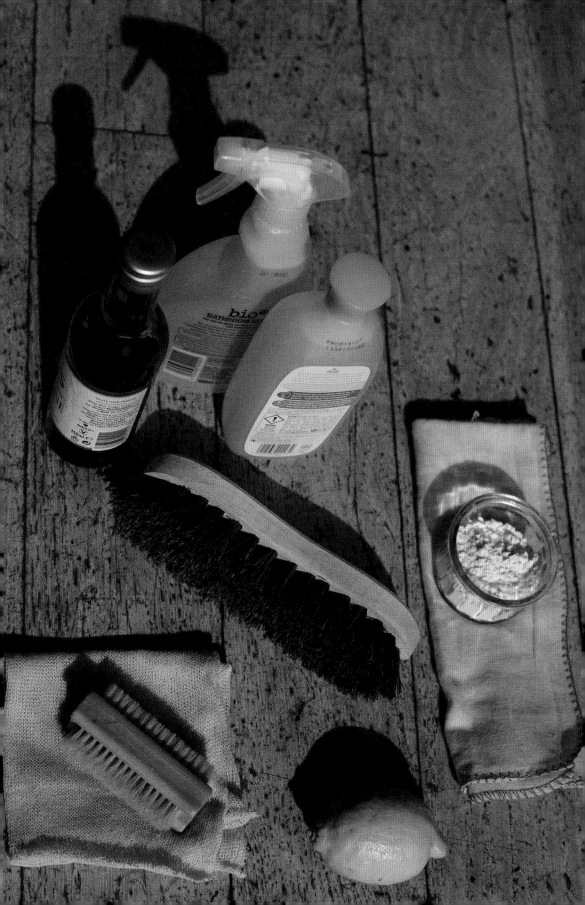

## Laundry

You can save yourself a small fortune by not buying conventional laundry products. You'll also find that your clothes last longer, that itchy rashes are a thing of the past, and you'll be reducing your carbon footprint. Choose eco brands, or better still ditch the detergents altogether and opt for laundry balls or soap nuts. Both are very cheap, eco-friendly and sustainable, and there's no need for fabric softener. With laundry balls you simply pop two into the drum of your washing machine with the clothing. They contain ionised pellets, which change the molecular structure of the water and draw off the dirt. Be sure not to overfill the machine, as the pummelling action helps the process. You can buy laundry balls as a pack of two, complete with natural stain remover (cost around £35 and guaranteed to do a minimum of 1000 washes).

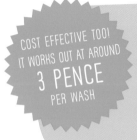

COST EFFECTIVE TOO! IT WORKS OUT AT AROUND **3 PENCE** PER WASH

THERE'S ALSO THE EXCELLENT ECO EGG, PACKED WITH SCIENTIFICALLY FORMULATED, HYPOALLERGENIC CLEANING PELLETS, WHICH NATURALLY ACTIVATE IN THE WATER TO LIFT AWAY DIRT AND GRIME GENTLY, WITHOUT USING ANY HARSH CHEMICALS. IT WORKS OUT AT AROUND 3 PENCE PER WASH.

Soap nuts have been used in India and Nepal as a natural detergent for centuries; they look a bit like dried-up conkers. You simply pop five or six little shells into a drawstring bag (a thin sock works even better, so that none can escape) and put it into the drum of your washing machine. When they come into contact with water they create saponin, which is soap. Use them three times before putting the soap nuts on the compost and refilling the little bag. You can buy a huge bag for around £5 or £6. You can also make your soap nut liquid by simmering two cupfuls of soap nuts in hot water for around two minutes, straining off the liquid, frothing it up (using a hand blender) and adding a couple of drops of essential oil (that's important, as they can smell unpleasant otherwise). This will make the most effective detergent for anything from washing the car to cleaning household surfaces – it's also a great shampoo.

## Fabric softener

This commercial product is in fact entirely unnecessary. Eco detergents (and obviously soap nuts and laundry balls) contain no optical brighteners, phosphates or harsh detergents to create the need for softening. If you do like a fragrance, then put a couple of drops of essential oil in the fabric-softener compartment of your washing machine, or treat yourself to some luxurious ironing water, which can enhance the natural fragrance of newly washed clothes. To soften towels, add a tablespoonful of vinegar to the softener compartment.

## A word about whites

Both laundry balls and soap nuts will do a great job of washing the clothes, but they won't remove stubborn stains. Always treat stains first with bicarbonate of soda, or try Ecover's excellent stain remover. And if you want your whites very white, then wash them separately and add in some eco laundry bleach.

## Steam cleaners

Don't underestimate how efficient steam cleaning is. Borrow one of these multi-purpose appliances from a friend, buy one from a general store or pick one up through Freecycle or eBay. You can transform curtains, carpets, furnishings, even cupboards and surfaces with a few hours' therapeutic blasting. And they are a great way to kill bugs, without using chemicals.

## Carpets and vacuum cleaners

In an ideal world we would all have sustainable flooring and live happily ever after. For the areas where you need carpet, however, avoid conventional carpet-cleaning products. I have already told you why: if you want to refresh a carpet, shake bicarbonate of soda over it and then vacuum. Add a spritz or two of essential oil if you like. When choosing a vacuum cleaner, opt for ones with Hepa filters, which are best if you have pets or allergies.

**To summarise**: ensure that any cleaning and personal-care products you bring into the home are 100 per cent natural. Your local independent health store is a good starting point as are some of the online stores listed in **Part Eight**, '**Resources**'. As the American futurist John Naisbitt wrote in his book *Megatrends* (1982):

> 'WE MUST LEARN TO BALANCE THE MATERIAL WONDERS OF TECHNOLOGY WITH THE SPIRITUAL DEMANDS OF OUR HUMAN RACE.'

## EMF Protection

This may seem like a shift in topic, but I believe that another important health hazard to address in our homes is that of electromagnetic fields (EMFs) that are integral to such human-made technologies as cordless and mobile phones, also to wi-fi. They have created yet another very worrying form of pollution. While not pretending to have enough of a scientific background to pass on full details of the negative aspects of EMFs, I can at least raise your awareness and point you in the direction of the scientific evidence and solutions. One of the best scientific resources for this area can be found at www.bioinitiative.org, which includes an incredibly well-referenced report by the key scientists at the forefront of exposing the dangers of radio frequency (RF) EMFs. I personally think it's one of the biggest health issues facing us today, and most people don't realise the extent to which our lives and homes are jammed with invisible 'electro-smog' (e-smog) that could, to a greater or lesser extent, be affecting both our short- and long-term health and wellbeing.

Electromagnetic radiation in and around your home presents a potentially serious health risk, depending on its type, its intensity, how long you are exposed to it and how susceptible you are. We can hardly escape e-smog due to the rapid development of technologies for wireless communication. The notorious atmospheric smogs that blighted London and other cities from Victorian times well into the twentieth century prompted people to do something about them because they could be seen; invisible e-smog, however, is much more insidious. There have been many scientific investigations looking at its likely impact on health, and the results have ranged from 'no apparent health risk', to e-smog being considered one of the 'big silent killers of the 21st century'.[4] There is no doubt that children are generally more sensitive to it than adults, and several governments have now accepted that normal usage of cordless and mobile phones might present an increased risk of particular types of cancer and malignancy.[5]

It is clearly not viable for most of us to give up our technological lifestyles: the vast majority of urban dwellers own mobile phones, cordless telephones, wi-fi, computers, laptops, microwave ovens and an array of electronic equipment. Then there are kitchen appliances, radio alarm clocks, and desk lamps that can produce alternating electric fields, even if switched off. Outside our windows there will often be a mobile phone transmitter within sight, and although the present UK government line remains (in 2015) that there is no proven health risk from exposure to mobile phone or TETRA masts, unfortunately their safety guidelines are based on the assumption that the only harmful effect of microwaves is that they will 'cook' you at high enough power levels. There is much research, however, claiming damaging (non-thermal) biological effects at well below the levels that cause heating.[6] The reality is that there is much disagreement as to where safe levels should be set, as well as much variation in different countries as to how levels are measured and what really is a safe level of exposure.

### Where are the EMFs in your home?
As well as the high frequency radiation from transmitters and wi-fi, rather worrying are the 'fields' created by seemingly innocent items in your house such as cordless (DECT) phones. Unlike mobiles, which transmit unwanted radiation only when in use, the base stations of cordless phones are transmitting powerful signals 24 hours a day, desperately trying to seek out their little receiver friends dotted around your house. It's been said that the radiation from cordless systems flying around our houses is 100 times more dangerous than using mobiles.[7] You may want to think about going back to a corded phone! There are also special, low radiation cordless phones available such as those made by Orchid.

Think carefully about where you put the wireless router in your house, and how long you keep it on. Keep it well away from children, especially babies, and anyone who's pregnant. If there's a baby in the house, think carefully about the risks and benefits of using a wireless baby monitor.

### Shield yourself

SITEFINDER

The first thing to do is to establish whether or not you have a problem. Find your nearest TETRA or G3 transmitter by visiting the 'Sitefinder' website; enter your own postcode and check your house for electro pollution. You can also rent or buy electric and magnetic meters. They are simple to operate, and you can run a fifteen minute check which will alert you to any possible problems.

Some people are affected by e-smog so badly that they can't live in certain areas near mobile phone masts or power lines. Some report headaches or 'hot ear' when using cellular phones. Many just notice a huge difference in their wellbeing when they get away from their usual environment – away from the electro pollution of their city or office, perhaps out into the countryside (though these days that's not necessarily an escape from EMFs either). In most domestic situations, it is impossible to escape from EMFs completely. Short of wrapping ourselves in a lead duffel coat or installing a Faraday Cage (a highly sophisticated EMF-screening system) what can we do?

If this is a serious concern for you, explore the possibility of metal fibre woven net screens for your mattress and around your bed; you could also buy radiation-shielding paint, but these are expensive measures.

The most important time to protect yourself is during sleep, as EMFs interfere with the delicate neurological balances and mechanisms necessary for your body to 'repair' itself. On average, we spend a third of our lives asleep. TVs, computers, radios, in fact anything that you plug in emits radiation that can affect your sleep patterns. Don't sleep on a bed with a metal frame, as this can amplify radiation; wood is good by contrast. Change your halogen bedside lamp for a standard one, because the transformers emit loads of EMFs; the chances are that they will be on the floor right under your head. Get an old-fashioned alarm clock and don't use your mobile to wake you up.

Again, this might sound too obvious, but try to minimise use of your mobile and cordless phone. Use an 'airtube' earpiece or speakerphone on your mobile, and try not to have it in direct contact with your ear or head. Avoid keeping your mobile in your pocket, bra or anywhere else within 10 mm of your body. Even the legal blurb hidden deep inside your iPhone tells you this: 'To reduce exposure to RF energy, use a hands-free option, such as the built-in speakerphone, the supplied headphones, or other similar accessories. Carry iPhone at least 10 mm away from your body to ensure levels remain at or below as-tested levels.' Remember to switch off your wi-fi at night. As a further precaution, use an anti-radiation cover on your mobile phone; these come in many different designs, sizes and colours, and use several very different approaches to lessening our RF load. You can also use various forms of protective device on your cordless phone base station and on all computers and laptops (see **Part Eight 'Resources'**).

To summarise: scientific communities are continuing to disagree in all areas, so revert to your own instincts, and ask yourself 'could there be a problem?' My view is that there definitely is, and precaution is the sensible option.

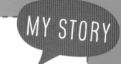

### Nuro Weidemann
Lymphoma survivor

*When I was 49 years old, I was diagnosed with an aggressive form of non-Hodgkin's lymphoma. The diagnosis came as a total surprise as I considered myself pretty healthy.*

*I decided against any conventional therapies and instead embarked on a diet to try to alkalise my body. This involved drinking several freshly pressed green juices a day and avoiding all processed food. In addition, I followed traditional naturopathic detoxification methods, chucked out all toxic house cleaners and cosmetics, and installed water filters for our drinking water and the shower.*

*After eighteen months of clean living, the tumour had disintegrated, and a PET scan could no longer detect any cancerous activities in my body.*

*I was overjoyed, to say the least!*

*Creating this shift in my body was a full-time job, but an enjoyable one. It required my full commitment and considerable support from my family and friends.*

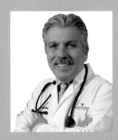

# CHAPTER 13

# DETOXIFYING YOUR BODY

## Dr Francisco Contreras

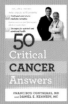

OASIS OF
HOPE

Stephie was a top-notch marathon runner. She never made the headlines but she had run the Boston Marathon, the New York City Marathon, the London Marathon and the Berlin Marathon. In each, she was able to traverse the gruelling 26 miles and 385 yards in under five hours. She was not setting world records but she was accomplishing what less than 1 per cent of humanity has ever done, and that makes her world class to me. I was surprised to see her in my office, recently diagnosed with breast cancer. Her lifestyle appeared to be perfect. Her exercise and nutrition were exemplary. She did not have the BRCA1 or BRCA2 genes that indicate a hereditary tendency, so her issue was not genetic, and it was difficult to see how it was metabolic. What was going on?

Cancer is an opportunistic disease. Malignant cells circulate in most, if not all, people alive in the twenty-first century. But tumours will not form and the disease known as cancer will not result unless it is provided an opportunity. All it takes to get a foot in the door is a malfunction in the immune system. There is no greater cancer prevention agent than the one we have had since birth. In fact, it is impossible to get cancer if the immune system is functioning fully. But when the immune system is not working at optimal levels, the door inches open and cancer can get a foothold. Malignant cells can begin to proliferate until they form tumours that can then spread to other organs. The immune system is the perfect shield. Unfortunately, it is under constant attack by stressors – physical, emotional and spiritual. The good news is that there are specific actions you can take to lower your exposure to stressors and to detoxify yourself. The topic of detoxification is one of the most important for cancer prevention and treatment because a good cleansing programme will allow a person's immune system to be restored and bolstered for the fight against cancer.

What is new about this chapter on detoxification is that it addresses how to detox the whole person – body, mind and spirit. Since 1963, we have been helping people cleanse themselves holistically at Oasis of Hope, a cancer centre that was founded by my father in Tijuana, Mexico. Medical science validates this approach, and the stories and testimonies of tens of thousands of patients are responsible for our conviction that a total care approach is essential for a person to beat cancer.

Take Stephie, for example. She was living close to a perfect lifestyle. But laboratory tests confirmed that her immune system was not functioning correctly. Through the course of her treatment, we identified a number of stressors in her life. She lived in an urban environment and was constantly exposed to the typical air pollution found in large cities. She also confided that when she was a child, an uncle had sexually abused her. She explained that she often felt uneasy with men. She associated this past traumatic event with her inability to be emotionally intimate with her husband, and her marriage ended in divorce. On the surface, Stephie's athletic and healthy nutrition lifestyle put her in a low-risk category for cancer. But the years of breathing polluted air, coupled with the emotional distress associated with her past and the loss of her marriage, allowed her immune system to drop its guard, and breast cancer ensued.

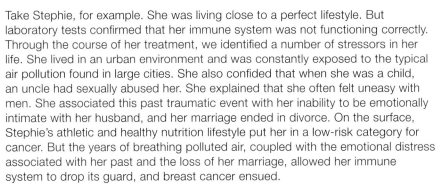

The following paragraphs identify the most common stressors on a person's body, mind and spirit. I also explain how we detoxify our patients in the three realms at Oasis of Hope. Some of what I share can be done on your own. Some of it will require you to seek a holistic treatment centre, such as Oasis of Hope, that really understands the connection between the body, mind and spirit.

Cancer incidence in the UK is projected to increase substantially by the year 2030.[1] While some of this increase is linked to growth in the ageing population, a substantial proportion will be attributable to currently known risk factors such as obesity, lack of exercise, smoking and poor nutrition. What does that mean? It means that we are making little progress in teaching and motivating people to change their lifestyles to prevent cancer. And although survival rates have improved slightly, in reality we are no closer to 'the cancer cure' than we were in the 1960s.

The true hope is to prevent or control cancer through detoxification and holistic protocols. Please keep yourself informed and make every effort to stave off cancer through detoxification. First, become aware of how many immune-depressing toxins you come into contact with in your daily life. Your body is constantly under assault. Now, more than any other time in history, you need your immune system functioning at its best in your defence. Most people have some idea, but really don't know just how toxic our world actually is. If you've not already read them, it is well worth spending time on taking in the information in **Chapter 11**, '**Environmental toxins**', and **Chapter 12**, '**Toxins in the home**'. **Chapter 9**, '**Managing stress**', describes how toxic stress can be in your life and how damaging this can be to your immunity; it also provides you with the foundations for a drive to reduce exposure to toxins as far as possible. This clearly makes complete sense, whether you have cancer or not. The rest of this chapter focuses on strategies for reducing or eliminating toxins that have already accumulated in your body.

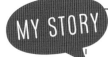

### Lynne
### Breast-cancer patient

*Following a severe allergic reaction to mercury amalgam dental fillings, initially thought of as rare, but now officially accepted as a toxin by a European Council Resolution, I was left completely bedridden, unable to function normally, due to damaged mitochondria. This in turn created an anaerobic environment that supports cancer.*

*Now that I have cancer, I know that my best chance of surviving is to reduce any further toxicity in my life as far as possible and to give myself the best organic food, along with the supplements recommended by my Functional Medicine practitioner. With my experience of the devastating effects of toxicity, I'd recommend cleaning up your life, cancer or no cancer, as I believe that toxins are the source of much chronic disease.*

## Detoxification

### Body

There are many supplements, protocols and interventions available for detoxification. Having spent over thirty years working with cancer patients, I can state that the three most powerful agents to rid the body of toxins are whole live organic food and juice, with exercise as a vital factor. The vegan diet can cut off the sugar supply line to cancers and it can also benefit people with rheumatoid arthritis, diabetes and heart disease.[2] Some of the best foods for detoxing include artichokes, asparagus, cucumber, leeks and watercress.[3] I would also like to highly recommend the anti-cancer properties of kale, cabbage, bok choy and cauliflower.

I often put patients on a two- to three-day juice fast, which is one of the best ways of kick-starting the detoxification process. We give a green juice consisting of romaine lettuce, kale, spinach, parsley and a slice of green apple. Not only does this drink provide nutrients that boost the immune system, but it cuts off the supply line to the cancer cell ketogenically (see '**The Ketogenic diet**', pp. 90-93, in **Chapter 5**, '**Diet as the foundation of good health**').

Daily aerobic exercise, for example a brisk half-hour walk, improves insulin sensitivity. Studies of those with breast and colorectal cancer, conducted at Harvard Medical School, Boston, USA (2005) and Dana-Farber Cancer Institute, Boston, USA (2006) showed that the risk of mortality was reduced by 50 per cent or more, because an exercised body produces less insulin and insulin growth factor (IGF).[4]

In addition to organic foods, juices, chelation, probiotics and exercise, I recommend that you look into treatment protocols that include intravenous vitamin C, ozone, ultraviolet blood irradiation and enzymes. Further information about how I use these therapies is available in my book *50 Critical Cancer Answers*.

## Mouth

Many health practitioners will tell you that illness starts in the colon. But I say it starts with the mouth. To detox, stop putting processed foods into your mouth. It is also important not to have permanent (or semi-permanent) metal dental materials put in your mouth. Fillings that are made out of amalgams containing mercury and other metals are very toxic and have been outlawed in many nations around the world.[5] As Dr Yoshiaki Omura wrote in a study of 1996: '...mercury exists in cancer and pre-cancer cell nuclei.'[6] He confirmed that mercury residuals break down the immune system, making the body susceptible to pathogens. Most people already have metal fillings. You may wish to run out now and have them removed, but consider this before you do anything: Dr Omura found that the removal of amalgams resulted in an increase in mercury levels in all the body's organs. Therefore, if you decide to have amalgams removed and replaced with non-toxic materials, it is critical that you work with a biological dentist and health practitioner who have effective pre-conditioning and post-removal detoxification protocols (see the BSMFD website).

BSMFD

## Colon

Given that a single exposure to a toxin is stressful to the body, I now ask: how much worse is being repeatedly exposed? The fact is that most of are in this situation – because the human race is constipated. You should be moving your bowels three times a day, just as a baby does. But most people move their bowels once a day at most, while many other move them only once every two or three days. This is especially true for cancer patients as constipation is one of the most common negative side effects of chemotherapy and painkillers. In one 2013 study from the *International Journal of Palliative Nursing*, 72 per cent of patients taking pain killers suffered from constipation.[7]

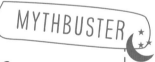

MYTHBUSTER

# "THE BODY NATURALLY DETOXIFIES, IT DOES NOT NEED ANY HELP"

The body's methylation pathways often struggle to cope with modern lifestyles. Toxins cause imbalances which can contribute to cancer. Furthermore, when faced with a barrage of toxic chemical treatment, our detoxification pathways can be overwhelmed and so will function better with support.[8]

The reason constipation is such an important topic is that, while the bowel is not moving, the toxins are absorbed into the bloodstream and will circulate through the body only to be deposited in the colon again. If the bowel doesn't move, the toxins will be absorbed again. In other words, toxins are recycled over and over again until the bowel moves. In order to detoxify yourself, you need to change your diet to one that is both high in fibre and low in animal proteins and white-flour products.

Many treatment centres offer colonic irrigation. Some practitioners indicate that constipation leads to a build-up of 'plaque'. As a surgical oncologist who has operated on thousands of colons, I can tell you that no such 'plaque' exists. However, a colonic irrigation can be very cleansing for people who are suffering from constipation. This treatment is also advised for those who are undergoing radiation that results in rectal bleeding; research has shown that this subsides after irrigation.[9] While I recognise the potential benefits of this technique, I do not use irrigation, preferring instead to rely on dietary change; this I see as essential. I try to teach my patients how to maintain proper colon health through diet and supplementation.

### Probiotics

Probiotics are essential to the health of the colon. They can help with nutrient absorption and toxin elimination, but their benefits extend well beyond that. One 2010 study from the National Dairy Research Institute, Karnal (Haryana), India found that probiotics promote immune responses, the augmentation of cytokine pathways, along with the regulation of tumour necrosis factors (TNF – one of our defences against cancer) and interleukins.[10] Probiotics help bind mutagens and inhibit mutagenesis and have benefited patients with colorectal and bladder cancer.[11] A study conducted in 2012 by the Department of Urology, North West London Hospitals NHS Foundation Trust, and the Department of Urology, University College London Hospitals NHS Trust reported that, compared with the control group not taking probiotics, the recurrence-free interval was longer in bladder patients who were taking probiotics.[12] I highly recommend probiotics as a part of a comprehensive detoxification programme.

### Liver

You may have heard the saying, 'Happy wife, happy life.' I have a saying that might yet catch on: 'Happy liver, happy life.' The liver filters the blood and removes chemicals and other toxins before they are circulated through the rest of the body. The better you support the health of your liver, the better your body can detox. One of the most widely embraced alternative therapies to stimulate optimal liver function is the coffee enema.[13] We have been using coffee enemas since the 1960s and have observed how our patients have benefited. They often joke with our nurses, asking for cream and sugar with the enema. This doubtless alleviates the anxiety associated with most treatments administered via the rectum. Coffee enemas provide powerful antioxidants that are readily absorbed through the rectum, and they also help evacuate the bowel.

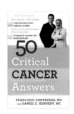

My absolute champion for liver health is extract of milk thistle *(Silybum marianum)*. The active nutrient is silymarin, which is described in several of my books, including *50 Critical Cancer Answers*. This antioxidant helps the liver regenerate itself like no other nutrient of which I am aware.[14] It is also a powerful immune-boosting agent (see 'The liver and detoxification, p. 180,' in Chapter 11, 'Environmental toxins').

# COFFEE ENEMAS

## Dr Bernard Willis

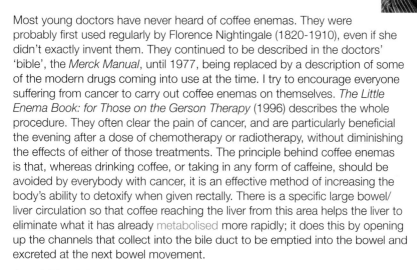

Most young doctors have never heard of coffee enemas. They were probably first used regularly by Florence Nightingale (1820-1910), even if she didn't exactly invent them. They continued to be described in the doctors' 'bible', the *Merck Manual*, until 1977, being replaced by a description of some of the modern drugs coming into use at the time. I try to encourage everyone suffering from cancer to carry out coffee enemas on themselves. *The Little Enema Book: for Those on the Gerson Therapy* (1996) describes the whole procedure. They often clear the pain of cancer, and are particularly beneficial the evening after a dose of chemotherapy or radiotherapy, without diminishing the effects of either of those treatments. The principle behind coffee enemas is that, whereas drinking coffee, or taking in any form of caffeine, should be avoided by everybody with cancer, it is an effective method of increasing the body's ability to detoxify when given rectally. There is a specific large bowel/liver circulation so that coffee reaching the liver from this area helps the liver to eliminate what it has already metabolised more rapidly; it does this by opening up the channels that collect into the bile duct to be emptied into the bowel and excreted at the next bowel movement.

An additional, important feature of a coffee enema is that it stimulates the liver to produce more of an enzyme called glutathione-S-transferase, the enzyme that helps to manufacture glutathione, which is the body's most important detoxification chemical. If your cancer is partly a result of a lifetime's accumulation of toxic chemicals, it is likely that you will long ago have used up all your supplies of glutathione. Making fresh supplies can therefore only be good for you. This function of coffee enemas is certainly important if you are jaundiced.

How often you carry out coffee enemas depends on how bad your condition is and how much better you feel when you start doing them.

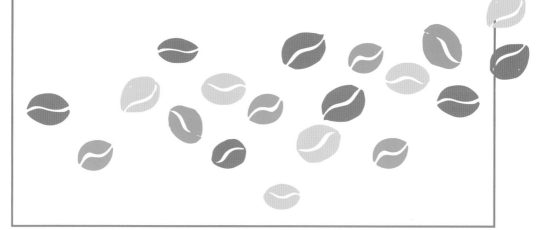

### Kidneys

In Mexico we drink a lot of 'Jamaica', which is a delicious tea made from hibiscus. We serve it regularly to our patients because it supports both kidney and bladder health and is an excellent addition to your detox programme.[15]

Another classic alternative medicine detoxifying agent is disodium EDTA. This is referred to as chelation therapy, in which heavy metals are pulled out of the tissues for elimination through the urine. It is effective for the removal of lead, nickel and mercury, which may have leached into your system from dental materials. In addition to the benefits of heavy metal detoxification, chelation therapy is thought to have anti-tumour qualities.[16, 17] Further research is required to understand how chelation may work against cancer.

### Mind

Many psychiatrists all over the world have developed ways of helping people detoxify from negative emotions and thoughts. In the context of cancer treatment, we have found that the most effective tool is cognitive restructuring – changing the way a person thinks about an event. You cannot always control your circumstances, but you can always choose how you will react to a situation. Most people believe that emotions happen to them, but that is not true. You choose the way you feel about any situation.

It is important to identify circumstances or events in your life that provoke feelings of anger, fear and other negative emotions. Once you have identified them, you need to reframe the situation so that you learn how to minimise negative emotions and nurture positive ones. For example, when a person is diagnosed with cancer, it often happens that he or she feels as if a death sentence has been pronounced. The paradigm with which many people live is, 'I am dying from cancer.' But that cognitive structure results in chronic negative thinking. To detox from that pattern of thought, you can practise developing new, hopeful paradigms, for example, 'I am living, and I am dealing with cancer.' 'Dealing with cancer' is an empowered approach to coping with cancer stressors.

### Spirit

The key to spiritual detoxification is surrender. The spirit soars when a person realises and accepts that he or she cannot control the universe. Faith is a curative substance and hope brings healing. Love of God, love of others and of oneself will generate contentment and peace. People experience spirituality in many different ways but to me, applying religious truths to one's life is the most powerful way of building spiritual fortitude. When a person is nourished by a diet of the fruit of the spirit, his or her soul will detoxify and purity will result.

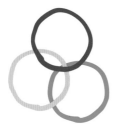
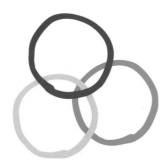
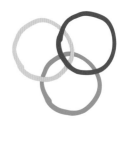

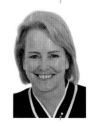

# DETOXING AT HOME

Detoxing the body isn't necessarily as intense or as difficult as it might sound. People often think of detox as a situation in which you massively deprive yourself of everything you enjoy. In fact, good detoxification can be an entirely normal part of your life. Whether you have cancer or not, gently and constantly including a detoxification element in your programme brings tremendous health benefits.

You can detox both internally and externally. The skin is a much underused detox organ and can help relieve the pressure on the liver and kidneys (I list four methods below). Detoxing internally will really boost your wellbeing. All forms of detox may increase the speed at which the body eliminates drugs, so make sure that you get advice on what is an appropriate and safe programme for you.

There are clinics where more intensive detoxing with support and help is available, but at home the following can form part of your programme:

### Internal detoxing
- Juicing, the most nutritious form of detox; it boosts your energy and sense of wellbeing (see 'Juicing for cancer', pp. 102-5, in Chapter 6, 'Concentrated nutrition: juicing, raw and superfoods')
- Liver flush, done regularly, will ensure your liver has the support to cope with any treatments; ask your practitioner about this
- Coffee enemas are part of many metabolic programmes; they flush the liver and remove toxins from the bowel (see 'Coffee enemas', p. 195)
- Epsom salts, taken orally, help to clear the bowel and raise magnesium levels; talk to your practitioner about this as there are some contraindications
- Bentonite clay has a high concentration of minerals and will remove toxins from the bowel
- Sodium bicarbonate not only alkalises, but kills yeasts and microbes

### Skin detoxing
- Epsom salt baths remove toxins and draw magnesium into the body; the most delightful way to detox
- Bentonite clay baths are highly effective at removing heavy metals from the body
- Dry skin brushing stimulates your lymphatic system and improves your circulation
- Personal infrared saunas are an inexpensive and enjoyable way to utilise the skin as a detox organ; build up slowly to around thirty minutes use a day

Filtering your water supply will ensure that you are not being subjected to toxic hormones daily and to the high level of chemicals that are used to clean the water. Drinking water regularly is a cheap and efficient method of detoxing.

Remember that cancer is a very complex disease. Although these are home strategies, they should be practised under the overall supervision of an expert, as your particular circumstances could mean that one or more of these approaches is unsuitable or may need to be adapted to suit you.

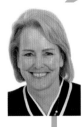

# LONG-TERM DETOXIFICATION PLANS

If you have been diagnosed with cancer only recently, you might be struggling to deal with all the implications simultaneously. Try not to worry. Once you are on the road to recovery, it may be time to take stock and consider if you wish to make further investigations.

Looking at the underlying factors that allow cells to multiply unchecked, there is a certain amount of evidence that viruses, bacteria and parasites can play a part.[18] The link between viruses and certain types of cancer is well established, both in contributing to and increasing the risk of recurrence. This is the case for lymphomas and cancers of the cervix, head and neck, throat, stomach, bladder and lung; further types will probably be revealed as research in this area progresses.

Clinical evidence on parasites and their relationship to cancer is a little more sporadic, but the links and potential are certainly real. We can pick up parasites from cattle, our water supply and all too often from yeasts, amoeba, fungi and microbes. I would be surprised if anybody came through chemotherapy or radiotherapy to the gut without suffering candida in the gut. Damage to the gut flora that control yeast overgrowth through these treatments or through accompanying antibiotics can give free rein to candida to convert into a fungus that can spread throughout the body.

Bacteria can also be associated with malignancy, although again, the evidence is in short supply; further research on this is needed urgently. The most established link is that between *Helicobacter pylori* and stomach cancer.[19] Long-term infection can lead to ulcers and then on to malignancy.

Viruses, bacteria or parasites can inhabit the body without producing any symptoms, but they can undermine your recovery and so deserve serious consideration. This is too large a subject to detail here, but dealing with these germs as part of your recovery detox programme is not difficult and need not be costly; if it is, get some advice from your support team. Consult your practitioner for information on testing, if appropriate, and on strategies to get rid of any infections.

# IN CONCLUSION

As you can see, there are many things you can do to detoxify and help prevent or overcome cancer. You may be wondering what happened to my patient Stephie. She is cancer free. I am sure that our Oasis of Hope therapies were helpful but the number one agent that detoxified her body, mind and spirit was her own attitude. She used the same determination needed to run marathons to discipline herself to make all the necessary changes needed to live a cancer-free life. She also understood that cancer treatment is not a sprint. It is a marathon that takes commitment, discipline and persistence.

Cancer is a race that can be won.

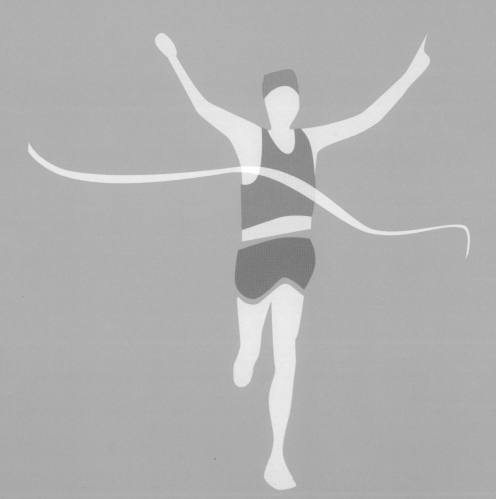

# PART FIVE

## HOSPITALS AND
# TESTING

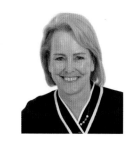

# INTRODUCTION TO PART FIVE

Patricia Peat

In the UK, an NHS oncologist represents a key player in most people's Integrative Medicine team, so it's wise to become as familiar as possible with what you should expect in dealing with the NHS and with oncologists. This part of *The Cancer Revolution* looks at the ways in which you can get the support you need from them.

An understanding of the tests used to detect, assess and monitor cancers is essential to keeping you informed and at the centre of your own treatment programme. The two chapters in Part Five include an overview of both those tests used by the NHS and others that are available within Integrative Medicine.

"NEVER FORGET THAT THROUGHOUT YOUR DISEASE PROCESS, IT IS YOU IN THE DRIVING SEAT MAKING DECISIONS, NOT THE ONCOLOGISTS."

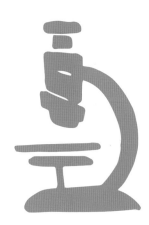

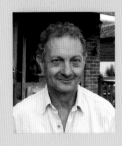

# CHAPTER 14

## BE INFORMED

### Dr Henry Mannings

STAR
THROWERS

A cancer diagnosis, whether it is for you, a child or another loved one, is a disorientating and frightening experience. It is likely to be have been preceded by a period of increasing concern, doctors' visits and diagnostic tests. And, hot on the heels of the diagnosis, comes the induction into the stressful and difficult life of the cancer patient. To call the experience life-changing is an understatement. This new world operates with different rules from those of the world you've experienced before. There is a new language to learn, new rules of engagement and, it feels, little time and space for you to adjust. But adjust you must, and this chapter is intended to equip you with some practical advice. I hope that it will help you to regain some measure of control and to ensure that you're not just a passive case number to be processed. The aim is to supply you with the knowledge required to build a partnership with your clinicians as you navigate your way through treatment.

### The oncologist

Generally, it is a physician or surgeon who, following a series of investigations, informs you that you have cancer. If it is a surgeon, you may be offered surgery to remove the tumour if it is operable; but even in these cases you will normally be referred to an oncologist to manage any additional treatment, usually chemotherapy, that is often included as part of a treatment protocol. Doctors each have a specialist field and so will pass you on to the oncologist for full analysis and communication of the full picture to you.

Some may deal with you in a warm and empathic manner, whereas others will adopt a more formal approach, which they see as professional; the latter often act as if they are the only experts and assume that you the patient will unquestioningly do as you are told. This may seem cold and impersonal, but doctors often feel that they have to place some emotional barriers between themselves and their patients, if only to safeguard their own wellbeing.

It is highly unlikely that you wil have had much say in the choice of your oncologist. For most of us, whether patients, parents or carers, we will have had no chance to think about who we'd like to choose; things are too frantic and scary for much deliberation. This is largely due to a system designed to meet people's needs in the panic and stress of diagnosis. You do, however, have options to slow things down and give yourself time to think. Before your first meeting, be ready to articulate what you would ideally want from an oncologist, who is, after all, generally the consultant in charge of your treatment.

Most oncologists specialise in two or three types of cancer. It is important to find out how much interest and experience they have in your type. For example, are they involved in research into your form of cancer? If so, they may be sufficiently knowledgeable to be aware of the most promising trials that are available. It is not just acceptable but vital that you ask these questions, so that you build a good relationship with your doctor; remember that it might last for many months or even years. You will have to place an enormous amount of trust in what he or she does, so asking some awkward questions is important from two points of view. First, because you want to know the answers, but, possibly more importantly, you want to see how the oncologist reacts to your questions. If the reponse you get is one of affront or if your questions are considered to have been insulting or impertinent, that does not bode well. It is obviously a much more promising start if your questions are answered honestly and without much fuss.

Of course, the answers themselves might matter most of all. It is not always possible, however, to work out what a good answer is. This is partly down to how well you ask the questions. For example, asking a question about how often the doctor treats cancer is not as good as asking how often he or she treats **your** type of cancer, and even that is not as good as asking for more detail about the specific sub-type of cancer with which you have been diagnosed.

Even more difficult to interpret is the question of research. On the face of it, having an oncologist who has a distinguished publishing record and is much in demand for conferences and lectures might seem a great idea. What could be better than being treated by a world-class expert? The downsides can be that your oncologist is so busy in the laboratory, in the conference hall or lecture theatre that he or she is not readily available to you, might skip clinics or delegate to junior colleagues.

## The first oncology appointment

At your first meeting with your oncologist you'll normally find him or her accompanied by an oncology nurse, and possibly one or more other doctors. At this moment you are probably feeling fearful, with little idea of what to expect. You have been told that you have cancer but have no real understanding yet of what this means. In your head, cancer means death, and you feel totally panicked as you are not ready to die.

These feelings, while often overwhelming, are completely normal and expected, yet in this situation you are likely to find it difficult to take in or comprehend the information supplied to you. It is therefore imperative that you bring at least one other person to this appointment, preferably someone who is clear-headed. You might choose your partner, a close family member or best friend – though beware of asking anyone who is even more freaked out than you are. If possible, try to find someone who has a medical, nursing or scientific background as well as a strong personal connection with you.

In terms of outlining your prognosis, the oncologist will recommend a treatment, which could be a hormone therapy, chemotherapy, radiotherapy or a combination of these, depending on the type of tumour. Typically you will be presented with an outline of a protocol – which drugs, how many cycles (treatment courses), the sequence of treatments and so on. If surgery is still an option, chemotherapy may be given either before surgery (neo-adjuvant), to reduce the size of the tumour, or after (adjuvant) to mop up any tumour cells that 'got away'. Common side effects, both minor and major, will probably also be discussed.

It is important to ask if the therapy is being given with curative or with palliative intent; unfortunately for many it will be the latter. It is vital to understand the standpoint from which you are being advised, as this provides the context of the treatment you are about to be given. Without this clarity, for example, a patient may accept a harsh treatment with marginal benefits in the hope of a cure, when in fact a cure is not even an intended outcome. In addition to the side effects of chemotherapy and radiotherapy, it is important to confirm that the stated improvements in survival have been established in the medical literature; some oncologists can overstate the benefits of the treatments.

At this stage, try to take in as much information as possible, but do not make any decisions. These are among the most important decisions you will ever have to make, so take as long as you need to digest the information calmly. The only exceptions to this are the rare situations in which any delay could lead to death, as in some leukaemias where a low platelet count could lead to severe haemorrhage. Most oncologists will appreciate that you need time before deciding on your next step. They might be happy for you to ring them to let them know if you want to proceed or not. In the meantime, you will want to research the treatment offered carefully.

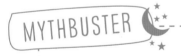

MYTHBUSTER

## "UNLESS EVERY CANCER CELL IN MY BODY IS KILLED OR CUT OUT I WON'T SURVIVE"

It is unlikely that orthodox approaches can kill off every cancer cell in the body – and they don't claim to do so. If that were the way to 'cure cancer', there would be little reason for any hope. What Integrative Medicine aims to do is to enable your body to provide long-term support for your whole being; it is intended to help you to control cancer, not to get rid of it at speed.

If you are a woman who has not yet reached menopause, you may want to discuss the possible impact of treatments on your fertility and consider freezing some eggs before commencing.

Some people feel the need to ask the oncologist how much longer they have to live, as they want to put their affairs in order and/or plan for the future of their families. Usually, if the patient does not request this information, it will not be volunteered, so don't ask unless you really want the doctor's opinion. The answer will be given on the basis of survival figures comparing rates of survival with and without treatment. This figure is derived from statistics relating to a large group of patients, most of whom have not considered an integrative path, and will not have looked at other ways of helping themselves. Given that you are reading this book, you are not part of that statistical group, and so the prognosis may have little relevance to you, other than as a benchmark to aim for and to beat.

Sometimes, the oncologist might tell you how effective the treatment is. This is described in terms of a 'complete' or 'partial' response. It is imperative that you understand what this means, as it can be easily misinterpreted. A complete response means either that the tumour has disappeared on a CT scan or that the tumour markers have normalised. A partial response means that the tumour has shrunk by at least 50 per cent; if it has shrunk less than that, it is classified as 'stable' disease, whereas if the tumour has continued to grow, the disease is referred to as 'progressive'.

Contrary to what you might think, a complete response means simply that there has been no evidence of a tumour for a month. So, if you have been told that you have had a complete response to chemotherapy, it does not necessarily mean that you are cured. In reality the tumour could be back in a few weeks or months, but you are currently in a state where there is no disease apparent.

If you have been told that your disease is incurable because your cancer is not amenable to surgery ('not resectable' is how your doctor might describe this), it is important to make certain that this really is the case. If the tumour has spread to other organs, the reality is that surgery is not an option, although occasionally this can change if the tumour turns out to be exceptionally sensitive to chemotherapy. If there is no evidence of spread or distant disease, you must ask why surgery is not an option. This decision has to come from a surgeon, not from an oncologist or radiologist.

Some tumours are localised, with no evidence of spread, but are deemed inoperable because the tumour has encased vital blood vessels. In that case, I would urge you to get a second opinion from a hospital known for performing surgery in the region of the body that is relevant to you. Again, do not rely on a referral to a second oncologist, as he or she might have insufficient knowledge of the surgical skills required; instead do some research on the internet to find a surgeon with an outstanding reputation and insist that you are referred.

## Subsequent meetings

Once a treatment plan has been agreed, you will be given a programme with details of dates and times for drugs, radiotherapy, surgery and/or various scans and tests to monitor how you are doing. There will be checkpoints where you will be 're-staged', and the plans will diverge depending on whether your disease is stable, increasing or decreasing.

Meeting doctors will be a regular event, but when you are having different forms of treatment, it's the major meetings with your oncologist that will assume the greatest importance, particularly when waiting for results from scans or examinations. On such occasions you will probably be stressed and apprehensive. No matter how much you like or respect your doctors, feeling tense and nervous is completely understandable. Sitting in the waiting-room can cause anxiety, especially if the clinic is running late. You can all too easily get so stressed that you forget the questions you've waited for ages to ask. You might be blindsided by news (good or bad), get diverted by some other train of thought or simply sit there passively while the doctor leads the discussion. Afterwards, you'll kick yourself for not having remembered to ask your questions, in which case you will either have to wait for the next appointment or find someone else to help you.

So, again, the first rule before you see your doctor, particularly for any big follow-up meetings, is to prepare in advance. First and foremost, take the time to sit down and go through what it is you want to know. If possible, don't leave it to the last minute. Discuss your questions with family or friends if you like, but make sure that you have a whole list written down on paper. You can hand this list to the doctor, stating that these are the points you would like covered during your conversation. Tick off the questions as they are answered to ensure that nothing is missed.

Having pen and paper to hand is always sensible: if your oncologist mentions a drug, treatment or side effect that you've never heard of, write it down immediately. As a lot of the drugs that are used in oncology have complicated names, never be afraid to stop and ask for the spelling. The drugs may just trip off the tongue of a specialist, but for most of us us they are new and strange. It's the same for treatments – such terms as intra-arterial chemoembolisation, photodynamic therapy and so on are difficult to remember, especially in the wake of bad news.

Some people even consider recording their meetings. While this is useful as a point of reference in the event of any disagreement, I would advise that you guard against putting your medical team in defensive mode. Get the consent of all concerned before making a recording.

Especially if the meeting has been a difficult one, recheck your list and go back to anything that has been missed. It takes a certain amount of courage and discipline to do this, and you may wish to avoid coming across as demanding, but it is always important that you get your questions answered. The default position is normally for the patient to be a passive receiver of treatment. That might be fine if you're dealing with a bit of an infection, but when you're dealing with cancer, you need to take control – believe it or not, you'll feel better as soon as you do so.

It is certainly worthwhile to get your oncologist's email address. Ask for it outright, or else find it on the hospital website. There will be times when you want to ask a quick question or to discuss something you've read about (for example a new drug or treatment) at the next appointment. Rather than just turning up at an appointment with an article for discussion with your doctor, send the article in advance and there will be more chance of having it read, with time for a detailed response. Some doctors will be more than happy to communicate via email, while others might be shocked. At worst your emails will be ignored; at best you can engage in a dialogue that enables you to access support outside a clinic or a hospital ward.

# TREATMENTS

First-line treatment – the first treatment recommended – has become standardised, and oncologists normally follow prescribed guidelines. As a result, therapy options can be limited.

## Chemotherapy

This is given in cycles, each of which usually corresponds to a three- or four-week period. For example, you may have one chemotherapy drug just once every three weeks, another drug weekly for three weeks and then a week off. Some chemotherapy is in tablet form, and this usually means taking it daily, but again often with a period of rest. If it is not included in your protocol by default, ensure that you and your oncologist agree to a reassessment after an allotted number of cycles, normally after the second or third cycle of treatment. At that point, investigations such as a repeat CT/MRI scan, chest X-ray or blood tests for tumour markers should be done to ensure that the tumour is responding to therapy.

If there is no response to chemotherapy by the end of the third cycle, the chances of response after that are small, and it is time to change tactics. I have seen patients being continued on chemotherapy despite tumour progression, either because they were not re-assessed properly after three cycles, or because the oncologist decided to continue for no valid reason – perhaps they had nothing else to offer. This is not acceptable, not only as it affects the patients' quality of life, but as it wastes valuable time when they could be looking at other possibilites, or simply enjoying their lives.

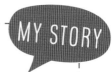

**MY STORY**

### Mara
Breast cancer, diagnosed in April 2011

*My experience has shown that one should always, always, always go for a second opinion. Not all consultants are alike. Don't assume that all the young ones will be innovative and the older ones will hark back to their days of study many decades ago. In my experience it has been completely the other way around.*

*It may be difficult to know where to go for a second opinion, so my advice is to look for a big hospital, a teaching hospital, a university hospital. Look at the credentials and photos of the consultants on their website – you will find some you like the look of and some you don't. Keep copies of all your notes so as to avoid delays in obtaining information from your current consultant. If you can afford it, pay to be seen as a private patient for your first consultation; that way you can be seen almost immediately. It's worth it for peace of mind – then you can join his/her NHS list later.*

*I spent two and a half years with a consultant who was the top man at my local hospital – what a mistake! When things got really bad for me, I found a consultant in a nearby city who was known to be sympathetic to Integrative Medicine. This new man has turned out to be about as good as you can get.*

*He is interested in me, I can talk to him and he is up to date. He has far more skills than the previous consultant, and clearly cares about me. He has offered me several options and has no intention of carrying out the extremely harsh treatment deemed essential by my previous consultant.*

*In my experience, getting a second opinion has been a life-saver. Hold out for what you want, or at least for someone you can have a rapport with. They are out there, and it makes the whole experience of having cancer, which is grim at the best of times, bearable. These 'super-specialists' really can change your whole life.*

*Don't give up. Lucky me; I wish you luck too.*

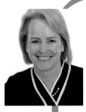

# FRONTIER NHS TREATMENTS

The NHS has several relatively unknown treatment approaches that, while possibly suitable in your case, will not necessarily be offered to you. Oncologists might not be that familiar with them or be aware of the range of cancers treated with them; perhaps they are not in the habit of recommending them. In some instances, mainly when cancer is not widespread, these treatments can offer fewer side effects or even an encouraging prognosis, so they are definitely worth investigating (see **Part Eight, 'Resources'**). Included in this category are CyberKnife (a sophisticated radiotherapy technique), photodynamic therapy or PDT (a laser treatment), NanoKnife (using electrical current), laser ablation, radio frequency ablation or RFA and high intensity focused ultrasound or HIFU.

At your re-assessment meeting, sit down with your oncologist and consider your next move. If the tumour has shrunk and you are not suffering the effects of treatment, then the obvious answer is to continue. If the tumour has increased in size, further discussion is certainly warranted. It may be suggested that you have a break from treatment, to give you time to recover from the effects of chemotherapy, and then to consider whether you want to try the second line. At this point, it is worth asking the oncologist a simple question: 'If your partner or child were in the same position as I am in now, would you go down this route?' If not, why not?' In most cases this will produce a truthful answer. Whether your doctors feel the second-line chemotherapy option is worth considering or not, they should be able to guide you on your next move.

## Tumour spread to liver and lungs

Tumours that have spread to the liver used to be considered untreatable. Now that surgeons have a better knowledge of liver anatomy (or more specifically understand that the liver can be divided into different sections, each with its own blood supply) it has become possible to treat these secondary cancers. As a result of this, certain sections of the liver can be resected, as long as there is enough of the organ left behind to carry out its normal functions.

If liver resection is not possible, however, all is not lost. There are procedures such as radio-frequency ablation (RFA), in which, under the guidance of a CT scan, a needle is placed directly into the tumour and a radio-wave passes down the needle, resulting in heating of the tumour and its death. New forms of ultrasound are capable of carrying out the same destructive process without the need for penetration through the skin, although this is not yet widely available. Not all lesions can be targeted this way: it depends on their position, size and quantity.

Therefore, if you have secondary tumours in your liver, ask for referral to a centre that has liver surgeons and radiologists. You have nothing to lose and everything to gain from an assessment for possible treatment. Once you are diagnosed with tumours in your liver, don't allow an oncologist to suggest waiting to see how you respond to chemotherapy.

Insist on urgent referral: the smaller the tumours, the easier they are to deal with.

A few interventional radiologists (the doctors who are using these new ablative therapies) will similarly ablate secondary tumours in the lungs, so if the spread of the tumour is limited to this area, ask about referral for RFA. Your oncologist might say that such a service is not available, at which point you and your support team set about finding the closest regional centre that does the procedure. It is your right to be referred there for a second opinion. If your oncologist refuses to refer you, you could approach your GP for a referral or even decide to change your oncologist.

# SEARCHING FOR CLINICAL TRIALS

## International options

If chemotherapy is no longer considered a worthwhile option for you, ask your oncologist for advice on what to do next. You might be told simply to go away and enjoy the rest of your life, or possibly to enter a trial. Looking for a clinical trial can be daunting. It is certainly crucial to review the available options. The first and most important thing to keep in mind is that clinical trials are conducted for different reasons, which are usually indicated by the phase that the trial has reached, whether Phase I, II or III.

Phase I trials are normally the first to test candidate drugs or other treatments for humans. To get to Phase I, a drug will have gone through 'pre-clinical' testing in the test tube (in vitro) or in animals (in vivo). Occasionally a drug is tested in tiny amounts in humans before going into a proper Phase I trial. The key aim of the latter is to find the appropriate dosing of the drug. The effectiveness of a treatment is of secondary importance. The researchers are convinced by the pre-clinical evidence that the

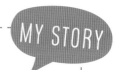

MY STORY

### Gordon
Oesophageal cancer, diagnosed in 2012

*Some specialists may have disappointed you with their neutral or negative reaction to your strategy, but it's important not to cast them off too soon. You may just need them further down the line. Keep the key members of your team informed, even if they don't all fully agree with your strategy. If they are at all professional, they will respect you for what you are doing, and will agree to meet you again when you want to discuss something with them later.*

*I had a few verbal battles with my oncologist, but she was very supportive when I decided to retire from my employment (thus releasing me from workplace stress). She was key to helping me get my employment pension enhanced to its maximum. I have since started working again part time for people I want to work for. I keep my oncologist fully informed of my progress with my European cancer specialist, as I may need her again. She may even become curious herself one day.*

drug has some effect, but they cannot establish how good it is in practice until a proper dosing schedule is in place. Also, Phase I trials tend to be on a small scale (there are only a few patients, often based at a single hospital or clinic and involving only a few members in the research team).

Phase II trials take things a step further. The dose has been established and there are often some indications of effectiveness. There is still an element of scrutinising the dosing schedule or treatment protocol, but the emphasis is now on finding out whether the positive effects seen in the pre-clinical studies hold true in humans. Phase II studies are often on a larger scale – more patients, more doctors, possibly multiple locations.

Phase III trials are generally the final stage of testing a treatment before it becomes widely accepted. It depends on the Phase II trial (or trials, in some cases), suggesting that a treatment is as good as (or better than) an existing one; these two could have the same overall effectiveness, but one of them might show certain benefits, for example fewer side effects or a lower cost. In the best cases a new treatment should give better results than an existing one and have fewer side effects. Phase III trials tend to involve significantly larger numbers of patients and clinicians as well as increased numbers and range of treatment centres. Given the substantially greater quantity of patients, the results are considered 'statistically significant'.

In terms of desirability, Phase III trials are clearly more of interest than Phase II, and Phase II more than Phase I. Having established that much, you now need to find out what trials are going on at the moment. Each hospital should have one or more doctors in charge of co-ordinating its clinical trials. They will know what is available, and the chances are that your oncologist will discuss your case with the relevant doctor.

NIH

If you want to cast your net wider, however, you could choose to consult the US National Institutes of Health Clinical Trials database. Despite this being run by the NIH, the scope is truly international. The user interface is simple, and you can input queries on your specific disease, on country of trial, phase of trial and much more, including queries on specific drugs (particularly useful if you are interested in following up on any details that you have found in researching the literature). You can also filter for trials that are currently recruiting as well as for those that have completed. For each trial there is a web page that shows details of the trial, relevant contact details and links to related papers or previous results and so on. If you wish to create RSS feeds you will be updated with new trials and updates to existing trials. It is a great resource.

PFIZER

Not all clinical trials are on the NIH database, however, (in particular some of the smaller Phase I trials are often omitted). Other places to look include some of the larger drug companies, whose Clinical Trials Officers are there to help direct candidates to the appropriate trials. Pfizer, for example, is among those to have a central site dedicated to oncology trials.

You might now be feeling overwhelmed by all this information. If so, just remember that it is a good source of contacts for you to consult when you are ready to find further details about anything you seriously want to explore. The people running the trials are ethically bound not to share results before a study is complete, but they can certainly offer advice at any time. If you strike up a good email relationship with one of the team, you could put your oncologist in direct contact with someone who is running a trial. Even if you do not participate directly in a trial (because it is in a different country, for example), your oncologist could possibly arrange for you to have access to the drug off-trial. At the very least you could print out the information about a trial or send your oncologist a link so you can discuss whether a trial or treatment is the right one for you or not.

## UK Clinical Trials Gateway

A recent addition to the tools available to those looking for clinical trials is the UK Clinical Trials Gateway. While not a central registry itself, it does enable the user to search a number of international registries through its website. You can look up specific types of cancer, drugs and various forms of therapy, both single and in combinations (e.g. 'celecoxib and cancer'). For each record returned by the search, you can find out whether the trial is recruiting patients and where the trial is taking place as well as details of the treatment itself. For patients wanting a trial, it is a really useful place to start.

UKCTG

## Other options

If you do not find any suitable conventional therapies or trials, it is time to explore alternative options. This search seldom includes your oncologists, as relatively few of them have relevant knowledge or experience; indeed, many of them will seek to warn their patients away from such approaches. It is important not to be lulled into spending enormous amounts of money on an unproven therapy without some sound advice. You could consult an organisation such as Cancer Options or Yes to Life that can help with specialised information in this area.

CANCER OPTIONS

## What is the web good for?

As far as medical research is concerned, where the internet comes into its own is in offering boundless opportunities to see what new treatments are being used throughout the world, with details of their results. You might decide to talk to doctors abroad or to track down the new treatments in your own country. It offers an overview of what treatments are still undergoing clinical trials and those that have pre-clinical evidence of efficacy. Furthermore, you could choose to contact researchers directly to ask questions about your own case.

YES TO LIFE

There is a wealth of information out there, both good and bad. The difficulty can be in establishing what is credible and what is not. The important thing is to remain sceptical at all times, but also to retain hope that you will find leads to help for your existing situation, whether involving new options in your country or abroad.

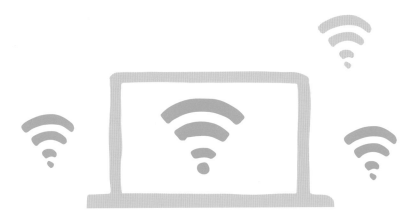

# CONCLUDING REMARKS

## Lines of communication

My contribution to *The Cancer Revolution* focuses on the relationship between patient and doctor, especially concerning areas where there are likely to be disagreements, for example in discussing alternative or complementary treatments. But this is not the only area where communications are often difficult. A recent study from the University of Athens, Greece found that 'managing communication around cancer diagnosis gives patients a sense of control in an otherwise uncontrollable situation'. The researchers found that: 'communication is an important factor in coping with cancer in that it enables people to exert control during a highly stressful and turbulent time. However, despite best efforts to structure and control that communication, cancer patients cannot always predict or control other people's reaction.'[1]

In my experience the need to communicate with friends and family can simply become exhausting. Particularly if you have just had bad news, the need to relay it multiple times almost always makes you feel worse. The constant repetition of such news is depressing, especially when you are aware that the person on the receiving end is likely to be distressed as well. You not only have to deal with your own reactions, but end up managing other people's too. It is not surprising that this adds to the stress you are already experiencing.

Of course your family and friends are not deliberately adding to your pressure. They are concerned and mostly want to help in some way, possibly by giving you a shoulder to cry on. What they often don't realise is that they are not the only people calling you, and that sometimes you need the space to think and absorb news (good or bad) on your own. Receiving a concerned phone call immediately after a difficult meeting with your oncologist or other doctor is especially exhausting. When you're uncertain how you feel after receiving scan results, or a new disease staging or diagnosis, having to relay the news is simply hard to do.

One way of solving this problem, at least to some extent, is to ask one – or perhaps better two – people to communicate with everyone else on your behalf. That way you can impose some control over the situation, so that you will have time and space to absorb news, to think about things and to focus your energies where you need them most. When you have something to report, you relay it only once or twice, and then let the news spread to your wider community of friends and family, without causing undue stress to yourself.

Finally and most importantly, it is vital to remember that, apart from infections, doctors do not cure diseases. On the other hand, surgeons can cure diseases, sometimes. To control such conditions as asthma, inflammatory bowel disease, diabetes or arthritis, the physician will prescribe drugs, but these therapies usually have to be taken continuously. Oncologists, when they know they can't cure you, switch to trying to control the rate of growth of the tumour.

Never forget that throughout your disease process, it is you in the driving seat making decisions, not the oncologists. They are there to advise you, but it is you who has to take control. The more informed you are, the better.

## To Summarise

- Put yourself in charge of your case
- Be sure that you trust and want to work with your oncologist
- Prepare well for meetings and take someone with you
- Make absolutely sure that you get all the answers you need
- Don't allow yourself to be rushed into important decisions
- You are entitled to second opinions – don't be put off pursuing them
- Be prepared to explore other options yourself
- Consider asking someone to manage your communications with friends and relatives

*N.B.: Some of this chapter is based on material by Dr Pan Pantziarka, and has previously appeared on www.anticancer.org.uk.*

## MYTHBUSTER

# "A CANCER DIAGNOSIS IS AN EMERGENCY – THERE JUST ISN'T TIME TO CONSIDER ALL THE OPTIONS CAREFULLY"

This myth has been well and truly busted. Apart from some exceptional cases, cancer is known to take many years to develop in the body. The urgency to rush into treatment within a matter of weeks, or even days, is nonsense. Take several deep breaths and step back from everyone who is concerned about when you are to begin your treatment. Give yourself time to educate yourself: take stock and approach the future with a full evaluation of what it is that what you want to do; ensure that you have a detailed, supportive programme in place.

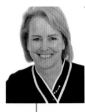

# WHAT DO I TELL MY ONCOLOGIST?

When it comes to discussing integrative approaches with doctors in the UK, reactions and responses vary tremendously. After you have spent time and effort researching and evaluating which strategies you want to incorporate in dealing with your cancer, you might then decide to discuss them with your oncology team. You might receive any of the following reactions:

- I have no idea about any of that, not my field, so do as you please
- Right, well, we don't like antioxidants or herbal stuff or supplements as they might interfere, so leave those out while you are on treatment
- The pharmacy will check what you are interested in and let you know if anything is likely to interfere with your treatment
- I will speak to the practitioners you are considering to provide your treatment and see if we can agree a strategy
- If you consider anything other than my method of treatment, I will refuse to treat or support you

If you get a really negative response from your team, you are certainly in difficult territory. Attitudes vary enormously between specific individuals and equally from hospital to hospital and department to department. There is no consensus of opinion from the medical profession. In contrast to the USA, in the UK there are no departments within the NHS that are set up to evaluate and provide doctors with standardised information; this means that the reaction you are getting is a completely individual one.

What needs to be established, if possible, is this: is the doctor providing a reasonable and professional opinion on something she or he knows about, or is it an opinion based on ignorance, perhaps even prejudice? It can be galling beyond measure to work hard at getting yourself motivated and positive about contributing to your recovery, only to be told that you are wasting your time and money on charlatans, that nothing you do can possibly make a difference.

If your doctor does know about the treatment you are having, and has concerns, of course you need to hear them. What you don't need is a consultation to turn into a battleground where the two viewpoints expressed are so polarised that you are never going to find any common ground. But it is vital to bear in mind that your doctor is fully qualified, knowledgeable and experienced in the relevant field; although he or she might have no interest in the other treatment options that you are pursuing, his or her expertise and support will probably form a cornerstone of your overall programme. So finding a constructive way to work with your doctor is definitely in your best interests.

Countless cancer patients who struggle with feelings of hopelessness and helplessness, on being told that their condition is not curable, can often resent their doctors' communication strategy. Those who are succeeding in surviving in good health, even if the eventual outcome is death, say that they come out of consultation of this kind totally deflated. They went in hoping for a crumb of support, only to have their efforts belittled by doctors who believe only in pharmaceuticals. If this is your experience, do not invite this type of comment in your discussions. Remember that doctors' views reflect only what they are able to achieve. In general they have no knowledge or experience of what you can achieve for yourself – yours is the only measure of that.

Integrative Medicine is about putting yourself in charge. You therefore need to evaluate:

- Is this person giving me an informed professional opinion that I need to pursue?

- Does my research into Integrative Medicine give me enough confidence to trust the source and everyone involved?

- If my doctor is not entirely behind my programme, can our relationship withstand my different viewpoint?; should I look for someone else to provide that element of my programme?

There is an increasing number of well-qualified and experienced people who can help you work out how you wish to deal with difficult situations and doctors (see **Part Eight, 'Resources'**). While no-one would advocate that you do not keep your doctor informed of important decisions that you are making about your care, it is vital that you place yourself at the centre of your team. Remember that each contributing person holds only one piece of the jigsaw; it is you who puts the entire puzzle together.

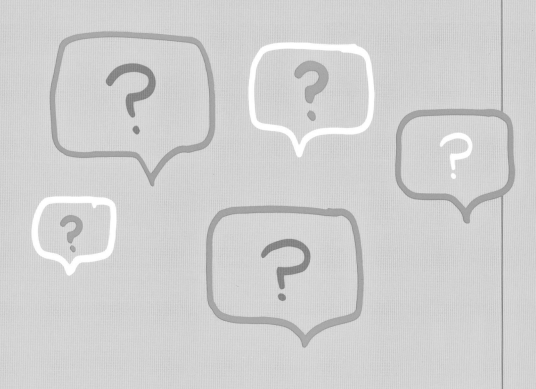

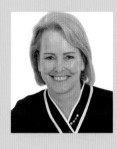

# CHAPTER 15

# TESTING: VITAL POINTERS TO SUCCESS

## Patricia Peat

When you are diagnosed with cancer, a great deal of analysis takes place before each step is decided. Once treatment is complete, type and level of analysis can vary tremendously, dependent on the specific cancer you have.

Tests fall into four broad groups:

- diagnostic scans
- cancer markers
- chemosensitivity tests
- functional tests

### Diagnostic scans

Scanning is the diagnostic technique with which we are most familiar (for an overview see **Appendix 2**, '**Understanding scans**'); but detecting any activity before it is large enough to be visible on a scan is obviously far more desirable. Scans are often used in tandem with biopsies – laboratory inspections of tumour tissue samples – to confirm a diagnosis.

### Cancer markers

Cancer or tumour markers are substances found in the blood or urine that are produced by the body in response to cancers, or indeed to some other benign conditions. There is no 'universal' tumour marker that can detect any type of cancer.

While initial analysis tells us a certain amount, in reality we learn most about someone's cancer in retrospect. Once treatment has been given, we have to wait to see how well it has worked. We largely lack the ability to predict how much the cancer might be resistant to treatment or how quickly it might come back if it has not been eradicated. Instead, practitioners attempt to track progress with tumour markers. In 2015 we have tumour markers for only a few of the known cancers, and interpretation of them needs to be made in relation to the wider picture. This is very much an area of scientific development – to have accurate and responsive markers for every case is an oncologist's dream, something for the future. So far, there are over twenty markers in clinical use, some associated with two or more cancer types. Your oncologist will guide you as to whether you have a marker and whether it is one that is responsive and reflective of the cancer state in your body.

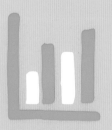

Doctors examine tumour-marker results with the following factors in mind:

- If you are diagnosed with a cancer that has a tumour marker, your cancer may not necessarily excrete those particular molecules; the marker will therefore remain low, even if you have active cancer
- Other elements in the body, such as viruses and inflammation, may cause an increase in a marker
- The cancer might at some point stop excreting the marker, even if it is active, and become independent of it
- Accuracy of some markers, for example the PSA (prostate specific antigen) for prostate cancer, is not entirely reliable

Markers therefore need to be interpreted with caution. It is all too easy to focus on them to such an extent that you become unduly stressed by mild fluctuations, which are actually not significant. It is usually the underlying trend that is important, and you need to notice a substantial rise occurring, several times, to justify concern. I often speak to people who are worried by an increase in a marker of three or four points; that is until I inform them that the upper levels can reach several thousands. Perspective is all-important here.

The PSA test is a prime example of how difficult this area is. It is deemed the 'gold standard' for assessing the progression of prostate cancer. Nevertheless, there are still major disagreements about its reliability, as the growth of prostate cancer can be independent of the test – or can become so. As already emphasised, there are no completely reliable methods to assess cancer, but I now describe some that I hope will add to your understanding of your cancer.

For on-going analysis of how dormant or active your cancer might be, there are a few options not currently used by orthodox doctors. One of the reasons for this is that, like drugs, they are subject to many years of scrutiny before the level of evidence for their use is accepted. Research in other countries as well as experience by practitioners in the UK is opening up options to access another level of monitoring, as used by integrative clinics around the world. Those to have proved most useful, all of which have applications for a wide range of cancers, are:

- Telomerase – over-expression rises with increased cancer activity; samples for testing can also come from a broad variety of tissues or body fluids
- Survivin – over-expression rises with increased cancer activity; an indicator of malignant activity for many cancers
- TM2-PK (or Tumour Marker 2 Pyruvate Kinase) – it shows the level of glucose being used by a tumour, hence also activity

Blood markers give us an advantage as they show activity well before a change becomes visible on a scan, and can therefore effectively monitor progress. They can indicate that you might need to increase your programme or that matters are stable or perhaps even improving. Among their disadvantages, however, is that finding an increased level might not be sufficient evidence to convince your oncologist to take action, if that is what you are wanting to do. Nevertheless, they can be useful for making informed adjustments to your integrative programme.

## Chemosensitivity tests

At the time of writing, the choice of anti-cancer drug depends on statistical analysis of large treatment trials. Chemosensitivity testing, in which chemotherapies are tested against cells isolated from a tumour sample or blood, has been in development for several decades. Such tests have one purpose – to identify agents that are likely to be effective against your cancer, based on trials with a sample of your tumour tissue.

It is obviously desirable to minimise the likelihood of chemotherapy being ineffective, and research continues in this area. It can take many years to evaluate whether the results are consistent and reliable. Testing is available privately and is widely advertised on the internet. In the UK, few doctors are entirely convinced that such tests are reliable. This is particularly frustrating for those who have a cancer from an unknown origin or of a rare type which has attracted little research.

My advice is that if you want to have chemosensitivity tests, it is important to consult your oncologist first in order to avoid the possibility of unnecessary expense. He or she might not agree to use the results for treatment and indeed might not be able to step outside approved treatment protocols to help you.

## Functional tests

Analysis in mainstream medicine focuses on three main aims:

- determining a diagnosis
- monitoring progress, ensuring that the body is functioning within acceptable ranges
- screening so that a medical condition can be identified at an early stage, before symptoms appear

It does not include identifying underlying elements that might have contributed to cancer development; nor does it involve any metabolic imbalances or **damage to your normal cellular environment** that might have arisen from treatment, such as gut symbiosis, inflammation and nutritional depletion. Furthermore it does not monitor **residual cancer activity or the state of your body's defences against further cells becoming** malignant.

**This is where functional testing comes in.** As a continuing theme in this book, integrative methods are recommended to restore normality and health to cells, thereby also helping to prevent recurrence.

### Areas to consider for testing

  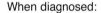

**When diagnosed:**

- gut symbiosis/candida
- viruses
- exposure to toxins
- vitamin and mineral balances
- inflammatory factors

**Following treatment, or if not having treatment:**

- gut symbiosis/candida
- balance of vitamins, minerals and essential fatty acids
- inflammatory factors
- hormonal profile, in the case of a hormone dependent cancer
- endocrine function
- oxidative stress; how well your body is coping with free radicals

## Gene tests

Genes, which indicate the level of repair to the body's defence mechanisms against cancer, can be tested through P53 (a blood protein test) and Bcl-2 (another blood test). Carried out regularly, these can give you a good indication of success, thus letting you know when you can afford to relax your programme. These tests fall outside the four categories listed above, but are important enough to warrant consideration.

For a table of tests and the reasons why you might use them, see thecancerrevolution.co.uk, Chapter 15.

THE CANCER
REVOLUTION

## Costs

Cost is an important consideration. In an ideal world we would all have a full analysis, but, realistically, most of us are restricted by cost. Testing, particularly if on-going, can soon run up a hefty bill. When choosing to work with someone who uses tests, ensure that he or she can give you good reasons for carrying them out; ensure that they are relevant to you and your condition. I am aware of some practitioners who just run the same tests on everyone, without underlying knowledge of each individual's specific needs.

Be sure to discuss with your practitioner:

• What is the aim of the tests?
• How much will they influence your health outcome?
• What are the on-going costs?

Beware of spending a lot on tests that are not sustainable in the long run or have little influence on important treatment decisions. If necessary, get another opinion from a different practitioner.

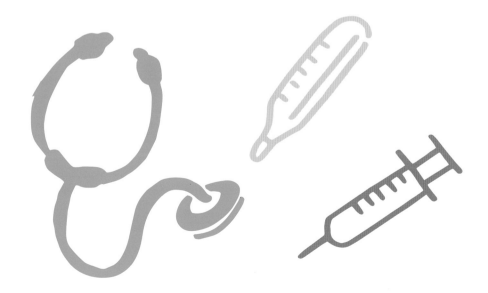

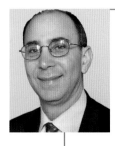

ROBERT
JACOBS

# FUNCTIONAL TESTING
## Robert H. Jacobs

Functional testing has evolved since the mid-1980s and is laboratory based. It focuses on measuring small changes in the body (i.e. quantifying the biochemical micro-environment). This type of testing can be used in several ways: to identify deficiencies or excesses of specific nutrients in the body that could lead to imbalances in its functioning; to show how (at a biochemical level) our diet affects our health; and to show how lifestyle, stress and environmental factors all affect our health. In Western society, there has been an increase in non-communicable chronic illness such as cancer, heart disease and diabetes, as mentioned in various contexts throughout this book.

These chronic illnesses have many complex contributory factors, among which a major one is nutrition;[1] see also **Part Two**, 'Nutrition'. Functional tests examine the micro-environment of our biochemistry, physiology and intracellular function, and the resulting information permits us, individually and specifically, to customise our diet and nutrition, to optimise each body's specific needs at any particular time. This enables us to participate in our health with a greater understanding of how our diet and lifestyle helps us to be healthy. We have a way to make informed choices and to understand the consequences of our actions upon our health. We can also help restore our health if we have been ill. These tests can enable us to ask and have specific answers to the questions: 'How can I stay healthy?' and 'What can I do to help prevent or minimise illness?'

## Why is testing important?

The biochemistry of the body is highly complex. We have approximately ninety trillion cells, every single one of which performs thousands of biochemical processes. To maintain health, the body makes constant adjustments through a stabilising process known as homeostasis. If this balance becomes disrupted, a biochemical, physiological or structural system is altered. The body usually recognises the alteration and automatically works to rebalance. For example, if we become overheated, our homeostatic mechanisms activate sweat glands to lower our body temperature; if we become chilled, a signal is sent to our muscles to shiver and produce heat. This regulation of body temperature happens automatically, naturally, day in and day out. If the body cannot rebalance or correct any disruption, however, imbalance occurs and could become a chronic condition. Depending on our genetics, age, environment, diet and many other factors, chronic imbalance can alter the basic biochemistry of our bodies with the development of symptoms that indicate the imbalance.

What causes such imbalances? What can we do about them? Can they be corrected before they increase and form the environment for illness within the body? Functional testing answers these questions. It offers a way of measuring the degree of balance in the body at a biochemical level and focuses on the areas of imbalance so that the imbalances themselves can be addressed.

Much laboratory-based functional testing uses blood, urine, saliva and stool to assess the level of healthy functioning of our body systems. It includes examining our ability to digest food, to assimilate nutrients, to metabolise nutrients and also to detoxify and metabolise hormones. This is done by measuring specific metabolites in the urine known as organic acids, amino acids in the urine and blood plus hormone levels in saliva and urine.[2]

With the results in hand, we can then focus on optimising our health, for example by individualising our diet in response to our nutritional needs; these can of course vary depending on the demands we might be making on our body, our current state of health and/or medications. If we are exposed to toxic chemicals, drugs, alcohol, radiation, cigarette smoke, stress, negative emotions, trauma or poor diet, our nutritional requirements might also vary. When we take antibiotics, for example, we often need to take probiotics afterwards to replace the beneficial intestinal bacteria killed by the antibiotics. The beneficial intestinal bacteria produce not only vitamins B2, B3, B6, B12, but vitamin K, biotin, folic acid and pantothenic acid; they also manufacture a number of natural antibiotics in our intestines. Destroying the beneficial bacteria causes nutrient depletions and decreases the immune response.[3] There are functional tests that identify and quantify the amount of both healthy and unhealthy bacteria in our digestive tract and can also identify fungi, parasites and worms. We can measure how well our food is being digested and assimilated and the amount of digestive enzymes our pancreas is producing, as well as assessing our ability to break down fats and assimilate nutrients.

Additionally, functional testing helps to ensure that we are not overloading our bodies with a nutrient or food which in itself can create an imbalance. Our biochemical requirements are individual, and through functional testing we can acquire enough information to individualise our diets and nutritional programmes. For example, a measurement of specific organic acids in the urine will show the overall antioxidant status of the body, including the deficiency or excess of such nutrients as vitamin E, vitamin A and coenzyme Q10.[4]

If our health is maintained by the natural constant adjustment of biochemical and physiological pathways – homeostasis – is there more that we can do to help maintain optimal balance? How can we find out?

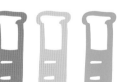

## Common functional tests

Listed below are the functional tests that are commonly used not only to evaluate our nutritional needs but to maintain homeostasis. To give a detailed view of the body's health, I usually recommend a combination profile that integrates many tests together. By combining the information from many tests, a very sensitive indication of deficiencies or excesses of nutrients can be obtained. The combination profiles I often include are:

- An organic acid profile, to evaluate gastrointestinal function, cellular energy production, neurotransmitter processing and our individual need for vitamins and minerals

- An antioxidant profile, to evaluate the body's antioxidant reserves, to make sure that we have enough antioxidants to prevent excessive free radical damage

- An amino acid profile, to measure dietary protein adequacy, digestion, absorption, and nutritional deficiencies, including essential vitamins, minerals and amino acids

- A red blood cell mineral profile, to measure intracellular nutrient mineral status

- A toxic heavy metal profile, to assess heavy metal exposure that can affect heath, including lead, mercury, arsenic, cadmium and tin

- A fatty acid profile to measure levels of the omega-3 and -6 essential fatty acids, the amount of saturated fats, trans-fatty acids and their ratios with each other, so that an optimal balance can be achieved in the diet to improve health and maintain good health

Further test profiles are available to measure the overall physiological burden of toxins, oestrogen metabolism and detoxification. A specialist laboratory of nutritional and environmental medicine offers a health-risk profile for measuring vitamins, elements, antioxidants, enzymes, fatty acids and other key indicators of inflammation.

## Food allergy testing

There are two main types of adverse immune reaction to foods, one known as IgE mediated and the other as non-IgE mediated allergy.[5] In both cases, the immune system is reacting by releasing substances that can lead to inflammation. Chronic inflammation is a significant contributory factor to the erosion of health and has been identified as underlying many non-communicable chronic illnesses such as cancer, diabetes and cardiovascular disease.[6] If a diet regularly presents the body with foods that create an allergic response, an underlying state of inflammation will result. Many people are aware of which foods trigger their allergies but sometimes these can be difficult to ascertain. With modern testing techniques, it is possible to accurately determine which foods or substances create allergic reactions; we can then remove those foods from our diets. Very sophisticated new testing systems for food allergies have been developed in response to the growing need to eliminate chronic inflammation from the body. These tests include IgE and non-IgE allergy testing, cellular antigen food testing and gluten antibody testing.

## Genomics and nutrigenomics

I introduce the subject of genomic and nutrigenomic testing here to show how research on nutrition and preventative healthcare is evolving. Medical science is developing rapidly in this area and it offers great promise for improved health, as well as an understanding of how our diet, lifestyle and environment have an impact on our health and gene expression. Nutrigenomics is an emerging field of science which examines how food interacts with our genes to affect our health. When this science is applied to the study of nutrition, many ways of optimising health through the personalisation of diet are opened up. This offers a way forward towards reduction in our risk of disease. The statement below from the US Center for Disease Control and Prevention summarises this well:

*A growing number of tests are being developed to look at multiple genes that may increase or decrease a person's risk of common diseases, such as cancer or diabetes. Such tests and other applications of genomic technologies have the potential to help prevent common disease and improve the health of individuals and populations. For example, predictive gene tests may be used to help determine the risk of developing common diseases, and pharmacogenetic tests may be used to help identify genetic variations that can influence a person's response to medicines. There is much we still need to learn about how effective these new tests are, and the best way to use them to improve health.[7]*

To conclude this section, I would like to emphasise the following: just as there is no single way of preventing heart disease or diabetes, it is equally clear that asking how we can prevent cancer, live with cancer or prevent a recurrence is always an individual matter. Chronic illness occurs for many reasons and must be approached taking many factors into account, including diet, lifestyle and genetics. There are many causes to the chronic disruption of homeostasis, including inflammation, diet, infection, toxicity and nutritional deficiency that impairs the body's ability to overcome the inflammation. Having introduced you to some of the methods of functional testing, I hope that you will be able to identify your individual needs, thereby enabling you to reduce risk factors and to restore and optimise health in your body.

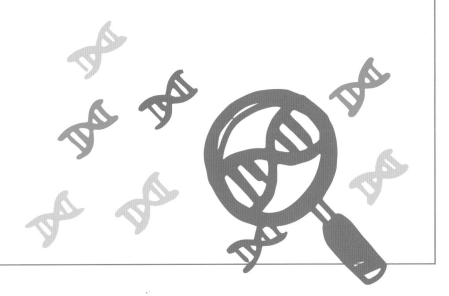

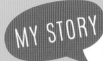

## Sue Taylor

### 6 years post-diagnosis

*After several weeks of heavy uterine bleeding, I was told I 'probably had cancer'. Rectal bleeding followed, and the detection of a breast lump that showed positive for cancer on a thermogram. I did not feel at all well. I refused biopsies as I understand they can be dangerous.*

*I consulted with Xandria Williams. Tests showed several toxins, as well as DNA damage, and many nutritional deficiencies. As a result I made immediate changes to my diet, followed her detox instructions and took her supplement programme. It was tough but effective. A month later we received the results from the tests Xandria describes in her book Detecting Cancer. The results were all abnormal and indicative of cancer. I repeated the tests every few months and my programme was adjusted accordingly.*

*After three years all my test results were essentially back to normal. Now, another three years later, I still feel terrific, have no worrying symptoms, no bleeding, and the breast thermogram remains clear. I honestly believe that without these tests and this carefully targeted recovery programme I would not be here now.*

## SOME KEY POINTS TO REMEMBER

If you are going to have any testing done, first ask yourself:

- 'What am I going to do with the result?'
- 'Will it really be useful to me?'

Discuss these questions, and also which tests are within your budget, with your practitioner. If you are hoping to use the results as a basis for orthodox treatment, first check with your doctor whether he or she will act on a result, thereby possibly saving you time and money and avoiding distress.

Tentatively feeling your way back into life after treatment can be very difficult. Rebuilding your fragile confidence after your body has let you down is a long-term project, requiring lots of time and patience. Tests can be vital pointers to the most constructive ways of regaining and maintaining full health, and can help enormously with re-establishing your self-confidence.

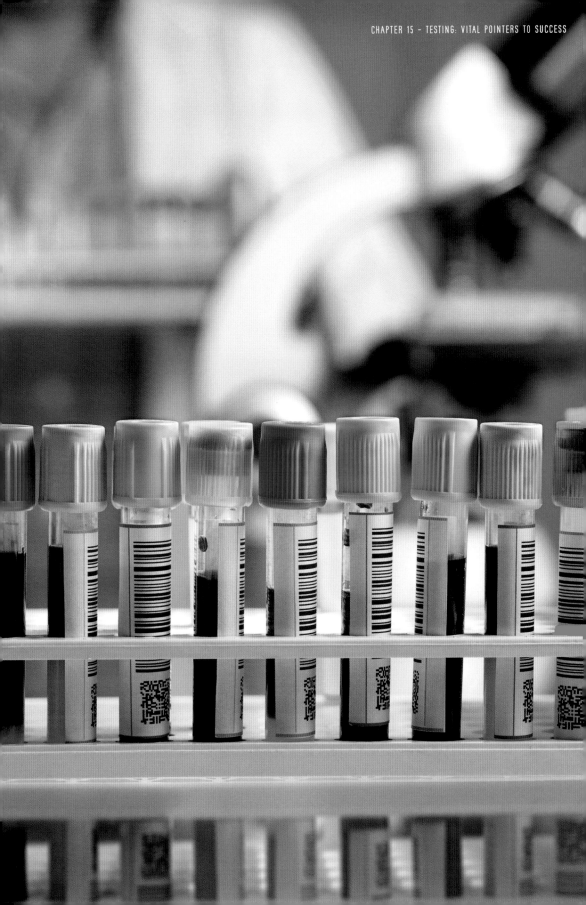

# PART SIX

# COLOPHON*

*The word colophon is derived from the Greek for 'summit'. As applied to an inscription at the end of a book or manuscript, the phrase *Colophonem adidi* is by Desiderius Erasmus (1466-1536): 'I have put a finishing touch to it.'

# CHAPTER 16
## FINAL THOUGHTS

Patricia Peat

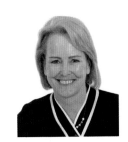

As I said at the outset, this book is designed to introduce you to the rapidly growing world of Integrative Medicine for cancer. I think we can conclude that although far from perfect, the underlying principles of Integrative Oncology are sound and are being increasingly supported by the latest research.

Those principles are:

- Cancer is a disease that is probably multi-factorial and therefore needs a multi-dimensional approach to maximise your chances of returning to good health

- Standard treatments do generally have a serious effect on the body's ability to function, and recovery can take some time. Integrative Medicine has strategies to offer that can prevent or minimise many side effects

- Standard treatments are merely a first step on the road to recovery; the next steps are the ones you take, which makes them even more important

- If you decide against standard treatments, aim to find the best information on holistic methods to help you build an effective programme

- Recovery should not be left to chance; there are many factors that contribute to developing cancer and careful investigation of these and of underlying imbalances is vital

- If anybody says that he or she has a 'cure', the 'answer' and that cancer is a 'simple disease', then that person is without doubt a charlatan. Cancer is an individual disease. Integrative Medicine does not have all the answers; in fact, nobody does

- Most important of all: you are the most crucial element in your recovery; spiritual, psychological and emotional elements all play as essential a role as your biochemistry

What is clear is that there is no single formula, no magic bullet. Instead you must begin the process of looking at health and recovery in a very different way from the one with which we were brought up. We have been taught that experts get us better, and that we 'receive' treatment. In order to recover from cancer, the experts can give us some effective help, but always remember that they specialise in cancer 'treatment' not cancer 'recovery'.

In order to help you prioritise your next steps after reading this book, I hope the following will be of help:

- Good nutrition is important but don't focus on it to such an extent that every day is spent worrying about everything you eat; it should be enjoyable, affordable and manageable

- Alkalise, oxygenate, exercise your body as much as you can

- Plenty of water and good detox helps physical repair, but take care not to stress the body by overdoing it

- Work out your budget and build your programme around what you can afford; simple cheap things can be extremely good

- Think about your current situation and what help you need for your next step; if you are in shock, emotionally exhausted or feeling very ill, you may need someone to support you and help with those areas before you can move on to major changes or treatment

- Establish what your principles are: what elements do you instinctively feel would be the ones to help you on your journey?; your intuition will serve you well in this respect

- There are countless supplements that may be helpful; ask someone knowledgeable to help you to prioritise your choices, ensuring that they are safe for you

- If you are considering wider treatment options, speak to someone impartial, or at least to people who have had the treatment you might choose before you commit yourself

- Stress and lack of sleep will undermine any strategies you undertake no matter how expensive; be sure to attend to the simple things as well

- Relaxation, meditation, mindfulness and EFT can all play vital roles; don't restrict yourself to medically based approaches

- Your programme should be exactly that – yours, not anyone else's! Putting yourself in charge and becoming your own healer is the real focus of Integrative Medicine

Returning to health is all about balance: balancing the body, balancing the mind; and the best way to achieve this is...a balanced approach!

I hope this book has been helpful in introducing you to the many positive ways you can influence your recovery and enable your mind, body and spirit to play a greater part in that than you previously thought possible. The power we have within us for healing, for genetically upgrading cells, for positively influencing a healthy future is immense. Integrative Medicine can give you the tools and empower you. You just have to believe and let it happen.

I wish you well.

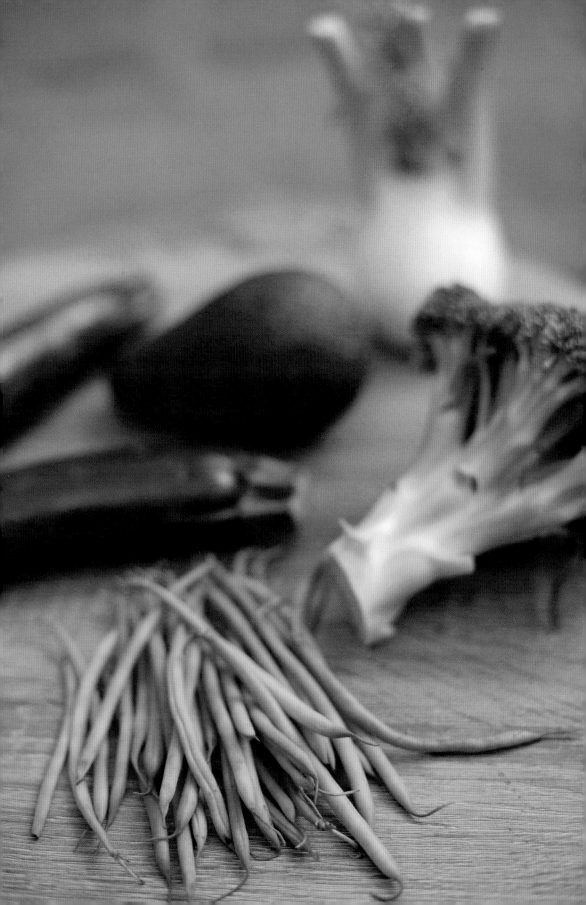

# PART SEVEN

## APPENDICES

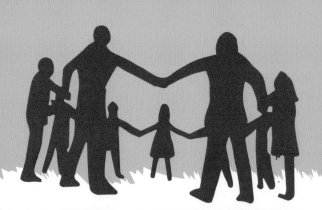

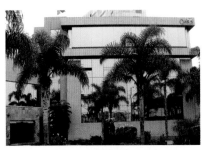

# APPENDIX 1

## INTEGRATIVE CLINICS AROUND THE WORLD

The following descriptions, presented by the various clinics' medical directors or senior physicians, represent only a sample of the approaches and organisations that are available internationally.

This appendix is intended to give you some idea of the breadth of techniques being used to help people with cancer. The clinics below have been selected as much for their differences in approach as for their status as treatment centres.

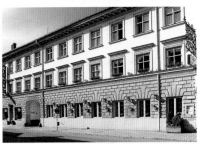

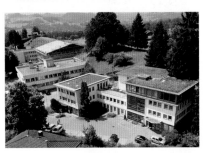

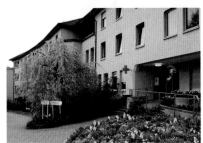

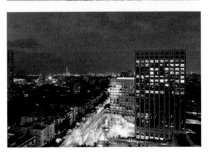

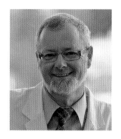

# PARACELSUS KLINIK, SWITZERLAND

The Biological Medicine Approach

## Dr Thomas Rau

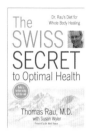

PARACELSUS
KLINIK

The Biological Medicine approach at the Paracelsus Klinik, Lustmühle, encompasses one central fact: every individual has his or her 'signature' pathway of response to cancer; our programme is therefore tailored to providing both specific and customised care.

There are three points of focus with regard to our Biological Medicine practice and supporting a patient's cancer protective capacity:

- enhancing detoxification
- removing obstacles to detoxification
- cleaning up the 'terrain'

Because cancer invariably takes 'advantage' of deficiencies in a person's immune system, the basic approach that the body uses to eliminate cancer cells is through cytotoxic/cytolytic activity and elimination pathways. When these pathways are blocked due to deleted detoxification genes in the liver, long-standing years of constipation, poor eating habits and/or other lifestyle issues, the capacity and functionality of the immune engine become stagnant from operating in such a poor 'terrain'. Moreover, the nutrient bath from which cells absorb – as well as eliminate into – is the terrain, technically referred to as the extracellular space. When this 'respiratory' and digestive capacity is diminished because of toxicity (similar to a house being consistently subjected to poor-quality air, eventually affecting the occupants), the inevitable outcome is cell dysfunction.

While body and teeth are seldom treated together, the two disciplines for body and dental medicine are in fact intimately connected. Because of this, at the Paracelsus Klinik we care for those who come to us at our Biological Dental and Medicine Departments. Furthermore, since body-centred medicine – i.e. organ toxicity or inefficiency, blood pathology, trauma and genetic loopholes – generally overlooks the teeth and dental history, we are often able to heal cancer and many other diseases through analysis and care of whole body. For example, there is now a well-established association between *Propionibacterium acnes*, a bacterium often found in an infected dental focus or foci, and prostate cancer. An article published in the Journal of Urology in 2005 found that 35 per cent of men who had undergone a prostatectomy (surgical removal of the prostate gland) due to cancer were infected with this bacterium, which had acted as a contributory cause to cancer development.[1] There are many other well-researched articles supporting this connection, which can be addressed with a treatment that is easy to provide: dental care as part of a Biological Medicine programme.

Among many others, the Paracelsus Klinik Biological Medicine cancer therapies include:

- whole body hyperthermia
- electromagnetic pulsed therapies
- mistletoe therapy
- hapten therapy against cell wall deficient bacteria, which frequently co-contribute to cancer development (as fungi used to do)
- fever therapy (exogenous or endogenous, i.e. from an external or internal source)
- endobionic therapies to address the 'terrain' and immune system
- Paracelsus-specific infusions to counteract cancer's acid-protecting 'milieu' and to enhance healthy granulocytic and lymphocytic function (granulocytes and lymphocytes are both types of white blood cell and form part of our immune system)
- mandatory dental appointments featuring a state-of-the art panoramic imaging system that can identify foci
- a cancer diet and nutritional counselling

I conclude this brief description of the Paracelsus Klinik by emphasising that there must always be integration between conventional and biological medicine, as they are often both needed to support the best outcome for cancer patients. Furthermore, and a point not to be overlooked, the biological forces of nature are omnipresent throughout the body, and the basic tenets of our Biological Medicine practices here support and further potentiate the best inherent immune defence possible against cancer development. Biological (or 'Biologic-Logical') Medicine offers the body a chance to resuscitate itself and to focus on its cancer-protective activities. We believe that it should be integrated into every cancer hospital in the world.

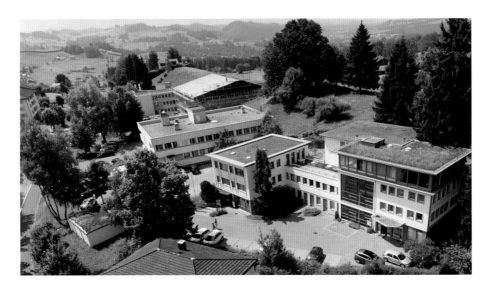

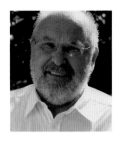

KLINIK ST
GEORG

# KLINIK ST GEORG, GERMANY

## Dr Friedrich Douwes

At the Klinik St Georg, Bad Aibling, we use three non-toxic treatment modalities to destroy cancer within the body and to promote its recognition by the immune system. These are hyperthermia, electro cancer therapy (ECT) and photodynamic therapy (PDT). With these three modalities we not only have the possibility of reducing the cancer mass gently within the body, but we can also change the immunogenicity (the ability to promote an immune response) of the cancer by inducing heat shock proteins, HSP70 for example, so that the tumour can be recognised and then destroyed by the patient's own immune system.

The phagocytes (white blood cells that protect the body by eating dirt, bacteria and dead or dying cells) help to dissolve the dead tumour material and present the immune system with the tumour antigens, so that it can start to function, and so that in future a restored, stimulated immune system will recognise malignant cells and respond appropriately.

Hyperthermia is an important modality in cancer therapy. While gentle, it is nevertheless an effective treatment and is one of the basic elements of the integrated approach practised at Klinik St Georg. During hyperthermia therapy, tumorous tissue is heated using various techniques. As a result of this heating:

• The cancer cells are damaged

• The supply of blood and oxygen is reduced, causing an increase of cancer-cell destruction

• The body's own immunological defence mechanisms are activated

Hyperthermia can be used alone or in combination with radiation, chemotherapy (sometimes insulin-potentiated; see below) and with non-toxic biological cancer therapies. It is also applied, very successfully, in aftercare or in prevention of secondary cancer. In particular, metastases and tumours that are inoperable or resistant to conventional treatments can be influenced favourably by hyperthermia.

In contrast to hyperthermia, electro cancer therapy (ECT) uses electrical current rather than heat. To create a standing electrical field, needles might be inserted directly into the tumour; or alternatively discs can be placed over the tumour tissue. The electrical field changes the pH value and the natural electrical charge of the tumour tissue. This disturbs the essential life processes of the tumour cells and causes them to die. This therapy is used at Klinik St Georg for the treatment of:

- breast cancer, especially rapidly spreading and inflammatory types

- tumours of the ear, nose and throat, especially throat

- gynaecological, urological carcinomas (prostate and bladder tumours) and sarcomas (soft tissue tumours)

- skin cancer such as basal cell carcinoma, spinocellular carcinoma and melanoma

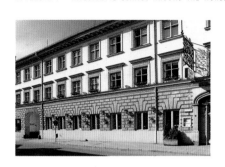

I founded the Klinik St Georg in 1991; we now have more than twenty years' experience with ECT and have achieved excellent results.

Photodynamic therapy (PDT) is a treatment in which a special dye or agent is used which accumulates specifically in the tumour tissue. By using a special light, usually a laser, this area is made fluorescent, thus producing damage to the tumour cells, resulting in cell death. These agents are named photosensitisers because they need a special light before the cytotoxic reaction is produced. Since the agent accumulates predominantly in tumour tissue, this provides a targeted and effective tumour therapy. This curative approach is mainly aimed at superficial cutaneous (skin) and mucosal tumours because of the limitation imposed by the depth of the light penetration. PDT is increasingly used in palliative oncology because it allows for interstitial (between organs) application of thin light applicators, which effectively destroy the tumour in a minimally invasive manner and with the least discomfort for the patient. Currently, PDT is especially used in bronchial, oesophageal and bladder cancers and in several types of skin tumour.

The three non-toxic treatment modalities can be used even in advanced cases of cancer for which conventional medicine has reached its limits. Parallel to this, we reduce the blood flow to tumours by inhibiting angiogenesis with a variety of natural compounds. Furthermore, we regularly employ insulin potentiation therapy (IPT), which is a simple medical procedure: it uses the hormone insulin, followed by chemotherapy and glucose to make chemotherapy drugs, in small doses, more effective with few or even no side effects. There are no double-blind, placebo-controlled studies for IPT, but a lot of experience and positive case reports, worldwide; after ten years of excellent results we have now included it in our Integrated Cancer Treatment Concept (ICTC). IPT was developed as a result of improved understanding of the cancer physiology and how the body works. It was shown that cancer patients can be treated with less toxicity than is the case with conventional medicine.

## Tailoring treatments to the individual patient

Whether or not we recommend IPT in combination with hyperthermia depends on the patient we are treating and their particular type of cancer. For instance, for lymphomas, leukaemias and testicular cancers we always choose conventional methods, but combine them with hyperthermia to reduce toxicity and increase effectiveness. Choice of chemotherapy is decided by individual chemosensitivity testing (see **Chapter 15**, '**Testing: vital pointers to success**') rather than by cancer type.

As another example, if a patient has previously had extensive conventional treatment and is consequently in bad shape metabolically – typically very catabolic with weight loss, anaemia or even cachexia – we would not use chemotherapy at the outset, but would start with an intensive support programme of nutrition, vitamins, minerals and bioactive substances. Even more important for these patients is detoxification and oxygen support, for instance with ionised oxygen or ozone.

We monitor results regularly with ultrasound and usually perform PET, CT or MRI scans (see **Appendix 2**, '**Understanding scans**') after six to twelve weeks of treatment. We also measure tumour markers (see 'Cancer markers', **pp.216-17**, **Chapter 15**, '**Testing: vital pointers to success**') and observe trends, which helps us to judge the treatment response.

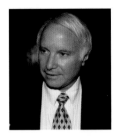

# INTERNATIONAL CENTRE FOR CELL THERAPY AND CANCER IMMUNOTHERAPY (CTCI), ISRAEL

CTCI

## Prof. Shimon Slavin

Treating cancer is like shooting a moving target: treatment may have to be changed depending on the status of the disease and the general condition of the patient. This is especially relevant for procedures that may be recommended at the International Centre for Cell Therapy and Cancer Immunotherapy (CTCI), because my team and I believe in fully personalised medicine. There are no two cancers that are the same and there are no two individuals that are the same; there is therefore no reason why treatment should be the same for all patients with the same disease.

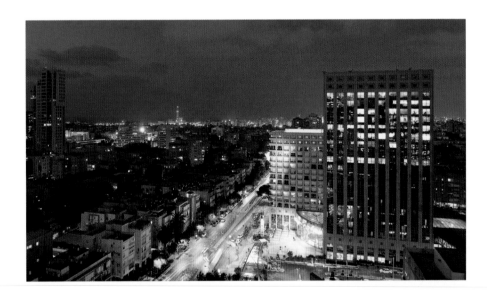

Our International Center in Tel Aviv offers innovative approaches to the treatment of all types of cancer, focusing on targeted and cell-mediated immunotherapy including vaccines, oncolytic viruses and especially using cancer-killer cells (T-cells, NK cells and macrophages), stem-cell-based anti-cancer modalities and other personalised tumour-targeted techniques. These can be particularly relevant to treating cancer patients who are at a clinical stage known to be resistant to standard anti-cancer treatments or who are at risk of tumour recurrence following conventional treatment.

It is obviously preferable to treat cancer at an early stage of the disease, ideally as soon as diagnosis is complete, so that optimal treatment can then be planned and tumour samples be cryopreserved (frozen). At the stage known as 'minimal residual disease', following initial tumour 'debulking' (physically removing as much malignant tissue as possible), a cure can be accomplished by combining conventional treatment with targeted immunotherapy. This can be effective even for patients at high risk of recurrent disease, unlikely to be cured by any of the conventional anti-cancer agents. Most patients with cancer reach a stage of minimal residual disease following initial surgery or first-line chemotherapy or radiation. At the time of writing, if no tumour is visible in their patients, oncologists tend to send them away with no further treatment recommendations. Yet, every cancer starts with a single cell. When such an abnormal cell escapes the surveillance of the immune system, continuous division results in tumour progression. At a stage of one million cells, the size of the cancer lesion is the size of a pinhead. No technology can detect such small cancer lesions. Patients might therefore have many such small lesions in different locations while being considered fully cured. Tumour progression might then occur later. Our goal, and the patients' best chance, sometimes their only chance of being cured, is to be treated at the stage of minimal residual disease.

Unfortunately, in our experience most patients seek help only when tumour metastases are diagnosed, when all other measures have failed, when it might be difficult or impossible to minimise the tumour burden due to multi-drug resistance. When cancer metastases progress, and when malignant cells are no longer responsive to available anti-cancer treatments, there is no real option for cure with any of the conventional anti-cancer agents; in such cases we aim to slow or stop the disease process on a fully personalised basis, using the unique procedures available at our clinic. While we are happy to treat any patient in need and offer several rational and innovative therapeutic approaches, we can never promise a successful outcome. Please remember that our treatment programme has to be regarded as an experimental approach, not yet considered 'standard of care'. To avoid false hopes, you must clearly understand that we cannot promise complete cure or even control of the disease, although we are committed to do our best to accomplish these goals.

Another important principle to take into consideration is that we always recommend using as many non-cross-resistant anti-cancer procedures as possible, each operating against a different target on resistant cancer cells. For example, if cancer cells become resistant to a particular anti-cancer treatment, and so escape unharmed, a subsequent treatment based on another principle will be applied, in an attempt to kill or block replication of such cells. This secondary treatment will use a different anti-cancer mechanism. Among other factors that may vary from patient to patient, the number of anti-cancer procedures that can be applied depends on cancer type, also on the period of time a patient can stay at our clinic and on any financial restrictions.

If we can keep the number of malignant cells under control and prevent or minimise tumour progression, patients may live for a long time with few or no symptoms. In most cases the danger is not from the current number of tumour cells, but from future tumour progression if treatment fails.

Bearing in mind the experimental nature of our treatment programme, we always recommend that our 'out of the box' methods be applied in addition to – not instead of – conventional ones, aiming to ensure that maximal possible treatment will be administered. If, however, all conventional methods have been tried but failed, clinical application of innovative procedures is fully justifiable.

Our approach consists of two steps.

## Optimal tumour debulking before attempting the use of immunotherapy

Unfortunately, despite the use of all available anti-cancer modalities, elimination of all malignant cells and prevention of tumour progression or recurrence might not be possible for two main reasons:

- The primary lesion might be in an inoperable location and/or there might be invasive residual malignant cells, invisible to the surgeon
- The fact that the cancer-initiating cells, the so-called cancer stem cells, are, a priori, resistant to chemotherapy and radiation

Based on the above, we recommend additional treatment in an attempt to further reduce the number of residual malignant cells, employing innovative methods and devices:

- oncothermia – targeted heat therapy to weaken cancer cell walls and to increase susceptibility to chemotherapy
- acoustic shockwave therapy (AST) – also to increase susceptibility to chemotherapy
- novel liposomal cisplatin chemotherapy – to deliver highly effective cisplatin as liposomal nanoparticles

## Treatment of minimal residual disease

Once the patient has exploited all possible approaches for minimising the tumour burden, our clinic will recommend innovative procedures, including targeted anti-cancer therapies and immunotherapy treatments. Immunotherapy attempts to activate a patient's own immune system against cancer; on the one hand using autologous immune-system cells, while on the other using allogeneic ones to kill cancer cells, since the patient's own cells may fail to do so. Other procedures, preferably including a combination of anti-cancer modalities to minimise the escape of cancer cells by developing resistance to conventional treatment, may involve some of our experimental procedures (for more details see **Appendix 1**, 'Additional materials' on thecancerrevolution.co.uk).

# ITA WEGMAN KLINIK, SWITZERLAND

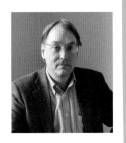

## Dr Maurice Orange

ITA WEGMAN
KLINIK

In 1917, Dr Ita Wegman (1876-1943), working as a gynaecologist in Zurich, started treating cancer patients with mistletoe at the suggestion of philosopher and polymath Dr Rudolf Steiner (1861-1925). The rationale and initial results were presented in medical conferences in 1921 and 1922.[2] Steiner regarded tumour growth as an imbalance between the physical and vitality body, where 'certain physical forces' overwhelmed the vitality leading to an inappropriate autonomy, fragmentation and enmity against the totality of the organism. He suggested that mistletoe could counter cancer, as well as re-establish integration by harnessing innate, healthy forces – now understood to involve the immune system.[3]

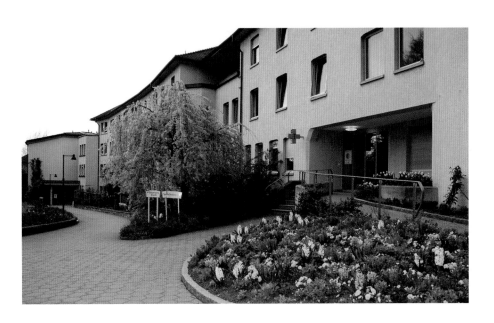

In 1921, Dr Wegman founded a hospital in Arlesheim, Switzerland (now named the Ita Wegman Klinik) where she continued to work closely with Steiner to develop anthroposophic medicine, a patient-centred approach that integrates spiritual insights with phenomenological, natural scientific and artistic methods. As well as being available in major hospitals in Germany and Switzerland, anthroposophic medicine is now current in general practice and consultant-led outpatient settings.[4] Cancer patients have access to a range of services, including psychological support (biographical counselling), dietary advice (using biodynamic produce where possible; see Chapter 4, 'How to buy good food'), additional bodily treatments (embrocation, massage, compresses) and artistic therapies.

Mistletoe *(Viscum album)* is a semi-parasitic plant. The extract is derived from a harvest twice a year and undergoes a complex manufacturing procedure. Extracts of mistletoe inhibit cancer-cell growth and enhance anti-cancer immunity. Treatment is medically supervised, typically given as subcutaneous injections with doses adjusted over time, and can last from several months to years. Experienced doctors also administer mistletoe as an intravenous drip and/or intratumourally.

Mistletoe-based preparations continue to be developed and improved; they form the backbone of anthroposophic cancer care. Furthermore, mistletoe therapies have been widely adopted as a supportive treatment by homeopathic doctors, naturopaths and mainstream doctors with a CAM interest. While Steiner foresaw the curative potential of this fascinating evergreen, mistletoe is of increasing importance in improving cancer patients' quality of life, as has been unequivocally shown through well-designed trials: patients tolerate and recover better from chemotherapy and radiotherapy.[5] The most likely reason for this is the well-documented effects on the immune system. Using mistletoe therapies for at least two years is associated with improved outcomes.[6]

Research has not yet produced convincing evidence of a direct impact of mistletoe on cancer itself or of improved survival. A recent trial (2013), however, demonstrated that mistletoe alone significantly increased survival time for pancreatic cancer, reduced disease-related symptoms and had no side effects.[7] Also, an increasing number of cases show that when mistletoe is used boldly, significant disease responses (including durable remissions) are possible.[8] There are several factors for this successful use, the most important of which seem to be:[9]

- starting treatment early – as soon as possible after confirmation of diagnosis and before surgery or chemotherapy
- using higher doses than is common
- eliciting fever at the beginning of treatment
- using more than one application – subcutaneous (the standard way of giving mistletoe) as well as intravenous and/or intratumoural (so-called 'off-label' use)

Fever strongly enhances the immunity and can be elicited with subcutaneous application alone. Experienced doctors often offer combination treatment.

Mistletoe therapy, also in higher doses, can be used safely alongside mainstream cancer treatments and most complementary modalities.[10] The only undesirable effects that might occur are allergy-type reactions, which are rare.[11]

UK centres and practitioners specialising in mistletoe therapy can be found in LIFE>, the Yes to Life searchable web directory.

LIFE>

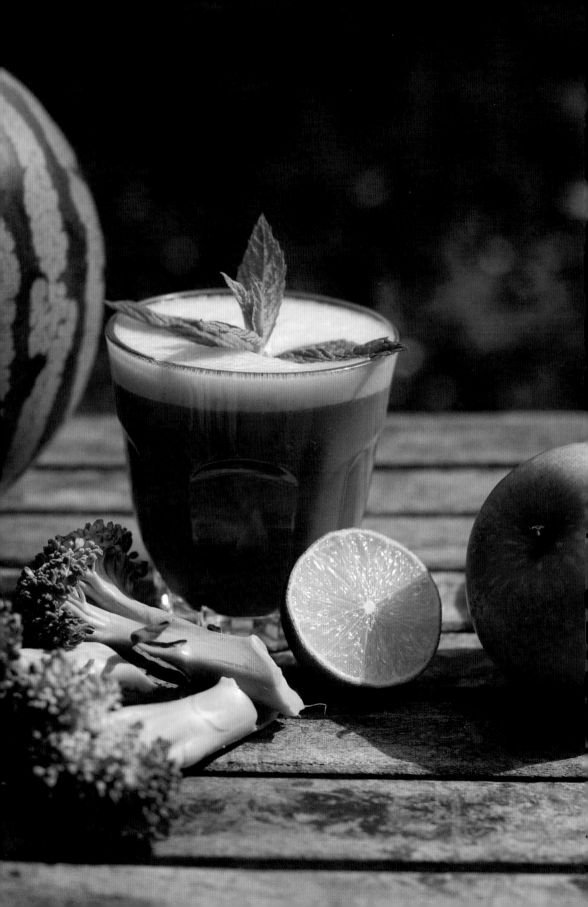

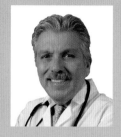

# OASIS OF HOPE HOSPITAL, MEXICO

## Dr Francisco Contreras

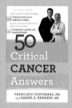

OASIS OF
HOPE

My father, Dr Ernesto Contreras, Sr, founded Oasis of Hope in Playas de Tijuana in 1963 with the vision of caring for the whole person – body, mind and spirit. In 1985, I began leading the hospital's multi-disciplinary team of oncologists, internists, nutritionists, nurses and counsellors. The treatment approach that has been offered to more than a hundred thousand patients from sixty nations since the 1960s is called Contreras Metabolic Integrative Therapy (CMIT).

CMIT is designed to destroy cancer cells, delay their growth and mutagenesis, and impede their spread as long as possible. It is also designed to maximise the time for which the patient enjoys a high quality of life. It consists of ten major elements:

- oxidative preconditioning
- cell signal transduction therapy
- immune stimulation therapy
- nutritional therapy
- emotional healing

- cytotoxic therapy
- redox regulatory therapy
- tumour acidity regulation
- exercise
- spiritual care

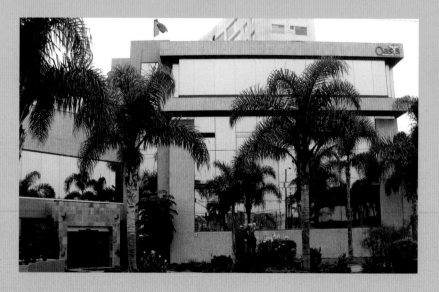

What sets Oasis of Hope apart is more than research: it is our half-century and more of clinical experience. While treating tens of thousands of people, we have explored critical cancer solutions to help patients achieve favourable outcomes. No single agent will cure cancer – winning takes an integrative approach that will intervene simultaneously in as many ways as feasible to promote the death of cancer cells and to halt the spread of tumours. CMIT represents a viable, innovative strategy to achieve this.

Oasis of Hope's survival rates are based on a five-year prospective study in stage 4 (late stage) breast, ovarian, lung and colorectal cancers and a review of decades of clinical data for stage 4 brain, oesophagus, kidney, melanoma of the skin, pancreas, prostate, stomach and bladder cancers. The data presented in the following table compare Oasis of Hope results with national averages as tracked by the National Cancer Institute SEER programme. The results make it clear that CMIT at Oasis of Hope offers a viable option to patients facing metastatic cancer, though naturally results vary from patient to patient.

## 5-Year Survival Rates for Stage 4 Cancers

| Cancer Type | Oasis of Hope | Conventional* |
|---|---|---|
| Breast (when Oasis CMIT was the first treatment received) | 75% | - |
| Breast | 45% | 20% |
| Ovarian | 54% | 18% |
| Lung | 9% | 1.6% |
| Colorectal | 16% | 7% |
| Brain | 50% | 50% |
| Oesophagus | 17% | 3% |
| Kidney | 20% | 12% |
| Melanoma of the skin | 20% | 15% |
| Pancreas | 25% | 2% |
| Prostate | 50% | 28% |
| Stomach | 15% | 4% |
| Urinary bladder | 17% | 6% |

* See the National Cancer Institute website seer.cancer.gov

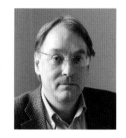

# APPENDIX 2
## UNDERSTANDING SCANS

Dr Maurice Orange

## IMAGING AND OTHER DIAGNOSTIC TOOLS

Different techniques of imaging (scanning) form an essential part of the early detection (screening), diagnosis and management of cancer. Combined with other diagnostic tools such as biopsy (taking a tissue sample), analysis of fluids and blood tests (e.g. tumour markers), imaging maps cancer and its progress and helps clinical decision-making. With some forms of imaging, however, there are collateral effects and associated risks that need to be considered. For example, some forms of imaging (including CT scans) increase radiation exposure; also, some forms of screening (for breast and prostate cancers) are associated with significant increase in unnecessary treatments. Newer, targeted and minimally invasive techniques aim to reduce the risk of radiation – and the amount of unnecessary scanning.

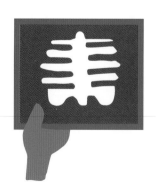
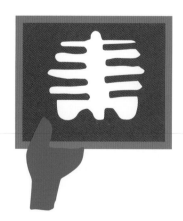

Patients often have concerns about the potential health damage of medical imaging. Ionising radiation has enough energy to damage cells, which can subsequently increase the risk of cancer. This is particularly relevant for children. These particular risks to health are actually low, however; every day we are exposed to natural radiation from sources in the environment, on average about 2.7 milliSieverts (mSv) a year. Many building materials contain low degrees of natural radioactivity and radon gas, so the largest exposure is to naturally occurring radiation in homes and workplaces. There is also naturally occurring radioactivity in food and from medical exposures, such as X-rays, gamma rays, neutrons, alpha particles and beta particles. For example, a simple dental X-ray is the equivalent of 0.005 mSv; a chest X-ray 0.1-0.2 mSv; a whole body CT scan gives 10-15 mSv. There are useful websites to consult for understanding and calculating radiation risk (see **Part Eight, 'Resources'**).

Each imaging technique has specific purposes, strengths and weaknesses. The choice of scan for any given situation would ideally be the one that gave the most or the best information. In practice, however, there are grey areas. An MRI is suitable for examining soft tissue (e.g. ligament and tendon injury, spinal cord injury, brain tumours) while a CT scan is better for bone injuries, lung and chest imaging as well as detecting cancers. An MRI usually costs more than a CT scan. An MRI does not use radiation, while CT scans do. Ultrasound does not use ionising radiation and so involves no risk of inducing cancer. While excellent for many things, MRI and ultrasound are often not the best test, and CT scans or X-rays are preferred. Talk to your healthcare provider about imaging options and what is best for you. If you can afford to do so, there might be a case for paying for a scan privately if it is impossible to get the one you want on the NHS.

## X-ray

The best-known, oldest and most common type of imaging, the X-ray, remains in regular use for early diagnosis, for example with lung and bone cancer. The information is sufficient for diagnosis, but more sophisticated CT and MRI scans are needed for accuracy. The radiation dose is small.

## CT (computerised tomography) scan

A CT scan uses X-rays to take a series of 'slice' pictures through the body at regular intervals; the computer puts these images together and can show a tumour in relation to its surroundings very clearly. The fact that a CT scan shows considerably more detail than a simple X-ray might prove critical to a treatment decision, for example whether or not to go ahead with surgery. CT scans are more expensive than X-rays and also expose patients to a higher quantity of radiation (one CT scan is approximately equal to two or more years' natural radiation exposure). Frequent scans should definitely be avoided in children. The radiation risk has to be weighed against the need for the information, which can be a difficult decision.

## PET-CT (positron emission tomography) scan

The most up-to-date – and most expensive – scanning technique is based on the fact that cancer cells have a much higher glucose uptake than normal cells. A PET-CT scan combines the two types of tomography to give detailed information about the localisation of metabolically active cancer sites, for example to track spread of the cancer. A PET scan uses a very small amount of an injected substance or radiotracer (FDG-18: a radioactive version of glucose) that shows the areas in which cells are active in the body. The radioactive glucose is excreted from the body quickly and does not cause any appreciable damage. This approach has the advantage that only malignant abnormalities are individually highlighted. Benign abnormalities or dead tumour tissue that might otherwise cause concern are clearly distinguished from active cancers. The amount of cancer activity is precisely indicated.

### MRI (magnetic resonance imaging) scan

MRI uses very high-strength magnetic fields to create the same type of 'slice' images as a CT scan, or it can build up 3D images. They are even more expensive than CT scans, can yield more detailed information – particularly in soft tissues and organs – and do not use ionising radiation. There are no recognised side effects from MRIs, although they are contraindicated for people who have pacemakers or some other metal implants. They are very noisy in operation and subject patients to long periods in a confined space, but most people are happy with the strategy of supplying piped music through over-ear headphones to make the experience bearable.

### Ultrasound scan

Ultrasound uses sound-waves for imaging and in many situations is a simple, non-invasive option. It is cheap and uses no radiation; in contrast to the four methods described so far, it is very compact and does not require a special environment. Indications of progress are often confirmed through ultrasound scans. In terms of the level of information it can provide and the number of applicable situations, however, ultrasound is far below the best of the above techniques. It is nevertheless useful for follow-up and first diagnosis.

### Bone scan

In cases where there may be lesions on the bone, these specialised scans use a technique similar to PET scans in that a radioactive 'dye' (isotope) is injected before the scan which then collects on the lesions and emits radiation that can be picked up by the scanner. The level of radiation exposure from a bone scan is about 6 mSv (ten times higher than a chest X-ray).

### Mammogram

Mammography is a specialised form of X-ray developed for breast scanning. It has been promoted as a regular screening technique for healthy women, but this is now in question, as it has led to the treatment of large numbers of pre-cancerous lesions in otherwise healthy women. The radiation is about 0.4 mSv (about four times that of a chest X-ray), although some sources suggest much higher levels of ionising radiation from mammography. In many instances, however, the negatives do have to be weighed against the need for information.

### Thermal image

Thermal imaging is not recognised by the NHS as a valid technique. It is completely harmless in that the process simply 'photographs' the heat coming off the body. Its particular strength lies in its ability to detect activity long before a tumour is visible on any other type of scan. Variations in temperature are an indication of activity below the skin; for example, a breast tumour will be associated with inflammation and so will display a 'hot spot'. A single scan has very limited application, since it is important to establish the normal pattern for an individual, and then to compare scans for signs of variation. To be useful, scans must be regular; this may present an issue of cost, but has no associated risks. As with other tests, it is advisable to consider the pros and cons of early detection and over-diagnosis carefully, as pattern changes in themselves are not specific enough to indicate cancerous changes. More time and further research are needed before thermal imaging will be widely accepted as a useful diagnostic tool that justifies the cost.

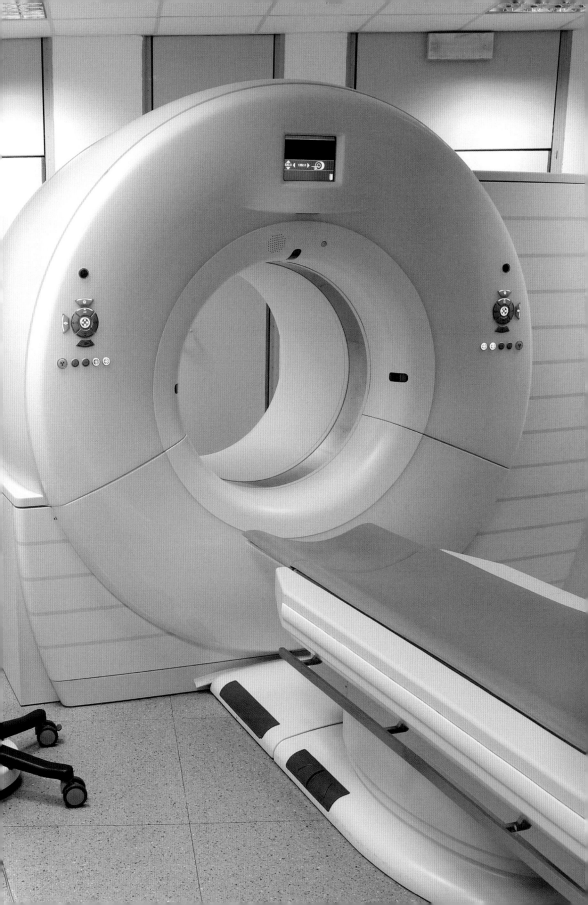

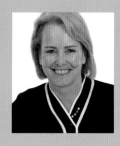

# APPENDIX 3

# WHEN DO YOU NEED A PRACTITIONER?

Patricia Peat

When embarking on any kind of integrative programme, there are certain times when consulting an appropriately trained professional is essential. There are also other times, of course, when you might feel in need of some expert input and when you are likely to benefit from being advised by a reliable practitioner. This book, however, offers guidance on the many ways in which self-help techniques can be a great resource, either instead of or combined with professional help. In time, you might well become enough of an expert in particular aspects of your programme, diet for example, that you can safely make all your own decisions, with only occasional need to refer elsewhere.

The chart below sets out some of the many possible situations in which you might find yourself, with appropriate specialists whom you could consult.

| When you need help | Who to go to |
| --- | --- |
| • building an integrative treatment programme<br>• reviewing an integrative treatment programme | integrative doctor, integrative specialist |
| • building a nutritional programme<br>• knowing what foods to eat and to avoid | nutritionist, integrative doctor, integrative specialist, naturopath, herbalist, Ayurvedic practitioner |
| • specialist diets, e.g. Budwig, ketogenic | appropriately trained specialist practitioner |

| When you need help | Who to go to |
|---|---|
| • preparing for standard treatments<br>• knowing what to eat during chemotherapy<br>• avoiding cachexia or weight loss | nutritionist, integrative doctor, integrative specialist, naturopath |
| • building a supplement programme | nutritionist, integrative doctor, integrative specialist, naturopath, Functional Medicine practitioner, herbalist |
| • building a supplement programme to support a specific treatment regime | integrative doctor, integrative specialist, some other practitioners – but check on their experience with cancer |
| • getting intravenous or other specialised treatment | integrative doctor |
| • being tested to establish vitamin and mineral levels, toxic imbalances and for hormone analysis | nutritionist, integrative doctor, integrative specialist, naturopath, Functional Medicine practitioner, herbalist |
| • being tested to monitor on-going cancer activity (in addition to standard testing/scanning) | integrative doctor, integrative specialist |
| • dealing with stress/shock or the effects of prolonged stress<br>• dealing with on-going pain<br>• dealing with side effects of standard treatments<br>• getting help with sleep | aromatherapist, acupuncturist, hypnotherapist, mindfulness teacher, Shiatsu practitioner, reflexologist, Reiki practitioner or healer, EFT trainer or massage therapist |
| • formulating a general on-going plan for your recovery and future, generating motivation | mentor/life coach |
| • planning and monitoring an exercise programme, particularly if your movement is restricted as a result of treatment | specialist coach with specific cancer rehabilitation training |
| • getting the support of an alternative medical system such as homeopathy or Ayurveda | an appropriately trained and qualified specialist |
| • dealing with fluid build-up resulting from lymph node removals | lymphatic drainage specialist |
| • getting psychological support | counsellor, psychologist, psychotherapist, cognitive behavioural therapist |
| • investigating and dealing with personal emotional issues that may be connected with your health | guided imagery/visualisation therapist, counsellor, support group |

For more details of the therapies offered by each type of practitioner see **Chapter 3**, **'Who's who in Integrative Medicine'**.

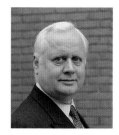

# APPENDIX 4

# MANAGING YOUR FINANCES WHEN YOU HAVE CANCER

CANCER
IFA

## George Emsden

Being told that you have cancer is a wake-up call. All those theoretical life-coaching questions 'What would you do if...?' are now real.

MAS

### Earnings and spending – Mr Micawber's view

Dreaming that 'something will turn up' is not helpful. It is vital to do some financial housekeeping – no rocket science there. Spending less than you earn is the key to managing your finances. Pencil, paper and a calculator are all you need. If income is more than you spend, fine. If income is less than you spend, there are only two choices: earn more or spend less – most people will try to do both.

To save on spending, you could start at the Money Advice Service. Avoid overdoing it, however; we are trying to reduce worry, not the opposite.

CAB

### What do you own? What do you owe?

Two sets of figures again, your assets and your debts. If making this calculation proves too much for you, get someone to help. Knowing exactly where you stand will remove a lot of stress. Ask yourself whether you can afford to pay any interest due and repay the loan(s). If the figures are bad, you could approach the Citizens' Advice Bureau, but it might take ages to get an appointment. Macmillan Cancer Support has a Financial Guidance service, but note that this charity does not give regulated advice.

MACMILLAN

If anyone owes you money, ensure that you get it back as soon as possible. Now that you are likely to need all your financial resources, don't allow yourself to be fobbed off. If you have a financial adviser, book a review meeting with him or her. If not, try the Chartered Institute for Securities & Investment (CISI) or Unbiased, a web directory of Independent Financial Advisers. Some financial advisers prefer to refer terminally ill clients to me. Two case studies may help understand what is on offer: on the CancerIFA website, click the Blogs tab and read Client Case Study (#01) and (#02).

CISI

UNBIASED

## An unexpected nest egg

If your cancer is deemed 'terminal' (a year or less), you can get your pensions paid out tax-free, provided a doctor confirms the medical details. There might be a charge for this. CancerIFA organises this service, and the process can take between one and four months. If you are one of the lucky ones who live much longer than expected, you need not worry about paying any pension money back. You can read about one lady who did beat the odds on my website: click the link to 'Dilys's Story' under 'Interesting Cancer Links' in the right-hand column of the home page.

PTS

People often forget about pensions from previous employment and billions of pounds lie unclaimed with insurance and pension companies and in old schemes. The reason for this is that these nest eggs are often small and difficult to trace when the employer or pension provider has been taken over or moved. If this applies to you, try the Pension Tracing Service or the Pensions Advisory Service. It is your money, and if you don't claim it, the insurance companies just end up paying tax on it. How daft is that?

PAS

Are you entitled to any state benefits? Applications are mostly done online these days, so you can find out quickly if you are entitled to them. You will need your National Insurance number. If your illness is terminal and you have less than six months to live, the application will be speeded up using a DS1500 form. A Macmillan Benefits Adviser can help you with this.

STATE BENEFITS

## Clear the decks and make a will

Coping with the financial stress of cancer can be helped by having a clear-out. Possessions you no longer need can be sold on eBay, taken to a charity shop, given away to family and friends directly or via your local Freecycle website. **Remember that you can't take any of your stuff with you.**

MACMILLAN

Most people hate the thought of making a will. Well, if you haven't done so already, now you have to, for the sake of your remaining family as much as for your own. Writing a will (or even having a Wish Book) can avoid practical complications (e.g. whether you wish to be buried or cremated) as well as arguments among your family and/or friends.

FREECYCLE

## What now?

Once you know where you stand financially, you will feel a sense of relief. It is time to look forward.

With your financial affairs tidy, you can plan some treats for yourself. How about a new wardrobe? Something you have always wanted to do? Telephone or email a friend with whom you haven't been in touch for ages. Find out whatever happened to your childhood sweetheart? Bury a hatchet? Resolve an old argument? Visit a familiar haunt or somewhere new? Have a reunion with your long-standing friends from school or work? Give some special presents to family, friends or charity?

Some of the above need not cost much. Having your finances organised will give you the resources to be generous both to yourself and towards others.

# PART EIGHT

# RESOURCES

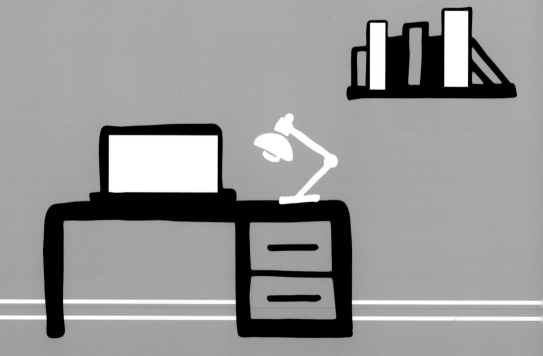

# SCIENTIFIC REFERENCES

This note is here for those of you who are expecting the scientific references, indicated by superscript numbers throughout the text, to be at the end of the book. As *The Cancer Revolution* is primarily aimed at a general readership, the references have been placed in the appropriate chapter sections of The Cancer Revolution website.

For the scientific references see **thecancerrevolution.co.uk**.

THE CANCER
REVOLUTION

# ADDITIONAL MATERIAL

The additional material listed below is grouped into chapters and sections to reflect the book's structure, with a 'General' section pn pp. 290-93.
You will therefore occasionally find the same resource mentioned more than once, if it is relevant to more than one chapter.

For each chapter or section, the material is separated into 'Further Reading' and 'Websites'. Material that relates to our contributors have been highlighted in green and in the 'General' section, titles with a blue 'R' icon are recommended for further exploration of various aspects of cancer and Integrative Medicine.

The lists are generally arranged in alphabetical order of title; items by our contributors, however, are always placed first in order of surname (Further Reading) or title (Websites).

# CONTRIBUTORS: FURTHER READING

| Title | Author | | Publisher |
|---|---|---|---|
| The Cook's Garden | Lynda Brown | 1992 | Vermilion |
| The New Shopper's Guide to Organic Food | Lynda Brown | 2002 | Fourth Estate |
| 50 Critical Cancer Answers | Francisco Contreras MD | 2013 | Authentic Publishers |
| Beating Cancer | Francisco Contreras MD | 2011 | Siloam |
| Hope, Medicine & Healing | Francisco Contreras MD | 2009 | Oasis of Hope Press |
| The Hope of Living Cancer Free | Francisco Contreras MD | 1999 | Creation House |
| Practical 12-Gram Keto Meal Plans for Cancer Patients | Patricia Daly | | patriciadaly.com |
| Practical Keto Meal Plans for Cancer | Patricia Daly | | patriciadaly.com |
| The Cancer Directory | Dr Rosy Daniel | 2005 | Harper Thorsons |
| PDQ Integrative Oncology | Barrie Cassileth PhD, Gary Deng MD PhD, Andrew Vickers PhD, K. Simon Yeung RPh Lac | 2005 | BC Decker |
| Daylight Robbery | Dr Damien Downing | 1988 | Arrow Books |
| Imperfectly Natural Baby and Toddler | Janey Lee Grace | 2007 | Orion |
| Imperfectly Natural Home | Janey Lee Grace | 2008 | Orion |
| Imperfectly Natural Woman | Janey Lee Grace | 2005 | Crown House Publishing |
| Look Good Naturally... Without Ditching the Lipstick | Janey Lee Grace | 2013 | Hay House UK |
| Living Food: A Feast for Soil and Soul | Daphne Lambert | 2016 | United Authors |
| The Organic Baby & Toddler Cookbook | Daphne Lambert, Tanyia Maxted-Frost | 1990 | Green Books |
| Beat Cancer: How to Re-gain Control of Your Health and Your Life | Prof. Jane Plant, Mustafa Djamgoz | 2014 | Ebury Digital |
| Prostate Cancer | Prof. Jane Plant | 2007 | Virgin Books |
| The Plant Programme | Prof. Jane Plant | 2001 | Virgin Books |
| Your Life in Your Hands | Prof. Jane Plant | 2000 | Virgin Books |
| Swiss Secret to Optimal Health | Dr Thomas Rau, Susan Wyler | 2009 | Berkley Trade |
| The Topic of Cancer | Jessica Richards | 2011 | Jessica Richards |

| Book Number | Description / Notes |
|---|---|
| ISBN-10: 0091775868<br>ISBN-13: 978-0091775865 | 'Grow your own' guidance |
| ISBN-10: 1841154253<br>ISBN-13: 978-1841154251 | 'Essential reading for anyone who cares about what they put in their and their children's mouths.' Nigel Slater, *Observer* |
| ISBN-10: 1780781075<br>ISBN-13: 978-1780781075 | 50 tangible tips, plans, and prescriptive measures for tackling cancer and finding renewed health. Dr Contreras' most recent book |
| ISBN-10: 1616381566<br>ISBN-13: 978-1616381561 | 20 natural, spiritual and medical remedies that can slow - and even reverse - cancer's progression |
| ISBN-10: 1579460011<br>ISBN-13: 978-1579460013 | How patients can live with cancer, managing it like a chronic disease |
| ISBN-10: 0884196550<br>ISBN-13: 978-0884196556 | Cancer is approached from the view of one's emotional and spiritual factors in dealing with it |
| | 'Hands-on' advice from nutritionist and cancer patient, Patricia Daly |
| | 'Hands-on' advice from nutritionist and cancer patient, Patricia Daly |
| ISBN-10: 0007154275<br>ISBN-13: 978-0007154272 | Comprehensive UK directory of integrative approaches to cancer |
| ISBN-10: 1550092804<br>ISBN-13: 978-1550092806 | Complementary therapies in cancer care |
| ISBN 0099567407 | One of the first books to highlight to problems around vitamin D deficiency |
| ISBN-10: 0752885898<br>ISBN-13: 978-0752885896 | How to be a green parent in today's busy world |
| ISBN-10: 0752885820<br>ISBN-13: 978-0752885827 | Everything you need to know to create a healthy, natural home, in a very readable format |
| ISBN-10: 1904424899<br>ISBN-13: 978-1904424895 | Getting life right the natural way |
| ISBN-10: 1848502036<br>ISBN-13: 978-1848502031 | Find your way through the minefield of toxic cosmetics |
| | Due for completion Spring 2016. A book that brings alive the connections between food, our health and the health of the planet |
| ISBN-10: 1870098862<br>ISBN-13: 978-1870098861 | Specialised advice for parents concerned about the giving babies and toddlers the best possible nutrition |
| ISBN-10: 0091947952<br>ISBN-13: 978-0091947958 | Prof. Plant's most recent book, written with Prof. Djamgoz, aimed at empowering anyone with cancer |
| ISBN-10: 075351298X<br>ISBN-13: 978-0753512982 | Understand, prevent and overcome prostate cancer |
| ISBN-10: 0753509520<br>ISBN-13: 978-0753509524 | Recipes for fighting breast and prostate cancer |
| ISBN-10: 0753512041<br>ISBN-13: 978-0753512043 | The classic from Prof. Plant detailing her findings regarding dairy produce and more |
| ISBN-10: 0425225666<br>ISBN-13: 978-0425225660 | Dr Rau's diet for whole body healing |
| ISBN-10: 0957064403<br>ISBN-13: 978-0957064409 | Straightforward, practical advice on navigating through cancer treatment |

| Title | Author | | Publisher |
|---|---|---|---|
| Shazzie's Detox Delights | Shazzie | 2006 | Rawcreation Limited |
| Detox Your World | David Wolfe, Shazzie | 2012 | North Atlantic Books,U.S. |
| Naked Chocolate | David Wolfe, Shazzie | 2012 | North Atlantic Books,U.S. |
| Evie's Kitchen | Shazzie, David Smith | 2008 | Rawcreation Limited |
| Lifestyle and Cancer: The Facts | Prof. Robert Thomas | 2011 | Health Education Publications |
| Jason Vale's 5:2 Juice Diet | Jason Vale | 2015 | Juice Master Publications |
| 7lbs in 7 Days | Jason Vale | 2014 | Harper Thorsons |
| Juice Yourself Slim | Jason Vale | 2014 | Harper Thorsons |
| Vital Signs for Cancer | Xandria Williams | 2010 | Piatkus |
| Cancer Concerns | Xandria Williams | 2011 | Xtra Health Publications |
| Detecting Cancer | Xandria Williams | 2013 | Xtra Health Publications |

# CONTRIBUTORS: WEBSITES

| Website | Web Address | |
|---|---|---|
| Cancer Options | canceroptions.co.uk | |
| The Cancer Revolution | thecancerrevolution.co.uk | |
| Yes to Life | yestolife.org.uk | |
| Dr Francisco Contreras, Oasis of Hope | www.oasisofhope.com | |
| Dorothy Crowther, Wirral Holistic | www.wirralholistic.org.uk | |
| Jo Daly | www.jodaly.com | |
| Patricia Daly | patriciadaly.com | |
| Dr Rosy Daniel, Health Creation | www.healthcreation.co.uk | |
| Lizzy Davis, CanExercise | www.canexercise.co.uk | |
| Dr Gary Deng, MSKCC Integrative Medicine Service | www.mskcc.org/cancer-care/doctors/gary-deng | |
| Dr Friedrich Douwes, Klinik St Georg | www.klinik-st-georg.de/en | |
| Dr Damien Downing, New Medicine Group | newmedicinegroup.com/practitioners/dr-damien-downing | |
| George Emsden, CancerIFA | www.cancerifa.com | |
| Dr Chris Etheridge | www.drchrisetheridge.co.uk | |
| Jane Fior, Cancer Counselling London | www.cancercounsellinglondon.org.uk | |
| Barbara Gallani | www.thelifecentre.com/teachers/barbara-gallani | |
| Janey Lee Grace | imperfectlynatural.com | |

| Book Number | Description / Notes |
|---|---|
| ASIN: B002MYB9HU | Raw-food starter guide |
| ISBN-10: 1583944508<br>ISBN-13: 978-1583944509 | Quick and lasting results for a beautiful mind, body and spirit |
| ISBN-10: 1556437315<br>ISBN-13: 978-1556437311 | The astonishing truth about the world's greatest food |
| ISBN-10: 0954397738<br>ISBN-13: 978-0954397739 | Raising an ecstatic child |
| ASIN: B004L2LJ30 | The second and updated edition from Britain's leading oncologist in the field of lifestyle, nutrition and cancer |
| ISBN-10: 0954766466<br>ISBN-13: 978-0954766467 | Jason Vale's most recent book - a 'juicing' take on the popular 5:2 diet |
| ISBN-10: 0007436181<br>ISBN-13: 978-0007436187 | The Juice Master diet |
| ISBN-10: 0007267142<br>ISBN-13: 978-0007267149 | The healthy way to lose weight without dieting |
| ISBN-10: 0749952474<br>ISBN-13: 978-0749952471 | How to monitor, prevent and reverse the cancer process |
| ISBN-10: 0956855202<br>ISBN-13: 978-0956855206 | A practical 10-step path towards recovery described and explained |
| ISBN-10: 0956855237 | Book 3 of Xandria William's planned Cancer Quintet |

| Description / Notes |
|---|
| Consultancy providing personalised information on Integrative Medicine options |
| Companion website to this book - further material and updates |
| The UK's integrative cancer care charity |
| Hospital in Mexico founded by Dr Contreras' father |
| Complementary therapies for people with cancer, established by Dorothy Crowther |
| Jo Daly's site for her work as a homeopath in the USA |
| Specialised information on the ketogenic diet for cancer |
| Integrative support, mentoring and much more |
| Supported exercise programmes for people with cancer |
| Dr Gary Deng is an Integrative Medicine Specialist at Memorial Sloan Kettering Cancer Center in New York |
| German integrative clinic |
| UK integrative doctor |
| Specialised financial advice for those with cancer |
| Herbalist specialising in supporting people with cancer |
| Highly experienced professional cancer counselling |
| Yoga for people with cancer |
| Natural alternatives for your home and lifestyle |

| Website | Web Address | |
|---------|-------------|---|
| Juliet Hayward | www.healthy.co.uk/about.html | |
| Tom Hoyland | www.reflexologyandmassageeastfinchley.uk | |
| Robert Jacobs | robertjacobshealth.com | |
| Daphne Lambert, Greencuisine | www.greencuisine.org | |
| Clare Mclusky, Mindful Choice | www.mindfulchoice.co.uk | |
| Dr Henry Mannings, Star Throwers | starthrowers.org.uk | |
| Dr John Moran, Holistic Medical | www.holisticmedical.co.uk | |
| Dr Maurice Orange, Ita Wegman Klinik | www.klinik-arlesheim.ch/en | |
| Jane Plant, Cancer Support International | www.cancersupportinternational.com/janeplant.com/index.asp | |
| Dr Thomas Rau, Paracelcus Klinik | paracelsus.ch/?lang=en | |
| Jessica Richards | www.jessicarichards.co.uk | |
| Margella Salmins | www.margellasalmins.com | |
| Patrizia Sergeant | www.patriziasergeant.co.uk | |
| Shazzie | www.shazzie.com | |
| Prof. Shimon Slavin, CTCI | www.ctcicenter.com | |
| Prof. Robert Thomas, Cancernet | www.cancernet.co.uk | |
| Jason Vale, Juicemaster | www.juicemaster.com | |
| Robert Verkerk, Alliance for Natural Health (ANH) | anhinternational.org | |
| Xandria Williams | www.xandriawilliams.co.uk | |
| Dr Bernard Willis | drbernardwillis.com | |
| Dr André Young-Snell, Vision of Hope Clinic | www.visionofhopeclinic.com | |

# CONTRIBUTORS: ASSOCIATED WEBSITES

| Website | Web Address | |
|---------|-------------|---|
| Pomi-T Trial | www.cancernet.co.uk/pomi-t.htm | |
| Academy of Nutritional Medicine (AONM) | www.aonm.org | |
| Association of Reflexologists (AOR) | www.aor.org.uk | |
| British College of Osteopathic Medicine (BCOM) | www.bcom.ac.uk | |
| British Society for Ecological Medicine (BSEM) | www.bsem.org.uk | |
| British Society for Integrative Oncology (BSIO) | www.bsio.org.uk | |
| CANCERactive | www.canceractive.com | |
| Federation of Holistic Therapists (FHT) | www.fht.org.uk | |
| Integrated Healthcare Trust | www.integrativehealthtrust.org | |
| Pfeifer Protocols | www.clearfeed.com/pfeifer | |
| Society for Integrative Oncology (SIO) | www.integrativeonc.org | |
| Soil Association | soilassociation.org | |

| | Description / Notes |
|---|---|
| | Juliet Hayward works as a consultant for the Really Healthy Co |
| | Complementary therapies for those with cancer |
| | Functional Medicine practitioner |
| | Trust working with the healing aspects of food |
| | Mindfulness and cancer |
| | Charity based in Norfolk giving direct support to people with cancer |
| | UK integrative doctor |
| | Swiss integrative clinic |
| | Site promoting the work of Prof. Jane Plant |
| | Dr Rau is Medical Director of the Paracelsus Klinik in Switzerland |
| | Jessica Richards' site for her work as personal transformation specialist and leadership mentor |
| | Margella Salmins' site for her work as a Traditional East Asian Medicine practitioner |
| | Patrizia Sergeant's site for her work as a Journey, Bowen and Reiki practitioner |
| | Life mastery, business mastery and all things raw |
| | Israeli specialist cancer centre |
| | Website built by the UK's leading oncologist in the field of lifestyle, nutrition and cancer |
| | Juice, juice and more juice! |
| | Leading not-for-profit working to protect natural medicines and their availability to the public |
| | Biochemist, naturopath, author and teacher with a specialist interest in cancer |
| | UK integrative doctor |
| | UK integrative doctor |

| | Description / Notes |
|---|---|
| | Prof. Robert Thomas' groundbreaking UK trial of nutrition for prostate cancer |
| | UK forum for advancing nutritional medicine |
| | Professional UK association providing benefits, advice and guidance to reflexologists |
| | Osteopathic training and accreditation |
| | UK professional body promoting the study and good practice of allergy, environmental and nutritional medicine for the benefit of the public |
| | The leading UK professional body for practitioners of Integrative Medicine for cancer |
| | Charity providing the latest information on developments in Integrative Oncology |
| | Largest professional association for therapists in the UK and Ireland |
| | Charity promoting Integrative Medicine |
| | Information site for the Pfeifer breast and prostate protocols |
| | The leading US professional body for practitioners of Integrative Medicine for cancer |
| | Promoting environmentally and animal friendly farming methods |

# INTRODUCTION: FURTHER READING

| Title | Author | | Publisher |
|---|---|---|---|
| PDQ Integrative Oncology | Barrie Cassileth PhD, Gary Deng MD PhD, Andrew Vickers PhD, K. Simon Yeung RPh Lac | 2005 | BC Decker |

# INTRODUCTION: WEBSITES

| Website | Web Address | |
|---|---|---|
| British Society for Integrative Oncology (BSIO) | www.bsio.org.uk | |
| Memorial Sloan-Kettering Cancer Center | www.mskcc.org/cancer-care/integrative-medicine | |
| Society for Integrative Oncology (SIO) | www.integrativeonc.org | |

# CHAPTER 1: WEBSITES

| Website | Web Address | |
|---|---|---|
| The Cancer Revolution | thecancerrevolution.co.uk | |
| Vision of Hope Clinic | www.visionofhopeclinic.com | |
| Xandria Williams | www.xandriawilliams.co.uk | |
| British Society for Integrative Oncology (BSIO) | www.bsio.org.uk | |
| Green Med Info | www.greenmedinfo.com | |
| Medline | www.nlm.nih.gov/bsd/pmresources.html | |
| NHS Health Records | www.nhs.uk/NHSEngland/thenhs/records/healthrecords/Pages/what_to_do.aspx | |
| Society for Integrative Oncology (SIO) | www.integrativeonc.org | |

# CHAPTER 2: FURTHER READING

| Title | Author | | Publisher |
|---|---|---|---|
| Hormone Solution | Dr Thierry Hertoghe | 2004 | Random House USA Inc |
| Knockout | Suzanne Somers | 2010 | Three Rivers Press |
| Stay Young & Sexy with Bio-Identical Hormone Replacement | Jonathan V., M.D. Wright, Lane Lenard | 2010 | Smart Publications |
| The Hormone Cure | Sara Gottfried | 2014 | Simon & Schuster |
| Waking The Warrior Goddess | Christine Horner | 2013 | Basic Health Publications |
| Womancode | Alisa Vitti | 2014 | HarperOne |

| Book Number | Description / Notes |
|---|---|
| ISBN-10: 1550092804<br>ISBN-13: 978-1550092806 | Complementary therapies in cancer care |

| Description / Notes |
|---|
| The leading UK professional body for practitioners of Integrative Medicine for cancer |
| The Integrative Oncology Department at MSKCC |
| The leading US professional body for practitioners of Integrative Medicine for cancer |

| Description / Notes |
|---|
| Companion website to this book - further material and updates |
| Integrative Medicine for people with cancer |
| Biochemist, naturopath, author and teacher with a specialist interest in cancer |
| The leading UK professional body for practitioners of Integrative Medicine for cancer |
| Research data on integrative approaches |
| Research data |
| About your health records |
| The leading US professional body for practitioners of Integrative Medicine for cancer |

| Book Number | Description / Notes |
|---|---|
| ISBN-10: 1400080851<br>ISBN-13: 978-1400080854 | Stay younger longer with natural hormone and nutrition therapies |
| ISBN-10: 0307587592<br>ISBN-13: 978-0307587596 | Interviews with doctors who are curing cancer - and how to avoid getting it in the first place |
| ISBN-10: 1890572225<br>ISBN-13: 978-1890572228 | The science of hormone replacement explained |
| ISBN-10: 1451666950<br>ISBN-13: 978-1451666953 | Reclaim balance, sleep, sex drive and vitality naturally with the Gottfried Protocol |
| ISBN-10: 1591203635<br>ISBN-13: 978-1591203636 | Dr. Christine Horner's programme to protect against and fight breast cancer |
| ISBN-10: 006213079X<br>ISBN-13: 978-0062130792 | Perfect your cycle, amplify your fertility, supercharge your sex drive, and become a power source |

# CHAPTER 2: WEBSITES

| Website | Web Address | |
|---|---|---|
| Holistic Medical Clinic | www.holisticmedical.co.uk | |
| Pfeifer Protocol in the UK | www.holisticmedical.co.uk/mens_Prostate_Cancer_Pfeifers_Protocol.htm | |
| Pfeifer Protocols | www.clearfeed.com/pfeifer | |

# CHAPTER 3: FURTHER READING

| Title | Author | | Publisher |
|---|---|---|---|
| Choices in Healing | Michael Lerner | 1996 | The MIT Press |
| Mindfulness for Health | Vidyamal Burch, Danny Penman | 2013 | Piatkus |
| The Journey | Brandon Bays | 2012 | Atria Books |

# CHAPTER 3: WEBSITES

| Website | Web Address | |
|---|---|---|
| Barbara Gallani | www.thelifecentre.com/teachers/barbara-gallani | |
| Cancer Options | www.canceroptions.co.uk | |
| CanExercise | www.canexercise.co.uk | |
| Center for Homeopathy | www.jodaly.com | |
| Chris Etheridge | www.drchrisetheridge.co.uk | |
| Jessica Richards | www.jessicarichards.co.uk | |
| LIFE> Yes to Life Web Directory | yestolife.org.uk/y2l/directoryintro.html | |
| Margella Salmins | www.margellasalmins.com | |
| Patrizia Sergeant | www.patriziasergeant.co.uk | |
| Wirral Holistic Care | www.wirralholistic.org.uk | |
| Yes to Life | yestolife.org.uk | |
| Academy of Nutritional Medicine | www.aonm.org | |
| Acupuncture Society | www.acupuncturesociety.org.uk | |
| Association for Nutrition | www.associationfornutrition.org | |
| Association of Reflexologists | www.aor.org.uk | |
| Association of Traditional Chinese Medicine | www.atcm.co.uk | |
| Ayurvedic Practitioners Association | www.apa.uk.com | |
| British Acupuncture Council | www.acupuncture.org.uk | |

| Description / Notes |
| --- |
| Integrative Medicine practice, specialising in hormones |
| Pfeifer prostate protocol: supervision in the UK |
| Information site for the Pfeifer breast and prostate protocols |

| Book Number | Description / Notes |
| --- | --- |
| ISBN-10: 0262621045<br>ISBN-13: 978-0262621045 | Classic on holistic approaches from the founder of the Commonweal Centre in California |
| ISBN-10: 074995924X<br>ISBN-13: 978-0749959241 | A practical guide to relieving pain, reducing stress and restoring wellbeing |
| ISBN-10: 145166561X<br>ISBN-13: 978-1451665611 | Inspiration account of the author's recovery from cancer which formed the basis of a now popular therapy for cancer: The Journey |

| Description / Notes |
| --- |
| Barbara Gallani's teacher page on the Life Centre website |
| Consultancy providing personalised information on Integrative Medicine options |
| Lizzy Davis' site offering exercise resources and support for those with cancer |
| Information and contacts for homeopathy in the USA |
| Herbalist specialising in supporting people with cancer |
| Jessica Richards' site for her work as personal transformation specialist and leadership mentor |
| Extensive searchable directory of therapies, practitioners and clinics worldwide |
| Margella Salmins' site for her work as a Traditional East Asian Medicine practitioner |
| Patrizia Sergeant's site for her work as a Journey, Bowen and Reiki practitioner |
| Complementary therapies for people with cancer, established by Dorothy Crowther |
| The UK's integrative cancer care charity |
| UK forum for advancing nutritional medicine |
| The Acupuncture Society is an association and register of professional acupuncture therapists, formed to promote the development of TCM, Acupuncture, Chinese Herbal Medicine and other Oriental Therapies |
| Registered Nutritionists |
| Professional UK association providing benefits, advice and guidance to reflexologists |
| UK regulatory body engaged in academic study, research and the clinical application of Traditional Chinese Medicine |
| The APA represents qualified and insured Ayurvedic practitioners, Ayurvedic therapists and students of Ayurveda in the UK |
| UK professional/self-regulatory body for the practice of traditional acupuncture |

| Website | Web Address | |
|---|---|---|
| British Association of Accredited Ayurvedic Practitioners | www.britayurpractitioners.com | |
| British Association of Art Therapists | www.baatmembers.org.uk | |
| British Association for Music Therapy | www.bamt.org | |
| British Council for Yoga Therapy | www.bcyt.co.uk | |
| British Health Qigong Association | www.healthqigong.org.uk | |
| British Homeopathic Association | www.britishhomeopathic.org | |
| British Naturopathic Association | www.naturopaths.org.uk | |
| British Society for Integrative Oncology (BSIO) | www.bsio.org.uk | |
| British Society of Clinical Hypnosis | www.bsch.org.uk | |
| British Wheel of Yoga | www.bwy.org.uk | |
| Be Mindful | bemindful.co.uk | |
| Be Mindful Online | www.bemindfulonline.com | |
| Biodynamic Association | www.biodynamic.org.uk | |
| Biofeedback | www.naturaltherapypages.co.uk/energetic_medicine/Bio_Feedback | |
| Cancer Counselling London | www.cancercounsellinglondon.org.uk | |
| CANCERactive - Support Groups | www.canceractive.com/cancer-active-page-link.aspx?n=2173 | |
| College of Practitioners of Phytotherapy (CPP) | www.phytotherapists.org | |
| Commonweal Centre | www.commonweal.org | |
| Complementary and Natural Healthcare Council (CNHC) | www.cnhc.org.uk | |
| Emotional Freedom Technique (EFT) | http://www.energypsych.org/search | |
| Federation of Holistic Therapists | www.fht.org.uk | |
| Federation of Nutritional Therapy Practitioners | www.fntp.org.uk | |
| GCMT (Massage) | www.gcmt.org.uk | |
| General Hypnotherapy Register | www.general-hypnotherapy-register.com | |
| General Naturopathic Council | www.gncouncil.com | |
| Gerson Institute | gerson.org/gerpress | |
| Guided Mindfulness Meditation Practices | www.mindfulnesscds.com | |
| Healing Trust | www.thehealingtrust.org.uk | |
| Health Creation Mentor | www.healthcreation.co.uk/mentors | |

| Description / Notes |
|---|
| Professional Ayurvedic Association devoted to voluntary service in spreading awareness and the establishment of an authentic, effective, safe and undiluted system of Ayurveda |
| Find therapist, courses, conferences, training |
| Professional body for music therapy in the UK, providing both practitioners and non-practitioners with information, professional support and training opportunities |
| An excellent resource to find a herbalist in your area |
| Official governing body and instructor training centre for Europe, the UK and Northern Ireland |
| Information, education and research on homeopathy. Find a medical homeopath |
| Professional body of practicing naturopaths who are registered with the General Council and Register of Naturopaths (GCRN) in the UK |
| The leading UK professional body for practitioners of Integrative Medicine for cancer |
| Promote and assures high standards in the practice of hypnotherapy |
| Sport England recognised national governing body for yoga |
| All about mindfulness. Find a teacher |
| Online mindfulness course |
| UK association of biodynamic growers |
| Find a practitioner |
| Highly experienced professional cancer counselling |
| CANCERactive listing of UK support groups |
| Professional membership organisation of phytotherapists |
| Complementary therapies centre in California set up by Michael Lerner, who was inspired by the UK Bristol Cancer Help Centre (now Penny Brohn Cancer Care) |
| UK voluntary register of complementary therapists. Find a practitioner |
| Find a practitioner |
| Largest professional association for therapists in the UK and Ireland |
| Professional organisation for practitioners of nutritional therapy in Europe |
| Aims to represent the views of the whole spectrum of massage and soft tissue practitioners by working collectively in the best interests of the profession |
| Find a hypnotherapist or a training course |
| Regulates the Naturopathic profession |
| Information on Gerson therapy, clinics, programmes |
| Official outlet for 3 series of guided mindfulness meditation practices by Jon Kabat-Zinn |
| UK organisation of Spiritual Healers |
| Health Creation's mentor scheme set up for people with cancer by Dr Rosy Daniel |

| Website | Web Address | |
|---|---|---|
| Hypnotherapist Register | www.hypnotherapistregister.com | |
| Hypnotherapy Association | www.thehypnotherapyassociation.co.uk | |
| Hypnotherapy Directory | www.hypnotherapy-directory.org.uk | |
| Independent Yoga Network | www.independentyoganetwork.org | |
| International Federation of Professional Aromatherapists | www.ifparoma.org | |
| Journaling | www.breastcancer.org/treatment/comp_med/types/journaling | |
| Journaling/Treatment Diary | www.treatmentdiaries.com | |
| Life Centre | www.thelifecentre.com | |
| Macmillan - Support Groups | www.macmillan.org.uk/howwecanhelp/cancersupportgroups/cancersupportgroups.aspx | |
| Mercola | eft.mercola.com | |
| National Council for Hypnotherapy | www.hypnotherapists.org.uk | |
| National Institute of Medical Herbalists (NIMH) | www.nimh.org.uk | |
| Oxford Mindfulness Centre | www.oxfordmindfulness.org | |
| Register of Chinese Herbal Medicine | www.rchm.co.uk | |
| Register of Exercise Professionals | www.exerciseregister.org | |
| Reiki Council | www.reikicouncil.org.uk | |
| Reiki Federation | www.reikifed.co.uk | |
| Shiatsu Society | www.shiatsusociety.org | |
| Society of Homeopaths | www.homeopathy-soh.org | |
| T'ai Chi at Maggie's Centres | www.maggiescentres.org/centres/ukmap.html | |
| The Journey | www.thejourney.com | |
| Wright Foundation | www.wrightfoundation.com | |
| Yoga for Survivors | www.laurakupperman.com/yoga-for-survivors | |

# CHAPTER 4: FURTHER READING

| Title | Author | | Publisher |
|---|---|---|---|
| The Cook's Garden | Lynda Brown | 1992 | Vermilion |
| The New Shopper's Guide to Organic Food | Lynda Brown | 2002 | Fourth Estate |
| In Defence of Food | Michael Pollan | 2009 | Penguin |
| Eat Your Heart Out | Felicity Lawrence | 2008 | Penguin |
| Molecules of Emotion | Candace B Pert | 1999 | Pocket Books |

| Description / Notes |
|---|
| Find a hypnotherapist |
| Professional UK body representing approved hypnotherapists in active practice |
| Find a hypnotherapist |
| Organisation for Yoga Teachers and Teacher Training Schools |
| UK professional body representing aromatherapists |
| Description of Journaling as a support to those with cancer |
| Anonymous online sharing of health diaries |
| Yoga courses, workshops, therapies and teacher training |
| Directory of support groups |
| In depth description of EFT and EFT techniques |
| UK hypnotherapy professional association |
| UK professional body representing herbal practitioners |
| Resources and courses for the public |
| Regulating the practice of Chinese Herbal Medicine (CHM) in the UK |
| Provides regulation for instructors and trainers to ensure that they meet the health and fitness industry's agreed National Occupational Standards |
| Wide range of resources for Reiki |
| Find a course, practitioner, teacher |
| Promotes Shiatsu and ensures safe practice, training and professional conduct of all Shiatsu practitioners |
| Professional body for homeopaths. Find a homeopath |
| Find a Maggie's Centre |
| Brandon Bays' website for her Journey therapy: seminars, practitioners, books, recordings |
| Provides specialist cancer rehabilitation exercise courses for professionals |
| Yoga for Survivors: specialised yoga for people with cancer |

| Book Number | Description / Notes |
|---|---|
| ISBN-10: 0091775868<br>ISBN-13: 978-0091775865 | 'Grow your own' guidance |
| ISBN-10: 1841154253<br>ISBN-13: 978-1841154251 | 'Essential reading for anyone who cares about what they put in their and their children's mouths.' Nigel Slater, Observer |
| ISBN-10: 0141034726<br>ISBN-13: 978-0141034720 | The myth of nutrition and the pleasures of eating: an eater's manifesto |
| ISBN-10: 0141026014<br>ISBN-13: 978-0141026015 | Why the food business is bad for the planet and your health |
| ISBN-10: 0671033972<br>ISBN-13: 978-0671033972 | Why you feel the way you feel. Groundbreaking book on the biology of emotion |

# CHAPTER 4: FURTHER READING

| Title | Author | | Publisher |
|---|---|---|---|
| **Not on the Label** | Felicity Lawrence | 2013 | Penguin |
| **What to Eat** | Joanna Blythman | 2013 | Fourth Estate |

# CHAPTER 4: WEBSITES

| Website | Web Address | |
|---|---|---|
| **Abel & Cole** | www.abelandcole.co.uk | |
| **Big Barn** | www.bigbarn.co.uk | |
| **Biodynamic Association** | www.biodynamic.org.uk | |
| **Pesticide Action Network** | http://www.pan-uk.org | |
| **Raw Milk** | www.raw-milk-facts.com | |
| **Riverford** | www.riverford.co.uk | |
| **Soil Association** | www.soilassocation.org | |
| **Weston Price Foundation** | www.westonaprice.org | |

# CHAPTER 5: FURTHER READING

| Title | Author | | Publisher |
|---|---|---|---|
| Practical 12-Gram Keto Meal Plans for Cancer Patients | Patricia Daly | | patriciadaly.com |
| Practical Keto Meal Plans for Cancer | Patricia Daly | | patriciadaly.com |
| Little Red Gooseberries | Daphne Lambert | 2001 | Orion Books |
| Living Food: A Feast for Soil and Soul | Daphne Lambert | | United Authors |
| The Organic Baby & Toddler Cookbook | Daphne Lambert, Tanyia Maxted-Frost | 1990 | Green Books |
| Beat Cancer | Prof. Jane Plant, Mustafa Djamgoz | 2014 | Vermilion |
| Prostate Cancer | Prof. Jane Plant | 2007 | Virgin Books |
| The Plant Programme | Prof. Jane Plant | 2004 | Virgin Books |
| Your Life in Your Hands | Prof. Jane Plant | 2007 | Virgin Books |
| Cancer Concerns | Xandria Williams | 2011 | Xtra Health Publications |

| Book Number | Description / Notes |
|---|---|
| ISBN-10: 0241967821<br>ISBN-13: 978-0241967829 | What really goes into the food on your plate. Classic exposé of the supermarket industry updated with extraordinary new material on the horse meat scandal |
| ISBN-10: 0007476469<br>ISBN-13: 978-0007476466 | Food that's good for your health, pocket and plate |

| Description / Notes |
|---|
| Organic food delivery |
| Directory of local food producers selling directly to the public, including those selling online |
| Events, resources, training, certification, books, videos |
| Campaigning group promoting safe and sustainable alternatives to hazardous pesticides |
| Information site specifically about raw milk |
| Organic farm and delivery |
| Link to blog to read more by Lynda Brown |
| Natural fats, raw milk, health and nutrition. Events, videos, resources |

| Book Number | Description / Notes |
|---|---|
|  | 'Hands on' advice from nutritionist and cancer patient, Patricia Daly |
|  | 'Hands on' advice from nutritionist and cancer patient, Patricia Daly |
| ISBN-10: 075283844X<br>ISBN-13: 978-0752838441 | Organic recipes from Penrhos |
|  | Due for completion Spring 2016. A book that brings alive the connections between food, our health and the health of the planet |
| ISBN-10: 1870098862<br>ISBN-13: 978-1870098861 | A comprehensive but easy-to-follow guide to feeding babies from weaning to toddlerhood |
| ISBN-10: 0091947952<br>ISBN-13: 978-0091947958 | How to regain control of your health and your life |
| ISBN-10: 075351298X<br>ISBN-13: 978-0753512982 | Understand, prevent and overcome prostrate cancer |
| ISBN-10: 0753509520<br>ISBN-13: 978-0753509524 | Recipes for fighting breast and prostate cancer |
| ISBN-10: 0753512041<br>ISBN-13: 978-0753512043 | Understand, prevent and overcome breast cancer and ovarian cancer |
| ISBN-10: 0956855202<br>ISBN-13: 978-0956855206 | A practical 10-step path towards recovery described and explained |

| Title | Author | | Publisher |
|---|---|---|---|
| Detecting Cancer | Xandria Williams | 2013 | Xtra Health Publications |
| Vital Signs For Cancer | Xandria Williams | 2010 | Piatkus |
| Atlas of Cancer Mortality in the People's Republic of China | | 1979 | Pergamon Press 1981 |
| Cancer as a Metabolic Disease | Thomas Seyfried | 2012 | Wiley |
| Eat to Outsmart Cancer | Jenny Phillips | 2015 | CompletelyNovel |
| Healing the Gerson Way | Charlotte Gerson | 2010 | Totality Books |
| Live Raw | Mimi Kirk | 2013 | Skyhorse Publishing |
| Medicinal Mushrooms | Martin Powell | 2013 | Mycology Press |
| Nutrition and Physical Degeneration | Weston A Price | 2009 | Price Pottenger Nutrition |
| One Man Alone | Dr Nicholas Gonzalez | 2010 | New Spring Press |
| The Biology of Belief | Bruce Lipton | 2011 | Hay House UK |
| The China Study | T. Colin Campbell, Thomas M. Campbell II | 2006 | BenBella Books |
| The Metabolism of Tumours | Otto Warburg, Trung Nguyen | 2015 | EnCognitive.com |
| The Oil Protein Diet Cookbook | Dr Joanna Budwig | 2006 | Apple Publishing Co. |
| The Uncook Book | Tanya Maher | 2015 | Hay House UK |
| The Water Puzzle and the Hexagonal Key | Dr Mu Shik Jhon | 2004 | Uplifting Press |
| Tripping Over the Truth | Travis Christofferson | 2014 | CreateSpace Independent Publishing Platform |

# CHAPTER 5: WEBSITES

| Website | Web Address | |
|---|---|---|
| Greencuisine | www.greencuisine.org | |
| Jane Plant, Cancer Support International | www.cancersupportinternational.com/janeplant.com/index.asp | |
| Live Raw | www.New2Raw.com | |
| Patricia Daly | www.nutritionchoices.ie | |
| Shazzie | www.Shazzie.com | |
| Xandria Williams | www.xandriawilliams.co.uk | |
| Budwig Diet | www.budwigcenter.com | |

| Book Number | Description / Notes |
|---|---|
| ISBN-10: 0956855237<br>ISBN-13: 978-0956855237 | Book 3 of Xandria Williams' planned Cancer Quintet |
| ISBN-10: 0749952474<br>ISBN-13: 978-0749952471 | How to monitor, prevent and reverse the cancer process |
| ISBN-10: 0080288502<br>ISBN-13: 978-0080288505 | Analysis of mortality by cancer type |
| ISBN978-0-470-58492-7 | On the origin, management, and prevention of cancer. Groundbreaking reassessment of the mechanism of cancer (for science readers only!) |
| ISBN-10: 1849147175<br>ISBN-13: 978-1849147170 | How to create optimal health for prevention and recovery |
| ISBN-10: 0976018624<br>ISBN-13: 978-0976018629 | Defeating cancer and other chronic diseases |
| ASIN: B00VAZUT00 | Raw-food recipes for good health and timeless beauty |
| ASIN: B00SLVLWX4 | The essential guide |
| ISBN-10: 0916764206<br>ISBN-13: 978-0916764203 | A comparison of primitive and modern diets and their effects |
| ISBN-10: 0982196512<br>ISBN-13: 978-0982196519 | An investigation of nutrition, cancer and William Donald Kelley |
| ISBN-10: 1848503350<br>ISBN-13: 978-1848503359 | Unleashing the power of consciousness, matter and miracles |
| ISBN-10: 9781932100662<br>ISBN-13: 978-1932100662 | The most comprehensive study of nutrition ever conducted and the startling implications for diet, weight loss and long-term health |
| ASIN: B015E7AT8Q | Original text |
| ISBN-10: 0969527225<br>ISBN-13: 978-0969527220 | An imaginative yet practical guide for healthy food preparation by seven-time Nobel Prize nominee |
| ISBN-10: 1781805644<br>ISBN-13: 978-1781805640 | The essential guide to a raw-food lifestyle |
| ISBN-10: 0975272608<br>ISBN-13: 978-0975272602 | Scientific evidence of hexagonal water and Its positive influence on health |
| ISBN-10: 1500600318<br>ISBN-13: 978-1500600310 | The return of the metabolic theory of cancer illuminates a new and hopeful path to a cure. Metabolic theory for general readers |

| Description / Notes |
|---|
| Consultations, courses and retreats with Daphne Lambert |
| Site promoting the work of Prof. Jane Plant |
| Shazzie's site to help you change to raw food |
| Specialised information on the ketogenic diet for cancer |
| Life mastery, business mastery and all things raw |
| Biochemist, naturopath, author and teacher with a specialist interest in cancer |
| Spanish centre offering Budwig protocol and other integrative treatments |

| Website | Web Address |
|---|---|
| Dr Nicholas Gonzalez | www.dr-gonzalez.com |
| Dr William Kelley | www.drkelley.com |
| Eating Academy | www.eatingacademy.com |
| Fight Cancer with a Ketogenic Diet | http://www.ketogenic-diet-resource.com/cancer-diet.html |
| Gerson Diet | www.gerson.org |
| Hippocrates Health Institute | www.hippocratesinst.org |
| Mercola - Ketogenics | www.mercola.com |
| Nutrition Facts | nutritionfacts.org |
| Otto Warburg | www.nobelprize.org/nobel_prizes/medicine/laureates/1931/warburg-bio.html |
| Soil Association | www.soilassociation.org |
| Weston Price Foundation | www.westonaprice.org |

# CHAPTER 6: FURTHER READING

| Title | Author | | Publisher |
|---|---|---|---|
| Detox Your World | Shazzie, David Wolfe | 2012 | North Atlantic Books, U.S. |
| Evie's Kitchen | Shazzie, David Smith | 2008 | Rawcreation Limited |
| Naked Chocolate | Shazzie, David Wolfe | 2012 | North Atlantic Books, U.S. |
| Shazzie's Detox Delights | Shazzie | 2001 | Rawcreation |
| 7lbs in 7 Days | Jason Vale | 2014 | Harper Thorsons |
| Jason Vale's 5:2 Juice Diet | Jason Vale | 2015 | Juice Master Publications |
| Juice Yourself Slim | Jason Vale | 2014 | Harper Thorsons |
| Crazy Sexy Juice | Kris Carr | 2015 | Hay House Inc |
| Juices and Smoothies | Amanda Cross, Fiona Hunter | 2003 | Hamlyn |
| Live Raw | Mimi Kirk | 2013 | Skyhorse Publishing |
| Mum's Not Having Chemo | Laura Bond | 2013 | Piatkus |
| New Pyramid Miracle Juices | Amanda Cross, Charmaine Yabsley | 2009 | Hamlyn |
| The Gerson Therapy | Charlotte Gerson, Morton Walker | 2005 | Kensington Publishing |
| The Uncook Book | Tanya Maher | 2015 | Hay House UK |
| The Wheatgrass Book | Ann Wigmore | 1987 | Avery Publishing Group Inc. U.S. |

| Description / Notes |
| --- |
| Dr Gonzalez's clinic: Dr Gonzalez has now died and his work is being carried forward by his colleague Dr Linda Isaacs. Clinic and treatment details, books, videos |
| Online book by Dr Kelley, Dr Gonzalez's mentor - One Answer to Cancer |
| Peter Attia's blog with much focus on ketogenics |
| Ellen Davis |
| Gerson Institute - information on clinics, programmes and the therapy. Videos, testimonials, books |
| Hippocrates Health Institute - programmes, events, videos, resources |
| Search for ketogenics interviews with Dr Thomas Seyfried and Dr Dominic D'Agostino |
| The latest in nutrition-related research delivered in easy to understand video segments |
| Details of Warburg and his Nobel Prize award |
| Promoting environmentally and animal friendly farming methods |
| Natural fats, raw milk, health and nutrition. Events, videos, resources |

| Book Number | Description / Notes |
| --- | --- |
| ISBN-10: 9781583944509<br>ISBN-13: 978-1583944509 | Quick and lasting results for a beautiful mind, body and spirit |
| ISBN-10: 0954397738<br>ISBN-13: 978-0954397739 | Raising an ecstatic child |
| ISBN-10: 1556437315<br>ISBN-13: 978-1556437311 | Uncovering the astonishing truth about the world's greatest food |
| ASIN: B002MYB9HU | Raw-food starter guide |
| ISBN-10: 0007436181<br>ISBN-13: 978-0007436187 | The Juice Master diet |
| ISBN-10: 0954766466<br>ISBN-13: 978-0954766467 | Jason Vale's most recent book, a 'juicing' take on the popular 5:2 diet |
| ISBN-10: 0007267142<br>ISBN-13: 978-0007267149 | The healthy way to lose weight without dieting |
| ISBN-10: 1401941524<br>ISBN-13: 978-1401941529 | 100+ simple juice, smoothie & nut milk recipes to supercharge your health |
| ISBN-10: 0600608433<br>ISBN-13: 978-0600608431 | Over 200 delicious drinks for health and vitality |
| ASIN: B00VAZUT00 | Raw-food recipes for good health and timeless beauty |
| ISBN-10: 0749958960<br>ISBN-13: 978-0749958961 | Cutting-edge therapies, real-life stories – a road-map to healing from cancer |
| ISBN-10: 0600619168<br>ISBN-13: 978-0600619161 | Over 50 juices for a healthy life |
| ISBN-10: 1575666286<br>ISBN-13: 978-1575666280 | The proven nutritional program for cancer and other illnesses |
| ISBN-10: 1781805644<br>ISBN-13: 978-1781805640 | The essential guide to a raw-food lifestyle |
| ISBN-10: 0895292343<br>ISBN-13: 978-0895292346 | How to grow and use wheatgrass to maximise your health and vitality |

# CHAPTER 6: WEBSITES

| Website | Web Address | |
|---|---|---|
| 97 Reasons to Eat Raw Food App | itunes.com/app/97reasonstoeatrawfood | |
| Jason Vale, Juicemaster | www.juicemaster.com | |
| Shazzie | www.Shazzie.com | |
| Shazzie, Raw Food | www.New2Raw.com | |
| Wheatgrass | www.juicemaster.com/live-wheatgrass | |
| Bobby's Healthy Shop | www.bobbyshealthyshop.co.uk | |
| Champion Juicers | www.championjuicer.com | |
| Detox Trading | www.detoxtrading.com | |
| Detox Your World | www.DetoxYourWorld.com | |
| Excalibur Dehydrators | www.excaliburdehydrator.com/dehydrators | |
| Juiceland | www.juiceland.co.uk | |
| Juices and Smoothies | www.mindbodygreen.com | |
| Live Wheatgrass | www.livewheatgrass.com | |
| Norwalk Juicers | www.norwalkjuicers.com | |
| Philips Juicers & Blenders | www.philips.co.uk | |
| Real Foods | www.realfoods.co.uk/shop/superfoods | |
| Pure Synergy | www.thesynergycompany.com | |
| Marvellous Superfoods | www.marvelloussuperfood.co.uk | |
| Standard UK Diet | www.food.gov.uk/multimedia/pdfs/nutguideuk.pdf | |
| Standard US Diet | www.health.gov/dietaryguidelines/dga2010/DietaryGuidelines2010.pdf | |
| Tonic Attack | www.tonicattack.com | |
| UK Juicers | www.ukjuicers.com | |
| Vitamix Blenders | www.vitamix.co.uk | |
| Wheatgrass | www.wheatgrass-uk.com | |

# CHAPTER 7: FURTHER READING

| Title | Author | | Publisher |
|---|---|---|---|
| Fatigue | Xandria Williams | 1996 | Ebury Press |
| Antioxidants Against Cancer | Ralph Moss | 2000 | Equinox Press |
| Cancer and Vitamin C | Ewan Cameron, Linus Pauling | 2011 | Camino Books |
| Herbs Against Cancer | Ralph Moss | 1998 | Equinox Press |

| Description / Notes |
| --- |
| Shazzie's app |
| Retreats, recipes, books, videos, juices and more |
| Life mastery, business mastery and all things raw |
| Shazzie's site to help you change to raw food |
| Frozen wheatgrass delivery |
| Excalibur, Champion, raw-food equipment etc |
| Masticating juicers, videos |
| Wide selection of superfoods |
| Nature's Living Superfood, Pure Synergy |
| Wide range of dehydrators |
| Stockli, Excalibur, Vitamix, Champion, Magimix, raw-food equipment, etc |
| Daily wellness, inspiration and news |
| Frozen organic field-grown wheatgrass |
| Juice presses, water filters, dehydrators |
| Juicers and blenders |
| Wide selection of superfoods |
| Whole food organic supplements |
| Superfoods and personal care products |
| |
| |
| Frozen wheatgrass and broccoli juice delivery |
| Stockli, Excalibur, Vitamix, Champion, raw-food equipment etc |
| Blenders, recipes |
| Variety of sprouts, growing kits, wheatgrass juice |

| Book Number | Description / Notes |
| --- | --- |
| ISBN-10: 0749320664<br>ISBN-13: 978-0749320669 | The secret of getting your energy back |
| ISBN-10: 1881025284<br>ISBN-13: 978-1881025283 | Definitive investigation into the role of antioxidants in cancer treatment and known interactions with conventional therapies |
| ASIN: B00OX8ZS4I | A discussion of the nature, causes, prevention, and treatment of cancer with special reference to the value of vitamin C. By the 'fathers' of vitamin C therapy |
| ISBN-10: 1881025403<br>ISBN-13: 978-1881025405 | Characteristically thorough investigation of the potential of herbs in cancer treatment |

| Title | Author | | Publisher |
|---|---|---|---|
| How to Prevent and Treat Cancer with Natural Medicine | Michael T. Murray, Tim Birdsall, Joseph E. Pizzorno, Paul Reilly | 2004 | Riverhead Books,U.S. |
| Medicinal Mushrooms | Martin Powell | 2013 | Mycology Press |
| New Insights on Vitamin C and Cancer | Michael J. Gonzalez and Jorge R. Miranda-Massari | 2014 | Springer |
| Vitamin C: The Real Story | Steve Hickey, Andrew W. Saul | 2008 | Basic Health Publications |

# CHAPTER 7: WEBSITES

| Website | Web Address | |
|---|---|---|
| Dr Bernard Willis | www.drbernardwillis.com | |
| College of Naturopathic Medicine | www.naturopathy-uk.com | |
| Institute for Functional Medicine | www.functionalmedicine.org | |
| Institute of Health Sciences | www.instituteofhealthsciences.com | |
| Low Dose Naltrexone | www.lowdosenaltrexone.org | |
| Medicinal Mushrooms | www.medicalmushrooms.net | |
| Mistletoe for Cancer UK | www.mistletoeforcancer.org.uk | |
| Ralph Moss | http://cancerdecisions.com | |

# CHAPTER 8: FURTHER READING

| Title | Author | | Publisher |
|---|---|---|---|
| Lifestyle and Cancer: The Facts | Prof. Robert Thomas | 2011 | Health Education Publications |
| Anti-Inflammatory Oxygen Therapy | Mark Sircus | 2015 | Square One Publishers |
| The Oxygen Prescription | Nathaniel Altman | 2007 | Healing Arts Press |

# CHAPTER 8: WEBSITES

| Website | Web Address | |
|---|---|---|
| Cancernet | www.cancernet.co.uk | |
| Canexercise | www.canexercise.co.uk | |
| Hyperbaric Oxygen Chambers | yestolife.org.uk/y2l/directoryintro.html | |
| Prof Robert Thomas | www.cancernet.co.uk/rthomas.htm | |
| Chi Machine | www.chi-machine.co.uk | |
| Hyperbaric Oxygen Chambers | www.hyperbaricoxygentherapy.org.uk | |
| Macmillan | http://www.macmillan.org.uk/information-and-support/coping/maintaining-a-healthy-lifestyle | |

| Book Number | Description / Notes |
|---|---|
| ISBN-10: 1573223433<br>ISBN-13: 978-1573223430 | A natural arsenal of disease-fighting tools for prevention, treatment, and coping with side effects |
| ASIN: B00SLVLWX4 | The essential guide |
| ISBN-10: 1493918893<br>ISBN-13: 978-1493918898 | A slim volume packed with the latest research into vitamin C and cancer |
| ASIN: B00CB5TUR6 | The remarkable and controversial story of vitamin C |

| Description / Notes |
|---|
| UK-based integrative doctor |
| Training at 7 colleges across the UK |
| The 'home' of Functional Medicine – information, events, training |
| Find a trained nutritionist |
| Information site |
| Information and sales |
| Information about mistletoe therapy and the latest news of trials and research on mistletoe therapy for cancer |
| Leading international authority on Integrative Oncology |

| Book Number | Description / Notes |
|---|---|
| ASIN: B004L2LJ30 | The second and updated edition from Britain's leading oncologist in the field of lifestyle, nutrition and cancer |
| ISBN-10: 0757004156<br>ISBN-13: 978-0757004155 | Your complete guide to understanding and using natural oxygen therapy |
| ISBN-10: 1594771774<br>ISBN-13: 978-1594771774 | The miracle of oxidative therapies |

| Description / Notes |
|---|
| Website built by the UK's leading oncologist in the field of lifestyle, nutrition and cancer |
| Lizzy Davis' website for cancer rehabilitation through exercise |
| LIFE>, the Yes to Life searchable web directory, lists HBOT centres in the UK |
| Profile of Prof. Thomas |
| Suppliers |
| Charity supporting HBOT. Find an HBOT centre |
| Advice and information on exercise and cancer - click 'Keeping active' |

| Website | Web Address | |
|---|---|---|
| **Oxygen Concentrators** | www.uk.airliquide.com<br>www.baywater.co.uk<br>www.dolbyvivisol.com/england/our-services/<br>oxygen-therapy/patients-and-carers.aspx | |
| **Rebounders** | www.bobbyshealthyshop.co.uk | |
| **Reviber** | www.reviber.co.uk | |
| **Specialist Health Centre** | specialisthealthcentre.co.uk | |
| **Wright Foundation** | www.wrightfoundation.com | |

# CHAPTER 9: FURTHER READING

| Title | Author | | Publisher |
|---|---|---|---|
| The Cancer Directory | Dr Rosy Daniel | 2005 | Harper Thorsons |
| Eat to Beat Cancer | Dr Rosy Daniel, Jane Sen | 2003 | Thorsons |
| Beating the Blues | Xandria Williams | 1999 | Vermilion |
| **Dying to Be Me** | Anita Moorjani | 2012 | Hay House |
| **Integrated Cancer Care** | Jennifer Barraclough | 2001 | Oxford University Press |
| **Mind-Body Medicine** | Alan Watkins | 1997 | Churchill Livingstone |
| **Molecules of Emotion** | Candace Pert | 1997 | Simon and Schuster |
| **Radical Remission** | Dr Kelly Turner | 2014 | Harper One |
| **Remarkable Recovery** | Caryle Hirschberg, Marc Barasch | 1995 | Riverhead |
| **The Biology of Belief** | Bruce Lipton | 2015 | Hay House |
| **The Cancer Whisperer** | Sophie Sabbage | 2016 | Coronet |
| **The Psycho-Immunology of Cancer** | Claire Lewis, R O'Brian, Jennifer Barraclough | 2002 | Oxford University Press |

# CHAPTER 9: WEBSITES

| Website | Web Address | |
|---|---|---|
| Cancer Options | canceroptions.co.uk | |
| Dr Rosy Daniel | www.drrosydaniel.org | |
| Health Creation | www.healthcreation.co.uk | |
| Specialised Cancer Counsellors | yestolife.org.uk/y2l/directoryintro.html | |
| Yes to Life | yestolife.org.uk | |

| Description / Notes |
| --- |
| Suppliers |
| Wide range of health supplies |
| Suppliers |
| Exercise and lifestyle for cancer |
| Specialist exercise training |

| Book Number | Description / Notes |
| --- | --- |
| ISBN-10: 0007154275<br>ISBN-13: 978-0007154272 | Comprehensive UK directory of integrative approaches to cancer |
| ISBN-10: 000714704X<br>ISBN-13: 978-0007147045 | Classic on the subject with both the rationale and the recipes |
| ISBN-10: 0091818060<br>ISBN-13: 978-0091818067 | Guide to avoiding and lifting depression |
| ISBN-10: 1848507836<br>ISBN-13: 978-1848507838 | 'My journey from cancer to near death to true healing' |
| ISBN-10: 0192630954<br>ISBN-13: 978-0192630957 | Holistic, complementary and creative approaches |
| ISBN-10: 0443055262<br>ISBN-13: 978-0443055263 | A clinicians guide to psycho-neuro-immunology |
| ISBN-10: 0684846349<br>ISBN-13: 978-0684846347 | Why you feel the way you feel. Groundbreaking book on the biology of emotion |
| ASIN: B00M0KPVKC | Surviving cancer against all odds. A summary of survey results investigating the top strategies of extraordinary cancer survivors |
| ISBN-10: 0747213135<br>ISBN-13: 978-0747213130 | What extraordinary healings can teach us about getting well and staying well |
| ISBN-10: 1781805474<br>ISBN-13: 978-1781805473 | Unleashing the power of consciousness, matter and miracles |
| ASIN: B01661YN0O | How to let cancer heal your life. Sophie Sabbage applies her extensive professional experience of supporting people through challenging circumstances to her own devastating diagnosis to produce a guide for others |
| ISBN-10: 0192630601<br>ISBN-13: 978-0192630605 | Mind and body in the fight for survival |

| Description / Notes |
| --- |
| Consultancy providing personalised information on Integrative Medicine options |
| Dr Rosy Daniel's practice in Bath |
| Dr Rosy Daniel's complete lifestyle programmes and mentoring scheme |
| LIFE>, the Yes to Life searchable web directory, lists specialised cancer counsellors in the UK |
| The UK's integrative cancer care charity |

| Website | Web Address | |
|---|---|---|
| Befriending Networks | www.befriending.co.uk | |
| Cancer Counselling London | www.cancercounsellinglondon.org.uk | |
| Cancer Counselling Trust | www.cancercounselling.org.uk | |
| Centre for Transpersonal Psychology | www.transpersonalcentre.co.uk | |
| Cognitive Behavioural Therapy | www.babcp.com | |
| Healing Trust | www.thehealingtrust.org.uk | |
| Institute of Psychosynthesis | www.psychosynthesis.org | |
| Macmillan | www.macmillan.org.uk | |
| Neuro-linguistic Programming | www.nlpuktraining.com | |
| Online CBT Register | www.cbtregisteruk.com | |
| Online EFT Practitioners Register | www.aamet.org | |
| Penny Brohn Cancer Care | www.pennybrohncancercare.org | |
| Reiki Federation | www.reikifed.co.uk | |

# CHAPTER 10: FURTHER READING

| Title | Author | | Publisher |
|---|---|---|---|
| Daylight Robbery | Dr Damien Downing | 1986 | Arrow books |
| The Healing Energies of Light | Roger Coghill | 2000 | Journey Editions |
| Vitamin D Revolution | Soram Khalsa | 2009 | Hay House |

# CHAPTER 10: WEBSITES

| Website | Web Address | |
|---|---|---|
| Nutrition Associates | www.naltd.co.uk | |
| British Society for Ecological Medicine (BSEM) | www.ecomed.org.uk | |
| Grassroots Health | grassrootshealth.net | |
| Sunfriend | sunfriend.com | |
| Vitamin D Article | updates.nutrigold.co.uk/assets/pdf/newsletters/NG-Education-Newsletter-VitaminD.pdf | |
| Vitamin D Council | www.vitamindcouncil.org | |

# CHAPTER 11: FURTHER READING

| Title | Author | | Publisher |
|---|---|---|---|
| Detoxify or Die | Sherry Rogers | 2002 | Prestige Pubs |

| Description / Notes |
| --- |
| Search for befriending in the UK |
| Highly experienced professional cancer counselling |
| Sadly closed, but the website contains information and links |
| Find a practitioner |
| Find a practitioner |
| Healing centres and groups |
| Find a practitioner |
| UK charity for cancer support |
| Training and information |
| Find a practitioner |
| Find a practitioner |
| Centre for cancer support, education and complementary medicine |
| Find practitioners, courses, teachers |

| Book Number | Description / Notes |
| --- | --- |
| ISBN: 99567407 | One of the first books to highlight to problems around vitamin D deficiency |
| ISBN-10: 1582900124<br>ISBN-13: 978-1582900124 | Research demonstrates that light plays a critical role in physical and emotional well-being. |
| ISBN-10: 1401924700<br>ISBN-13: 978-1401924706 | How the power of this amazing vitamin can change your life |

| Description / Notes |
| --- |
| Dr Downing's website |
| Promoting the study of allergy, environmental and nutritional medicine |
| All things vitamin D |
| Wearable sun monitor |
| By nutritionist Kirsten Chick |
| Latest vitamin D news and research. Type cancer in the Search box and it links you to many of the most common cancers and the research linked to each |

| Book Number | Description / Notes |
| --- | --- |
| ISBN-10: 1887202048<br>ISBN-13: 978-1887202046 | The steady silent accumulation of toxins over a lifetime that produces most diseases, including cancer |

| Title | Author | | Publisher |
|-------|--------|--|-----------|
| **Eat, Drink and Be Healthy** | Walter Willet | 2005 | Free Press |
| **Enzymatic Basis of Detoxi-fication Vol 2** | William Jacoby | 1980 | Academic Press |
| **Natural Detoxification** | Jacqueline Krohn, Frances Taylor | 2001 | Hartley & Marks |
| **Textbook of Functional Medicine** | Sidney Macdonald, Peter Bennet et al | 2010 | Gig Harbor |
| **The Paleo Diet for Athletes** | Loren Cordain, Joe Friel | 2012 | Rodale Books |
| **Toxic Beauty** | Samuel Epstein, Randall Fitzgerald | 2010 | BenBella Books |

# CHAPTER 11: WEBSITES

| Website | Web Address |
|---------|-------------|
| Alliance for Natural Health | www.anh-europe.org |
| **Cancer Prevention Coalition** | www.preventcancer.com |
| **Collaborative on Health and the Environment** | www.healthandenvironment.org/tddb |
| **Environmental Working Group** | www.ewg.org |
| **Institute for Functional Medicine** | www.functionalmedicine.org |
| **International Agency for Research on Cancer** | www.iarc.fr |
| **Natura Foundation** | www.naturafoundation.org |
| **Pesticide Action Network** | www.pan-international.org |
| **Physicians for Social Responsibility** | www.psr.org |

# CHAPTER 12: FURTHER READING

| Title | Author | | Publisher |
|-------|--------|--|-----------|
| Imperfectly Natural Baby and Toddler | Janey Lee Grace | 2007 | Orion |
| Imperfectly Natural Home | Janey Lee Grace | 2008 | Orion |
| Imperfectly Natural Woman | Janey Lee Grace | 2005 | Crown House Publishing |
| Look Good Naturally... Without Ditching the Lipstick | Janey Lee Grace | 2013 | Hay House UK |
| **Cleaning Yourself to Death** | Pat Thomas | 2001 | Newleaf |
| **Geopathic Stress and Subtle Energy** | Jane Thurnell-Read | 2006 | Life-Work Potential |

| Book Number | Description / Notes |
|---|---|
| ISBN-10: 0743266420<br>ISBN-13: 978-0743266420 | The Harvard Medical School guide to healthy eating |
| ISBN-10: 0123959187<br>ISBN-13: 978-0123959188 | Reviews the state of knowledge on foreign compound metabolism at the level of what specific enzymes can do |
| ISBN-10: 0881791873<br>ISBN-13: 978-0881791877 | A practical encyclopedia. The complete guide to clearing your body of toxins |
| ISBN-10: 0977371379<br>ISBN-13: 978-0977371372 | The latest edition of this textbook from the Institute for Functional Medicine |
| ISBN-10: 160961917X<br>ISBN-13: 978-1609619176 | The ancient nutritional formula for peak athletic performance |
| ISBN-10: 1935251724<br>ISBN-13: 978-1935251729 | How cosmetics and personal-care products endanger your health... and what you can do about it |

| Description / Notes |
|---|
| Campaigning organisation for natural medicines founded by Robert Verkerk |
| Advocates and supports the prevention and early detection of cancer through research, education, advocacy and community outreach |
| Sharing environmental research and facilitating actions to improve health |
| Environmental health research and advocacy organisation |
| The 'home' of Functional Medicine – information, events, training |
| The specialised cancer agency of the World Health Organization |
| Training and news re psychoneuroimmunology and nutritional therapy |
| Working to minimise the negative effects and replace the use of harmful pesticides with ecologically sound alternatives |
| Working to prevent the use or spread of nuclear weapons and to slow, stop and reverse global warming and the toxic degradation of the environment |

| Book Number | Description / Notes |
|---|---|
| ISBN-10: 0752885898<br>ISBN-13: 978-0752885896 | How to be a green parent in today's busy world |
| ISBN-10: 0752885820<br>ISBN-13: 978-0752885827 | Everything you need to know to create a healthy, natural home, in a very readable format |
| ISBN-10: 1904424899<br>ISBN-13: 978-1904424895 | Getting life right the natural way |
| ISBN-10: 1848502036<br>ISBN-13: 978-1848502031 | Find your way through the minefield of toxic cosmetics |
| ISBN-10: 0717131629<br>ISBN-13: 978-0717131624 | How safe is your home? |
| ISBN-10: 0954243943<br>ISBN-13: 978-0954243944 | If you suffer from tiredness, headaches, irritability, miscarriages, or chronic ill health that doesn't respond to treatment, you may be suffering from geopathic stress |

| Title | Author | | Publisher |
|---|---|---|---|
| **Living Dangerously** | Pat Thomas | 2003 | Newleaf |
| **Wireless Radiation Rescue** | Kerry Crofton | 2012 | Global Wellbeing Books |
| **Zapped** | Ann Louise Gittlemen | 2006 | HarperOne |

# CHAPTER 12: WEBSITES

| Website | Web Address | |
|---|---|---|
| Imperfectly Natural | www.imperfectlynatural.com | |
| **Allergy Cosmos** | www.allergycosmos.co.uk | |
| **Bobby's Healthy Shop** | www.bobbyshealthyshop.co.uk | |
| **Ebay** | www.ebay.co.uk | |
| **EMF Research** | www.bioinitiative.org | |
| **Freecycle** | www.freecycle.org | |
| **Healthy House** | www.healthy-house.co.uk | |
| **Sitefinder** | www.sitefinder.ofcom.org.uk | |
| **Wireless Protection** | www.wireless-protection.org | |

# CHAPTER 13: FURTHER READING

| Title | Author | | Publisher |
|---|---|---|---|
| Beating Cancer | Francisco Contreras MD | 2011 | Siloam |
| 50 Critical Cancer Answers | Francisco Contreras MD | 2013 | Authentic Publishers |
| Hope, Medicine & Healing | Francisco Contreras MD | 2009 | Oasis of Hope Press |
| The Hope of Living Cancer Free | Francisco Contreras MD | 1999 | Creation House |
| **The Little Enema Book** | Gerson Support Group | | The Gerson Insitute |

# CHAPTER 13: WEBSITES

| Website | Web Address | |
|---|---|---|
| Oasis of Hope Hospital | www.oasisofhope.com | |
| **British Society for Mercury Free Dentistry** | www.mercuryfreedentistry.org.uk | |

| Book Number | Description / Notes |
|---|---|
| ISBN-10: 0717136000<br>ISBN-13: 978-0717136001 | Are everyday toxins making you sick? |
| ISBN-10: 0986473537<br>ISBN-13: 978-0986473531 | How to use cell phones more safely and other safer-tech solutions |
| ISBN-10: 0061864285<br>ISBN-13: 978-0061864285 | Why your cell phone shouldn't be your alarm clock and 1,268 ways to outsmart the hazards of electronic pollution |

| Description / Notes |
|---|
| Janey Lee Grace's website |
| Information and products for allergies |
| EMF protection supplies |
| Online auction site |
| Biologically-based exposure standards for low-intensity electromagnetic radiation |
| Get and give stuff for free |
| Information and products for allergies |
| Find the location of mobile phone base stations |
| EMF protection supplies |

| Book Number | Description / Notes |
|---|---|
| ISBN 1616381566<br>ISBN13: 9781616381561 | 20 natural, spiritual and medical remedies that can slow - and even reverse - cancer's progression |
| ISBN 1780781075<br>ISBN13: 9781780781075 | 50 tangible tips, plans and prescriptive measures for tackling cancer and finding renewed health. Dr Contreras' most recent book |
| ISBN13: 9781780781075 | How patients can live with cancer, managing it like a chronic disease |
| ISBN-10: 0884196550<br>ISBN-13: 978-0884196556 | Cancer is approached from the view of one's emotional and spiritual factors in dealing with it |
| ASIN: B0037CNFN2 | A practical guide |

| Description / Notes |
|---|
| Dr Contreras is the Medical Director of the Oasis of Hope Hospital in Tijuana, Mexico |
| Practitioners and information regarding mercury removal and biocompatible dental materials |

# CHAPTER 14: FURTHER READING

| Title | Author | | Publisher |
|---|---|---|---|
| The Topic of Cancer | Jessica Richards | 2011 | Jessica Richards |
| Questioning Chemotherapy | Ralph Moss | 1995 | Equinox Press |
| The Cancer Journey | Dr Pam Evans, Polly Noble, Nicholas Hull-Malham | 2011 | Antony Rowe Publishing Services |

# CHAPTER 14: WEBSITES

| Website | Web Address | |
|---|---|---|
| Cancer Options | canceroptions.co.uk | |
| Starthrowers | www.starthrowers.org.uk | |
| CaringBridge | www.caringbridge.org | |
| Cyberknife | www.cyberknife.com | |
| HIFU (High-Intensity Focused Ultrasound) | www.hifu-planet.co.uk | |
| Killing Cancer | www.killingcancer.co.uk | |
| Laser Ablation | www.macmillan.org.uk/Cancerinformation/ Cancertypes/Liversecondary/ Treatingsecondarylivercancer/Newertreatments. aspx#DynamicJumpMenuManager_6_Anchor_1 | |
| Nanoknife | www.totalhealth.co.uk/clinical-experts/professor-edward-leen/new-cancer-treatment-nanoknife | |
| Nanoknife | www.theprincessgracehospital.com/hospital-services/services/nanoknife | |
| National Medical Laser Centre | iris.ucl.ac.uk/iris/browse/researchGroup/1394 | |
| PDT (Photodynamic Therapy) | www.macmillan.org.uk/Cancerinformation/ Cancertreatment/Treatmenttypes/Othertreatments/ Photodynamictherapy.aspx | |
| PDT Norfolk | www.pdtnorfolk.co.uk | |
| Pfizer Oncology Clinical Trial Information Service | www.pfizercancertrials.com | |
| RFA (Radiofrequency Ablation) | www.macmillan.org.uk/Cancerinformation/ Cancertreatment/Treatmenttypes/Othertreatments/ Radiofrequencyablation.aspx | |
| UK Clinical Trials Gateway | www.ukctg.nihr.ac.uk | |
| US National Health Trial Database | clinicaltrials.gov | |

# CHAPTER 15: FURTHER READING

| Title | Author | | Publisher |
|---|---|---|---|
| Detecting Cancer | Xandria Williams | 2013 | Xtra Health Publications |

| Book Number | Description / Notes |
|---|---|
| ISBN-10: 0957064403<br>ISBN-13: 978-0957064409 | Straightforward, practical advice on navigating through cancer treatment. Includes advice on working with your medical team |
| ISBN-10: 188102525X<br>ISBN-13: 978-1881025252 | A critique of the use of toxic drugs |
| ISBN-10: 1907571248<br>ISBN-13: 978-1907571244 | Positive steps to help yourself heal. Includes advice on working with your medical team |

| Description / Notes |
|---|
| Consultancy providing personalised information on Integrative Medicine options |
| Charity based in Norfolk giving direct support to people with cancer, set up by Dr Henry Mannings |
| A place to share health updates, photos and videos with the people who care about you |
| Cyberknife information site |
| HIFU for prostate cancer – information site |
| Charity promoting PDT – now closing due to the death of the founder. Website still has information |
| Description of laser ablation |
| Nanoknife information site |
| Description of nanoknife |
| PDT research and treatment |
| Description of PDT |
| Charity promoting PDT |
| Search for clinical trials |
| Description of RFA |
| Search for clinical trials |
| Search for clinical trials |

| Book Number | Description / Notes |
|---|---|
| ISBN-10: 0956855237<br>ISBN-13: 978-0956855237 | Book 3 of Xandria William's planned Cancer Quintet |

| Title | Author | | Publisher |
|---|---|---|---|
| Laboratory Evaluations in Molecular Medicine | Bralley & Lord | 2001 | The Institute for Advances in Molecular Medicine |

# CHAPTER 15: WEBSITES

| Website | Web Address | |
|---|---|---|
| Robert Jacobs Health | www.robertjacobshealth.com | |
| Biolab | www.biolab.co.uk | |
| Institute for Functional Medicine | www.functionalmedicine.org | |

# APPENDICES: FURTHER READING

| Title | Author | | Publisher |
|---|---|---|---|
| Beating Cancer | Francisco Contreras MD | 2011 | Siloam |
| Biological Medicineh | Dr Thomas Rau | 2011 | Semmelweis-Institut |
| 50 Critical Cancer Answers | Francisco Contreras MD | 2013 | Authentic Publishers |
| Hope, Medicine & Healing | Francisco Contreras MD | 2009 | Oasis of Hope Press |
| The Hope of Living Cancer Free | Francisco Contreras MD | 1999 | Creation House |
| German Cancer Therapies | Dr Morton Walker | 2003 | Kensington |

# APPENDICES: WEBSITES

| Website | Web Address | |
|---|---|---|
| CancerIFA | www.cancerifa.com | |
| George Emsden | www.georgeemsden.co.uk | |
| International Center for Cell Therapy and Cancer Immunotherapy (CTCI) | www.ctcicenter.com | |
| Klinik Arlesheim (Ita Wegman Klinik) | www.klinik-arlesheim.ch/de/ita-wegman-ambulatorium.html | |
| Klinik St Georg | www.klinik-st-georg.de/en | |
| Oasis of Hope Hospital | www.oasisofhope.com | |
| Paracelsus Klinik | www.paracelsusclinic.com | |
| Breast Thermography | www.breastthermography.com | |
| Chartered Institute for Securities & Investment (CISI) | www.cisi.org/cisiweb2/cisi-website/cisi-financial-services-professional-body | |
| Citizen's Advice Bureau | www.citizensadvice.org.uk | |

| Book Number | Description / Notes |
|---|---|
| ISBN-10: 0967394910<br>ISBN-13: 978-0967394916 | Nutrients, toxicants and cell regulators (for science readers only!) |

| Description / Notes |
|---|
| Website of Functional Medicine Practitioner Robert Jacobs |
| London-based testing lab |
| The 'home' of Functional Medicine – information, events, training |

| Book Number | Description / Notes |
|---|---|
| ISBN 1616381566<br>ISBN13: 9781616381561 | 20 natural, spiritual and medical remedies that can slow - and even reverse - cancer's progression |
| ISBN-10: 3925524649<br>ISBN-13: 978-3925524646 | he future of natural healing |
| ISBN 1780781075<br>ISBN13: 9781780781075 | 50 tangible tips, plans and prescriptive measures for tackling cancer and finding renewed health. Dr Contreras' most recent book |
| ISBN-10: 1579460011<br>ISBN-13: 978-1579460013 | How patients can live with cancer, managing it like a chronic disease |
| ISBN-10: 0884196550<br>ISBN-13: 978-0884196556 | Cancer is approached from the view of one's emotional and spiritual factors in dealing with it |
| ISBN-10: 1575666103<br>ISBN-13: 978-1575666105 | Natural and conventional medicines that offer hope and healing |

| Description / Notes |
|---|
| George Emsden's site with specialised financial advice for those with cancer |
| George Emsden's financial advice site under his own name |
| Prof. Slavin is the Medical and Scientific Director of the CTCI in Tel Aviv |
| Dr Orange is developing Integrative Oncology at the Ita Wegman Klinik in Arlesheim |
| Dr Douwes is the Medical Director of the Klinik St Georg in Bad Aibling |
| Dr Contreras is the Medical Director of the Oasis of Hope Hospital in Tijuana, Mexico |
| Dr Rau is the Medical Director of the Paracelsus Klinik in Lustmühle |
| Dedicated to providing information on breast thermography, risk assessment, breast cancer, early detection, prevention and ultimately the preservation of the breast and the survival of women |
| Find a financial adviser |
| Find a Citizen's Advice Bureau near you |

| Website | Web Address | |
|---|---|---|
| Freecycle | www.uk.freecycle.org | |
| Macmillan Financial Support | www.macmillan.org.uk | |
| Mistletoe for Cancer UK | www.mistletoeforcancer.org.uk | |
| Money Advice Service | www.moneyadviceservice.org.uk | |
| NCI SEER Program | seer.cancer.gov | |
| Patient.co.uk | www.patient.co.uk/health/benefits-for-the-terminally-ill | |
| Pensions Advisory Service | www.pensionsadvisoryservice.org.uk | |
| Pension Tracing Service | www.pensiontracingservice.com | |
| Radiation Risk Assessment Tool | dceg.cancer.gov/tools/risk-assessment/radrat | |
| The Promise (Film) | www.thepromisefilm.net | |
| Unbiased | www.unbiased.co.uk | |
| X-Ray Risk | www.xrayrisk.com | |

# GENERAL READING

| Title | Author | | Publisher |
|---|---|---|---|
| The Cancer Directory | Dr Rosy Daniel | 2005 | Harper Thorsons |
| The Topic of Cancer | Jessica Richards | 2011 | Jessica Richards |
| Lifestyle and Cancer | Prof. Robert Thomas | 2011 | Health Education Publications |
| Anticancer: A New Way of Life | David Servan-Schreiber | 2012 | Michael Joseph |
| Antioxidants Against Cancer | Ralph Moss | 2000 | Equinox Press |
| Cancer Therapy | Ralph Moss | 1993 | Equinox Press |
| Crazy Sexy Diet | Kris Carr | 2010 | Globe Pequot Press Life |
| Crazy Sexy Cancer Survivor | Kris Carr | 2008 | The Lyons Press |
| Crazy Sexy Cancer Tips | Kris Carr | 2007 | The Lyons Press |
| Crazy Sexy Kitchen | Kris Carr | 2012 | Hay House UK |
| Doctored Results | Ralph Moss | 2014 | Equinox Press |
| How to be a Cancer Maverick | Nina Joy | 2015 | Solopreneur Publishing Ltd |
| Life Over Cancer | Keith Block | 2009 | Random House Inc. |
| Mum's Not Having Chemo | Laura Bond | 2013 | Piatkus |

| Description / Notes |
| --- |
| Get rid of unwanted stuff, or find things you need free |
| Click the tab 'How We Can Help' at the top of the home page, and then 'Financial Support' on the left |
| Information about mistletoe therapy and the latest news of trials and research on mistletoe therapy for cancer |
| Free and impartial money advice, set up by government |
| National Cancer Institute Surveillance, Epidemiology and End Results Program |
| Summary of benefits for the terminally ill |
| Find lost pensions from past employers |
| Find lost pensions from past employers |
| Calculate lifetime cancer risk from a range of exposures |
| Prof Ken Young, Consultant Physicist, National Coordinating Centre for the Physics of Mammography. Start viewing at 26:40 |
| Find a financial adviser |
| Calculate the risk of cancer from medical imaging |

| Book Number | Description / Notes |
| --- | --- |
| ISBN-10: 0007154275<br>ISBN-13: 978-0007154272 | Comprehensive UK directory of integrative approaches to cancer |
| ISBN-10: 0957064403<br>ISBN-13: 978-0957064409 | Straightforward, practical advice on navigating through cancer treatment |
| ASIN: B004L2LJ30 | The second and updated edition from Britain's leading oncologist in the field of lifestyle, nutrition and cancer |
| ISBN-10: 0718156846<br>ISBN-13: 978-0718156848 | One of the best and most popular general books on science-based Integrative Oncology |
| ISBN-10: 1881025284<br>ISBN-13: 978-1881025283 | A reference for all those considering using antioxidants, particularly along-side orthodox approaches |
| ISBN-10: 1881025063<br>ISBN-13: 978-1881025061 | The independent consumer's guide to non-toxic treatment. A classic on the subject from one of the most important writers in the field |
| ISBN-10: 1599218011<br>ISBN-13: 978-1599218014 | Eat your veggies, ignite your spark, and live like you mean it! |
| ISBN-10: 1599213702<br>ISBN-13: 978-1599213705 | More rebellion and fire for your healing journey |
| ISBN-10: 1599212315<br>ISBN-13: 978-1599212319 | A very different kind of 'personal journey' book that many have found enormously inspiring |
| ISBN-10: 1401941044<br>ISBN-13: 978-1401941048 | 150 plant-empowered recipes to ignite a mouthwatering revolution |
| ISBN-10: 1881025527<br>ISBN-13: 978-1881025528 | The suppression of laetrile at Sloan-Kettering Institute for cancer research. For those interested in the politics of cancer research and treatment |
| ISBN-10: 0992784069<br>ISBN-13: 978-0992784065 | After being diagnosed with Stage 4 cancer in 2012 and told she had 3 months to live, Nina decided to not just accept the diagnosis but to go out and investigate all the choices |
| ISBN-10: 0553801147<br>ISBN-13: 978-0553801149 | Keith Block's inspiring account of the approach he has developed in over thirty years' practice |
| ISBN-10: 0749958960<br>ISBN-13: 978-0749958961 | Extremely readable mix of personal experience and expert opinion from blog writer Laura Bond |

| Title | Author | | Publisher |
|---|---|---|---|
| **Radical Remission** | Dr Kelly Turner | 2014 | Harper One |
| **Say No to Cancer** | Patrick Holford | 2010 | Piatkus |
| **Tripping Over the Truth** | Travis Christofferson | 2014 | CreateSpace Independent Publishing Platform |
| **The Cancer Whisperer** | Sophie Sabbage | 2016 | Coronet |

# GENERAL WEBSITES

| Website | Web Address | |
|---|---|---|
| Cancer Options | canceroptions.co.uk | |
| LIFE> Yes to Life Web Directory | yestolife.org.uk/y2l/directoryintro.html | |
| UK Health Radio - The Yes to Life Show | http://ukhealthradio.com/blog/program/yes-to-life-show/ | |
| Yes to Life | yestolife.org.uk | |
| **Bite the Sun** | bitethesun.org | |
| **British Society for Integrative Oncology (BSIO)** | www.bsio.org.uk | |
| **CANCERactive** | www.canceractive.com | |
| **Cansurviving** | www.cansurviving.com | |
| **Inspired Nutrition** | www.inspirednutrition.co.uk | |
| **Maggie's Centres** | www.maggiescentres.org | |
| **Mercola** | www.mercola.com | |
| **Penny Brohn Cancer Care** | www.pennybrohncancercare.org | |
| **Rainbow Valley** | www.rainbowvalley.org.uk | |
| **Specialist Health Centre** | specialisthealthcentre.co.uk | |
| **The Haven** | thehaven.org.uk | |
| **Together Against Cancer** | togetheragainstcancer.org.uk | |
| **Wirral Holistic Care Services** | www.wirralholistic.org.uk | |

R  Recommended for further exploration of various aspects of cancer and Integrative Medicine

| Book Number | Description / Notes |
|---|---|
| ASIN: B00M0KPVKC | Surviving cancer against all odds. A summary of survey results investigating the top strategies of extraordinary cancer survivors |
| ISBN-10: 9780749954116<br>ISBN-13: 978-0749954116 | Updated version of one of the most popular manuals for 'looking outside the box' |
| ISBN-10: 1500600318<br>ISBN-13: 978-1500600310 | The return of the metabolic theory of cancer illuminates a new and hopeful path to a cure. Metabolic theory for general readers |
| ASIN: B01661YN0O | How to let cancer heal your life. Sophie Sabbage applies her extensive professional experience of supporting people through challenging circumstances to her own devastating diagnosis to produce a guide for others |

| Description / Notes |
|---|
| Consultancy providing personalised information on Integrative Medicine options |
| Extensive online searchable directory of integrative therapies and practitioners worldwide |
| Weekly show hosted by Yes to Life Chairman, Robin Daly, investigating all aspects of Integrative Oncology |
| The UK's integrative cancer care charity |
| All round health site: set goals, track progress |
| Leading UK professional body for practitioners interested in Integrative Oncology |
| Integrative Oncology information charity |
| Supportive forum for anyone looking for integrative approaches |
| Jenny Phillips and Jeraldine Curran - courses, classes, consultations and more |
| Located at hospitals around the UK, Maggie's offer a range of support, including complementary therapies |
| The web's most popular natural health site |
| Pioneering charity that introduced diet and lifestyle methods to the wider public now offering extensive education and support programmes |
| Charity supporting choice in cancer care |
| Exercise and lifestyle approaches |
| Support, education and complementary therapies for those with breast cancer |
| Charity with a centre in Leicester which supports Integrative Medicine and runs events for the public |
| Complementary therapies |

# INDEX

The List of Abbreviations can be found on pages 27-29.

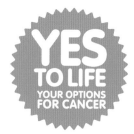

YES TO LIFE

CANCER
OPTIONS

LIFE>

## Yes to Life

I sincerely hope that you have found *The Cancer Revolution* both helpful and inspiring.

Yes to Life is the UK's integrative cancer-care charity. It offers direct support to people with cancer through a helpline staffed by a dedicated team of highly trained volunteers, all of whom have some first-hand experience of cancer that enables them to empathise and connect with callers in the most supportive way. Those who call are offered a personalised report of the Integrative Medicine options they could consider for their situation. The charity commissions recommendations from the Cancer Options consultancy. The charity provides these free of charge. Furthermore, Yes to Life runs a small grants scheme through which those in financial difficulties can receive support in obtaining Integrative Medicine.

The charity's website (yestolife.org.uk) features LIFE>, a unique searchable directory of integrative therapies, practitioners and organisations, all interlinked to provide users with quick access to relevant information. The directory is constantly being maintained, improved and updated. A recent addition is a forum where people can share their knowledge and experience of therapies detailed in the directory.

Yes to Life is rapidly becoming better known and is answering the needs of the increasing number of people with cancer who decide to look 'outside the box' of standard treatments alone. We've reached this point almost entirely through public support. To maintain our services, and indeed to develop further services, we need many more friends and donors.

If you choose to join us, you will be among those who make it possible for Yes to Life to give significant direct help and resources to people with cancer and their families at their time of greatest need. There are several ways of contributing, ranging from a monthly donation to a bequest in your will, from a one-off gift to support for a major project. However large or small the amount, you will be helping to create a legacy that is changing the face of cancer care in the UK.

Various options are detailed on our website. If you prefer to call our office, one of our team will be pleased to help you find the best way ahead for you to support our work.

Robin Daly
Chairman and Founder

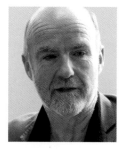

WE WISH
YOU WELL

HOPE THE BOOK
IS HELPFUL

## Charity Details

Contact Office
020 3222 0587
office@yestolife.org.uk

Helpline
0870 163 2990
helpcentre@yestolife.org.uk

Website
yestolife.org.uk

Charity No
1112812

Yes to Life Radio Show
ukhealthradio.com

 Like us on Facebook
Yes to Life

 Follow us on Instagram
Y2LIFE

 Follow us on Twitter
@yestolife

 Find us on Blogspot
www.yestolifecharity.blogspot.co.uk

# GLOSSARY

Within the Glossary, the primary term is followed by related words in parentheses, in alphabetical order, e.g. alkalise (alkali, alkaline, alkalinity). Words that are included in the Glossary generally appear more than once in the book and are highlighted in blue.